Keystone Flap for Complex Orthopaedic Problems

Springer Nature More Media App

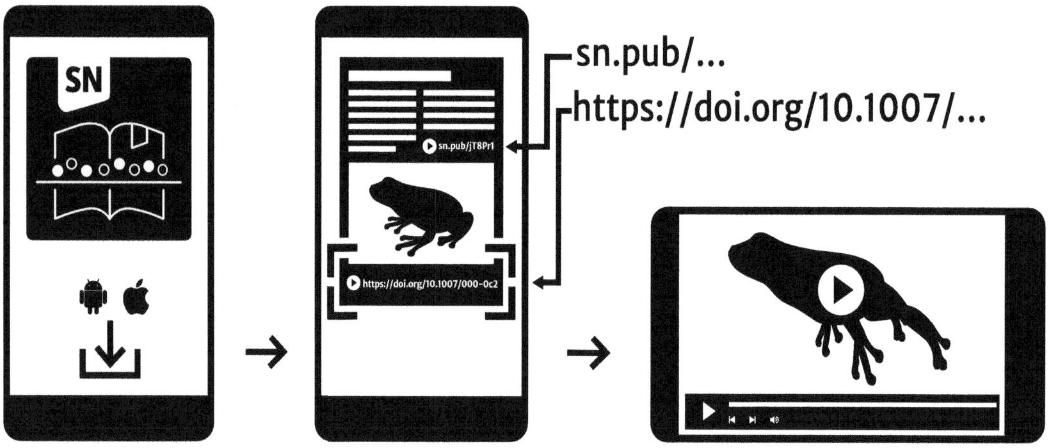

1. Download
2. Scan Link
3. Enjoy Video

Support: customerservice@springernature.com

Felix Behan

Keystone Flap for Complex Orthopaedic Problems

Reconstructive Surgery with Audiovisual Guidelines

Foreword by
Rollin Daniel
Wayne Morrison
Peter Choong

Springer

Felix Behan
Department of Surgery, St. Vincent's Hospital
University of Melbourne
Parkville, VIC, Australia

This work contains media enhancements, which are displayed with a "play" icon. Material in the print book can be viewed on a mobile device by downloading the Springer Nature "More Media" app available in the major app stores. The media enhancements in the online version of the work can be accessed directly by authorized users.

ISBN 978-3-031-76701-2 ISBN 978-3-031-76702-9 (eBook)
https://doi.org/10.1007/978-3-031-76702-9

This Springer imprint is published by the registered company Springer Nature Switzerland AG
The registered company address is: Gewerbestrasse 11, 6330 Cham, Switzerland

Foreword

Keystone Flaps for Complex Orthopaedic Problems authored by Felix Behan represents a major milestone with a wide ranging impact on surgery of the extremities. For reconstructive surgeons and their patients, it offers proven solutions to difficult clinical cases for which no alternative exists other than a prolonged open wound or an amputation.

From personal experience, I can attest to the validity of Hallock's acronym PACES to describe the characteristics of the Keystone island flap (hereinafter KIF). A year ago, I had a 3 × 4 cm defect on my back following excision of a melanoma, which required a flap closure. The procedure was done under local anaesthesia, and I had no pain in the OR nor afterwards. When shown an intraoperative photo sequence of the surgery, I simply could not understand how it was done—truly a magic trick. In order to understand what I was seeing, I went on the Internet and discovered the 'Keystone flap' and its originator, Felix Behan. Subsequently, I have had the opportunity to read numerous articles and watch multiple videos by Dr. Behan. The KIF is truly a revolutionary approach to skin flaps as it violates virtually every traditional rule of skin flap design. There is little adherence to classical dimensions, orientation, or specific blood supply. Flaps on the lower extremity can be distally based and rotated almost 90° with immediate excision of dog ears. The 'proof of concept' is both Dr. Behan's 25-year experience in 3000 cases and that of other colleagues throughout the world. The range of cases shown in this text should impress the reader but not lull them into a false sense of simplicity. Rather, they should adopt the same classification as if they were at the top of an alpine peak—are they a beginner, intermediate, or expert? Pick appropriate cases to start with and then continue the journey as one gains experience. Every operation has both a 'learning curve' and revisions/complications for the uninitiated.

For plastic surgeons, KIF represents a major advance in the evolution of skin flaps and forces a reassessment of treatment alternatives. Traditionally, major defects of the extremities were closed with pocket flaps for the upper extremity and cross-leg or tube pedicle flaps for the lower extremity. These multi-staged procedures were replaced with the advent of microvascular free flaps as the latter provided well-vascularised coverage in a single operation [1, 2]. The inception of free flaps stimulated the search for multiple donor sites and reawakened interest in defining the blood supply to the skin [3, 4]. Taylor performed extensive cadaver dissections defining the angiosome concept of the cutaneous blood supply [5]. These findings led directly to the development of perforator flaps [6]. In 1985, the author watched Marko Godina dissect out an anterior lateral thigh perforator flap for free tissue transfer. Although initial interest focused on identifying free flap donor sites, the use of perforator flaps to close locoregional defects became popular and reached their zenith in the 'propeller flap' [7]. Simultaneously, Ponten [8] popularised the use of fasciocutaneous flaps, demonstrating their value in closing difficult wounds, especially in the lower extremity. Extensive applications of fasciocutaneous flaps were summarised in Hallock's definitive text [9]. It is at this point that Behan began his truly revolutionary approach to skin flap design. The original applications were for closure of defects following the excision of melanomas [10].

In conclusion, KIFs will become the starting point for closure options of many extremity defects. Surgeons will no longer think first of a perforator flap or a free flap, but rather ask—'how can I close this defect with a KIF?' Why make the solution more complex, riskier, and expensive than necessary? Thus, Felix Behan's brilliant design and set of principles for the KIF flap have revolutionised the management of extremity defects, benefiting both patients and surgeons.

Rollin K. Daniel

Suggested Reading

1. Daniel RK, Taylor GI. Distant transfer of an island flap by microvascular anastomoses. Plast Reconstr Surg. 1973;52:111.
2. Daniel RK. Direct transfer of skin flaps by microvascular anastomoses. McGill University. MSC Degree in Experimental Surgery; 1972.
3. Daniel RK. The anatomical and hemodynamic characteristics of the cutaneous circulation and their influence on skin flap design. In: Grabb WC, Myers B, editors. Skin flaps. Boston: Little Brown; 1975.
4. Daniel RK, Cunningham DM, Taylor GI. Toward an anatomical and hemodynamic classification of skin flaps. Plast Reconstr Surg. 1975;56:330.
5. Taylor GI, Palmer JH. The vascular territories (angiosomes) of the body: experimental study and clinical applications. Br J Plast Surg. 1987;40:113–41.
6. Taylor GI. The angiosomes of the body and their supply to perforator flaps. Clin Plast Surg. 2003;30:331–42.
7. Teo TC. The propeller flap concept. Clin Plast Surg. 2010;37:615–26.
8. Ponten B, The fasciocutaneous flap: its use in tissue defects of the lower leg. Br J Plast Surg. 1981;34:215–20.
9. Hallock GG, editor. Fasciocutaneous flaps. Boston: Blackwell Scientific Publications; 1992.
10. Behan FC. Fasciocutaneous island flap for orthopaedic management in lower limb reconstructions using dermatomal precincts. ANZ J Surg. 1994;64:155–66.

Foreword

To quote Churchill, 'I don't collect first editions but prefer to wait to see if it is worthy of a second'. So too with Felix Behan's recent book, *Keystone Flap for Complex Orthopaedic Problems*, although a first, it feels like an eagerly awaited next in a series of magician's reconstructive tricks for all comers. This book follows earlier publications on repair of melanoma defects and an atlas of Keystone flaps. Its worth is already affirmed by the publishers, who have requisitioned this edition by popular demand.

Felix has been proselytising his Keystone flap principles as a reconstructive alternative for many years, but like most prophets, his message was slow to be adopted. The Keystone flap was new, intuitively wrong according to our plastic surgical principles, and created a secondary defect larger than the primary one, which was repaired by direct closure under tension. The flap audaciously boasted closure of holes hitherto un-closable by local flaps, the legitimate realm of microsurgery. It surely couldn't work. As a contemporary and long-time believer, I witnessed the justifiable scepticism and fear that stayed the hand of the conservatives and the burnt fingers that tempered the naively bold. But now, thanks to this book for orthopaedists and a wider audience, we can confirm with our own eyes that seeing is believing and begin to participate in the flap's ecumenical bounty.

Chapter 1: Principles is an insightful, meandering tale of the Keystone flap's gestation, intuitive dermatomal design principles, historical precedents, and the science, along with characteristic Behan-esque random anecdotes of personalities and events that have led to his enlightenment. Chapters 2 and 3 offer us a dazzling display, through colour photos, movies, and voice, of how the tricks are done. Case after case, we see challenging defects closed by various manipulations and modifications.

This book demonstrates the versatility of this method of reconstruction and loosens the chains of our microsurgical imprisonment and its cost implications. It democratises reconstruction to a much larger surgical audience and thereby, to patient recipients. This is a boy's (and girl's) own manual for reconstructive surgeons, but even if reconstruction is not your passion, marvel at the discovery of wondrous and seemingly impossible cases solved as if by magic and delight in the pictorial format that illustrates them.

Wayne Morrison
Department of Surgery
St Vincent's Hospital Melbourne, University of Melbourne
Parkville, VIC, Australia

Foreword

In the ever-evolving field of plastic and reconstructive surgery, innovation and practical application are the cornerstones of progress. The keystone perforator island flap represents one such revolutionary paradigm. In this specialised text, *Keystone Flap for Complex Orthopaedic Problems*, Felix Behan meticulously documents a ground-breaking approach that redefines reconstructive strategies for orthopaedic patients, combining scientific rigor, clinical precision, and patient-centred outcomes.

Felix Behan's keystone concept transcends conventional boundaries, offering a locoregional solution that eliminates the extensive time, costs, and complications often associated with microsurgical reconstruction. Through its simplicity and adaptability, the keystone flap provides an effective, aesthetic, and resource-conscious alternative, democratising access to high-quality surgical care in diverse clinical settings.

This text serves as a comprehensive guide, not only elucidating the technical principles underpinning the Keystone flap but also offering real-world case studies and audiovisual supplements to bridge the gap between theory and practice. The detailed inclusion of embryological underpinnings, design principles, and procedural innovations ensures a robust understanding of the technique, while the accompanying multimedia enriches the learning experience.

The significance of this work extends beyond its practical applications. It challenges long-standing surgical dogmas, advocating for a paradigm shift in reconstructive surgery where simplicity and functionality align seamlessly with aesthetic outcomes. In doing so, it empowers surgeons across the globe to achieve superior results, irrespective of the limitations imposed by their practice environments.

As a practicing surgeon, educator, and advocate for surgical innovation, I recognise the immense value this book brings to our field. Felix Behan's dedication to refining and disseminating the Keystone flap technique has established a new standard of care, one that prioritises patient satisfaction, surgical efficiency, and the principles of Occam's Razor in solving complex clinical challenges.

For surgeons, educators, and trainees alike, this text is more than a resource—it is an invitation to engage with an impactful methodology that reshapes the landscape of reconstructive and orthopaedic surgery. It is with great admiration and anticipation that I welcome you to explore the insights, techniques, and inspirations contained within these pages.

Peter F.M. Choong
Department of Surgery
Melbourne Medical School
Parkville, VIC, Australia

Faculty of Medicine, Dentistry and Health Science
St. Vincent's Hospital Melbourne, University of Melbourne
Parkville, VIC, Australia

Preface

This book's preface, which is really on reconstructive orthopaedic surgery as its subject, has a scope covering all regions of the body. Its single aim is to teach this cost-containment technique as an alternative to microsurgical reconstruction, which has dominated orthopaedic reconstruction for long periods of time. Surgical teams in hospital units that are disadvantaged therefore can find another method of closure, without the need of microsurgical techniques, yet both techniques have their applications depending on the circumstances and the clinical problem (e.g. diabetics sometimes create problems).

The patient's willing acceptance of the good outcomes is consistently illustrated throughout the text. In simple terms, this book shows how it is done, with the added advantage of operative videos and the voiceover PowerPoint presentation that explains the technique and its refinements in detail.

I recently penned a synopsis of the Keystone principle for the uninitiated who have trouble understanding my thinking and technique of the Keystone Perforator Island Flap. It was titled 'The Keystone Enigma', where I tried to explain the unexplainable from a wide clinical experience and perspective about 'how it works' and the basis of its success. In synoptic terms, we have tried to reduce surgical reconstruction from complexity to simplicity, as exemplified by pianist Einaudi and his portrayal of compositional presentations. Many have difficulty in emulating its success and the video PowerPoint presentation in this text goes a little way in overcoming this problem.

There are umpteen surgeons around the world doing variations of the Keystone design—why is this so? In simplistic terms, the younger generation who have not seen me operate have tried to put into practice and writing what they perceive to be my success. But before publication, as one of the overseas authors observed, the review process for the established journals is done by those who are not aware of this technique and its applications, slowly emerging as it is. So, they converted to lay language for the uninitiated.

I have transgressed certain principles in plastic and reconstructive surgery and removed the mindset of hunting for a perforator with its limitations, likened to a garden hose which we know often kinks. The island flap, based on random perforators in the suprafascial and infrafascial distribution, is the lifeline governing its success. The fascia is never repaired in closure, it is the epidermal closure, sometimes under tension, which creates the optimal aesthetic outcome and wound seal.

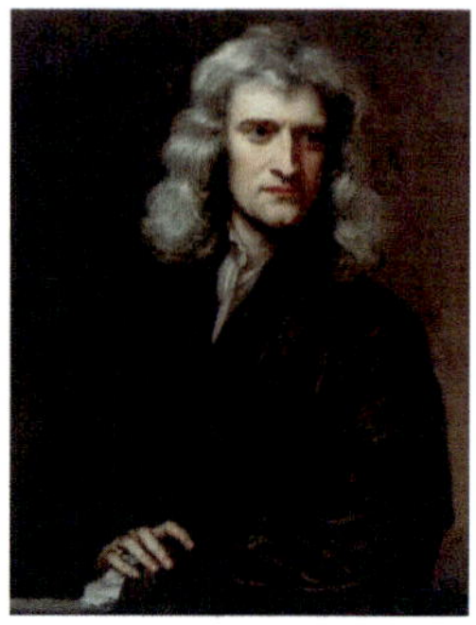

Fig. 1 Godfrey Kneller, portrait of Sir Isaac Newton (1643–1727), public domain

I have had to hark back to embryological principles to offer some basis for my scientific reasoning and use the dermatomal mark outs as an aide memoir for design, with the laxity of the tissues facilitating any advancement, rotation, or transposition. This embryological basis retains neural, autonomic, somatic, arteriovenous and lymphatic links—but yet not defined. Thanks to Professor Geoffrey Hallock in the USA, who synopsised the Keystone characteristics with the acronym P.A.C.E.S, now others are communicating with me worldwide looking for an answer, as Professor Rollin Daniel in California recently emailed me about my concepts, reflecting his inquisitive mind and using the word 'brilliant' to describe it in principle. All my findings have been observational and recorded scientifically with digital images and videos which helps to paint the full picture, repeating the edicts of Sir William Osler who noted that the advances in medicine are all based on observation.

Creating an island has a sympathectomy effect to explain the hypervascularity and pink flare which occurs, allowing us to close under tension.

This random overview that allows the suprafascial and infrafascial circulation of Saint Cyr—which must not be undermined—but the superior epidermal cover can be closed under tension while avoiding any fascial tear and the epidermis creates the wound seal. During this clinical series, my highlight moment came to the surface when I thought as an overview, I feel like a locksmith that has picked the lock. It can be universally applied because of these principles originating from basic sciences.

In summary, for plastic surgical literature since the times of Esser and Dieffenbach are filled with clinical successes and repetitive eponyms for flap repairs to try to universalise flap design, before the microsurgical development which focuses on individual anatomical units. The Keystone word has gone some little way to unifying all these ideas in locoregional repair.

Standing on the shoulders of giants, as Newton (Fig. 1) said about his discovery of gravity in 1666 and a year earlier when a beam of light shone through a prism creating a spectrum when he was a student at Cambridge—all part of Newton's philosophy in his text *Philosophiæ Naturalis Principia Mathematica*, thankfully translated by Voltaire on escaping the politics of Paris who went to England, befriended Newton so the translation accurately conveyed Newton's ideas. Let us not forget that French was the official diplomatic language in Europe at the time, thus Newton could correct translations, which no doubt would have some questionable transitions which would have been corrected by Newton.

More importantly, few have contacted me from around the world about my concepts and asking for my explanation for the clinical success of the Keystone 'enigma' when others venture into this field with new designs and different theories—one asks why? My work over 30 years has all been documented, covering over 3000 cases, leading to publications of six textbooks and umpteen chapter inclusions. I would not be publishing if this technique was not standing up to the rigours of time. Now microsurgery, with a boot on the other foot, has put a different cost factor and time factor in locoregional repair.

No wonder Newton and Darwin had their problems.

Parkville, VIC, Australia Felix Behan

Contents

List of Videos

1 Principles of Keystone Reconstruction

Contents

Core Messages
Clinical observation becomes the basis of research development as Osler quoted.

In orthopaedic reconstructions, soft tissue defects are easily closed using Keystone perforator island loco-regional flaps, avoiding the need for microsurgical free flap transfers and the time and cost restraints implied.

Based on experiences, repetition of the use of the technique increases the range of reconstructive options.

Supplementary Information The online version contains supplementary material available at https://doi.org/10.1007/978-3-031-76702-9_1. The videos can be accessed individually by clicking the DOI link in the accompanying figure caption or by scanning this link with the SN More Media App.

1.1 Keystone Technique and Characteristics

The Keystone [1] management in orthopaedic reconstruction employs the same principles as in any closure of a soft tissue defect often encountered in orthopaedic injuries. The soft tissue defect closure in oncological management can be applied

F. Behan, *Keystone Flap for Complex Orthopaedic Problems*,
https://doi.org/10.1007/978-3-031-76702-9_1

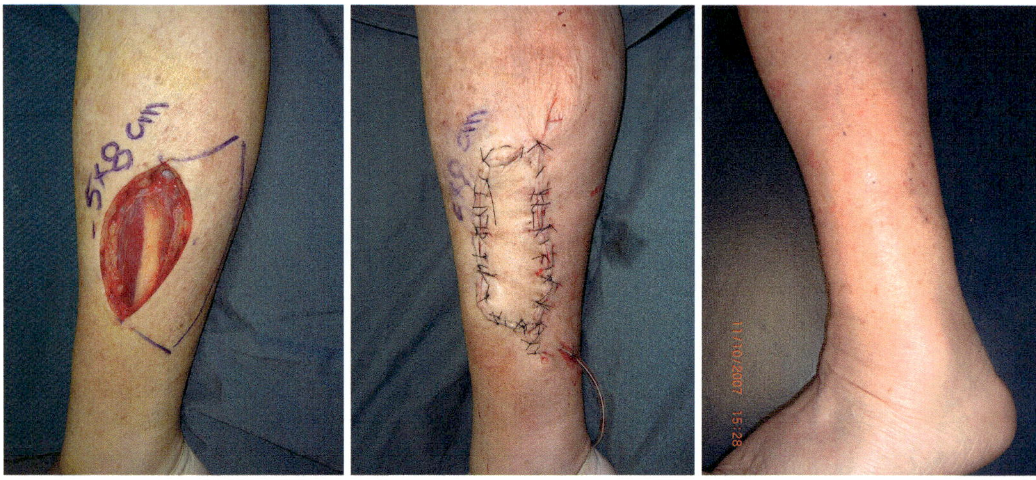

Fig. 1.1 Clearance Closure Conclusion

in similar integumentary losses based on orthopaedic injuries, and all variations of the Keystone have their applications and have made an important contribution in the surgical repair of major integumentary defects. Some have even asked 'is there such a thing as scarless surgery?' This case series about a melanotic lesion on the calf of a 65 year old, treated with clearance, and a Keystone island flap repair illustrates these principles (Fig. 1.1):

As neurovascular island flaps came into prominence in the 1990s and with the introduction of the Keystone concept, first published in the *ANZ Journal of Surgery* in 2003, this island design of reconstruction entered a new phase, avoiding microsurgical repairs.

My experience since 1995 over 20 years of over 3000 Keystone flaps universally applied all over the body is the basis of this publication. Additionally, soft tissue defects are included to show the range of applications of the Keystone flap, which is really a conjoined V–Y flap originally designed by Dieffenbach [2] in the 1850s. This surgical experience, documented photographically, is the basis of the surgical applications of the Keystone island perforator loco-regional flap for orthopaedic patients for closure of soft tissue defects.

As long as these reconstructive principles apply in raising the Keystone, there should be universal success.

1.1.1 Keystone Flap Technique

1. **Fascial lining**: This is an absolute prerequisite to line the deep surface of the Keystone, the source of the perforator supply, including neurovascular support and the accompanying autonomic, somatic and lymphatic input. The division of the deep fascia allows the unit to swing in a collateral method, and this single Keystone flap closes this double defect (the lesion and the flap) under tension.
2. **The dermatome roadmap—a random source of perforators**: The Keystone is designated within the dermatomal mark-out, and an axiomatic rule applies as random perforators embryologically follow the neural patterns of the dermatome, thus ensuring viability with arterial, venous and lympho-venular anastomoses
3. **Undermining is contraindicated beneath the Keystone**: Undermining the Keystone arc is totally contraindicated as this is the source of the random perforators from these embryonic axial sources. Even when undermining is necessary for a loco-regional repair, one-third of deep attachment must be maintained to achieve a viable outcome, should undermining be deemed necessary help to advance, rotate and transpose island

flaps. Drainage is essential and a single Redivac drain tube bent in the shape of a U can lie within both defects, the initial surgical problem and the subsequent Keystone flap, while discretely placed beneath the island avoiding perforators

4. **Like-for-like**: This reconstructive principle of using like-for-like, acknowledging Gillies contribution, is thus continued to optimise the aesthetic outcome
5. **3-Phase suturing technique**: The single layer closure using a locking mattress nylon suture at the points of tension stay in situ for three weeks and used throughout most cases, if not every one. The ordinary mattress sutures to complete the wound closure stay in situ for two weeks. And the epidermal closure is done with a continuous 3/0 nylon to provide perfect epidermal seal, and these sutures can be even cut from the seven-day period to avoid cross hatching. Absorbable subcutaneous sutures as a layered closure technique are thus avoided allowing the locking mattress suture to compensate for any deeper defect. Additionally, the absorbable sutures often leave a subcutaneous line of wound healing reactions and these lumps tend to be permanent, an observed clinical finding in spite of published material stating they are absorbable.

The emergence of microvascular surgical repair concepts has played an important part since Ian Taylor's [3] publication in 1973. However, when the Keystone island flap concept is used, cognisant of its listed characteristics, compares favourably when tissue match, low complication rate, a shorter operative timeframe, with recovery of sensory somatic supply in an aesthetic outcome, thus its value is continuing to be reassessed as an alternative to microsurgical repair in orthopaedics.

The **clinical characteristics** of the Keystone are summarised by the acronym P.A.C.E.S. as an aide memoir:

Pain: The **pain free** characteristic is a remarkable finding in the Keystone application in its postoperative phase. In simplistic terms, this may be explained that the cutaneous somatic supply divided around the arc of the Keystone creates an anaesthetic surface which recovers in some weeks as experienced in all linear surgical wounds. The only symptom the patient notices is a feeling of tightness which is one of the keynote features when wounds are closed under such tension.

Aesthetics: The Gillies principle of using **like-for-like** is standard reconstructive idea entrenched in history and producing outcomes which are most satisfying to the patient, particularly on exposed sites. The normal attractive appearance of the integument is lost when large defects are grafted or microvascular free flaps, without tissue match, fill the soft tissue defects as part of the orthopaedic repair.

Complications: Complications and adverse outcomes are not frequent. Wound breakdown when tension sutures are removed prematurely by an outside clinic may occur. Vascular complications are rare because the perforators are not individually skeletonised. Such technique may strip away the filamentous autonomic, somatic and lymphatic supports along the axial channels of such vascular perforator of the suprafascial and infrafascial perforators. Irradiated tissue is not a contraindication in the Keystone applications because of the hypervascularity principles established by this design concept. In the diabetic lower limb where the microcirculation is the centre of pathology, the elements of partial necrosis have occurred in type II diabetics and as a consequence closure must be done without tension and a generous use of skin grafting.

Expeditious in Execution: Time is money is a Benjamin Franklin quote from Fisher's book of 1748. If one can operate in a reduced timeframe, this has benefits for all modalities in the treatment and care of patients, particularly the elderly. It has also an economic factor and theatre throughput, whereas long reconstructive sagas may produce an adverse alternative. The implications for staff allocation need no elaboration in microsurgical team procedures. We need not repeat that the longer the operative procedure, particularly with microsurgical techniques, then pressure areas amplify the co-morbidities.

Somatic Recovery and **S**welling with the Resolution of Oedema: These final characteristics of the Keystone go hand in hand. As in any surgical wound, the division of the filamentous cutaneous branches creates a temporary anaesthetic field around the operative site. This may recover in the weeks that follow when the integument has healed and the scar is maturing. A final characteristic in observation is the resolution of swelling and oedema (cases 3.1.7 and 3.1.10) which goes hand in hand over this recovery period of up to 8 weeks.

Thus, clinically in any applied reconstructive situation, anything that offers advantages listed above are worthy of consideration.

Acquiring the technique, as in the author's experience, takes time hence the video supplement of cases explains the background and the refinements in the thinking behind the surgical technique, really a radical alternative to the established way of treating under the microsurgical domain.

Start small and then metamorphose into larger cases. In the main the Keystone can cover the majority of soft tissue defects in the upper and lower limbs.

In the various sections, cases reveal preoperative to the postoperative phase to illustrate the applications and unifying principles of reconstructive surgery using the Keystone—simplicity in surgery is always welcome—the Keystone is simple to apply once mastered when the basic principles are followed. Satisfaction becomes evident at the patient level, including that for the operator. This benefit of looking almost normal has a psychological benefit as well.

My experience in surgery as a plastic and reconstructive surgeon goes back to my mentor Sir Benjamin Rank in the 1970s and my colleagues in London, Ian Wilson and Charlie Westbury at the Westminster, Marsden and St George's Hospitals, London.

The standard skin grafting technique for large defects led me to develop island flap reconstructions, and based on my research, the Bezier [1] island flap was published in 1995 which is a curvilinear ellipsoidal V–Y flap in the Dieffenbach manner. For larger melanoma defects of the back one day, I doubled the size of the V–Y flap and ended up with a curvilinear arc flap, all based on intercostal random perforators. This arc flap came under the terminology of a Keystone. Geometrically, when one joins the opposite points of the curvilinear Keystone design, it suddenly appears like two conjoined double V–Y flaps and with underlying suprafascial and infrafascial perforator support [4].

DUET performances in surgery with the orthopaedic units were conducted as the Keystone solution for soft tissue defects did not have the restrictions of microsurgical repairs when re-manipulation and realignment orthopedically were absolutely contraindicated, as illustrated in this Atlas reflecting the value of this DUET surgery and its reliability was confirmed. Without the input of these combined referrals of complex cases needing complex reconstructions, the range of cases in the orthopaedic atlas would be insignificant.

All photographic illustrations are my own preoperative, intraoperative and postoperative phases and the advantage of the simple photographic digital camera allowed me to discuss cases during the intraoperative phase. My London experience with Ralph Hutchens, the Chief Photographer at the Royal College of Surgeons in the early 1970s was the introduction to my photographic developments and future expertise.

Thus, in conclusion, these orthopaedic cases from the Western Hospital in Melbourne and from private practice of orthopaedic consultants, who eventually appreciated the value of this technique without the contributions of referrals from my surgical colleagues Ray Crowe, Bob Pianta, Chris Haw and Ian Harris, have been the basis for this clinical series.

Difficult problems create solutions while observing the principles of Occam's Razor [5], i.e. something simple to initiate a solution.

The loco-regional Keystone flaps provide an attractive aesthetic alternative with its diverse architectural variations but still an island flap and perforator based, aligned within the dermatomes, based on suprafascial and infrafascial circulation, sourced from regional perforators.

1.2 How the Keystone Island Flap Evolved

The basis of the Keystone originally began with the Angiotome concept [6] of flap vascularity based on neuro-dermatomal patterns. This is defined as a system of linked axial pattern flaps using the dermatomes as an *aide memoir* for alignment and design. This developed from research into flap vascularity at the Royal College of Surgeons in London in 1971 when the importance of the fascial layer in loco-regional flaps became self-evident when doing vascular injection studies. The study of the blood supply of the integument led to certain anatomical conclusions of the importance of this fascial layer concept in loco-regional repairs. This was presented to the 6th International Congress of Plastic and Reconstructive Surgery in Paris, 1975 [7], having the support of the international surgical community including Professor William Manchester.

The pioneering German surgeon **Dieffenbach** (1792–1847) **in 1845 established** the principle of the V–Y flap and this became the hallmark of a lot of the reconstructive flaps used in clinical practice from the nineteenth to the twentieth centuries. The V–Y advancement loco-regional flap concept has been refined, and I developed the ellipsoidal V–Y variant which I call the **Bézier flap to facilitate tight closures and soften the aesthetic line, particularly in the management of melanoma.** Bézier curve is an ellipsoidal V–Y flap. The Keystone is a conjoined architectural shape of two V–Y flaps with V–Y points at extreme (joining the diagonals produces the shape in a conjoined manner). I had my arc flap, fascially based, totally islanded and leaving any communicating venous links where possible all based on supra- and infrafascial random perforators. My original terminology of the curvilinear arc design was superseded by the word Keystone thanks to my colleague Alan Breidahl FRACS of Melbourne. This name with its architectural Moorish connotations has led to the development of observational findings leading to further clinical applications, even closing under tension because of its reliability. Even **design variations,** as illustrated in Fig. 1.2, from squares to rectangles have been used but always governed by the size and dimensions of the soft tissue defect. But, the principles of varying the design are still based on the dermatomal alignment with its intact neurovascular and lymphatic support. These embryological principles are respected in all Keystone designs as long as they are fashioned in the dermatome and undermining leaving at least one third of deep attachment is a basic prerequisite in

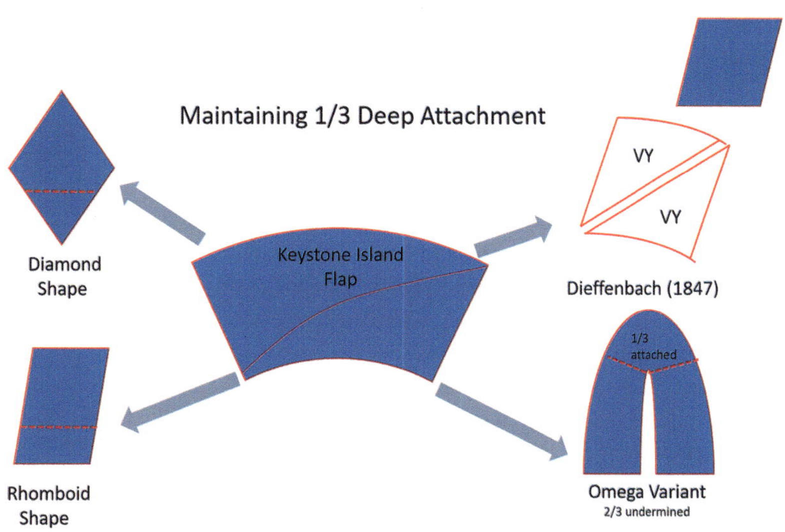

Fig. 1.2 Design variations of the Keystone flap governed by the defect

Keystone applications. Specific vascular investigations of perforators with angiography have not been found necessary—another financial benefit in minimising cost—if the above principles are followed in raising Keystone reconstructive flaps. Such is the reliability of the vascularity, closure under tension is an accepted norm and even undermining, retaining the fascial base ensures its viability as long as there is one third of deep attachment retained throughout and as long as there is an intact nerve supply aligned within the dermatomes, there must be a vascular support system accompanying the nerves. In the **Omega variant**, the middle third deep attachment follows the same rule and allows the arm of the Keystone to close variations in anatomical sites. It has applications for closing defects of the lower limb where the flaps can be bent in the shape of a U, as illustrated, hence the eponym the Omega variant. The other clinical observation as summarised below is the hyperaemic phase if these design precepts are followed where the Red Dot Sign is a characteristic finding of all Keystone closures in spite of wound apposition under lines of tension. The cases included, which illustrate these points, will be noted throughout. As the perforators are not skeletonised and therefore not stripped of fine elements of autonomic and somatic nerve supply and lymphatic drainage support, one can only assume hypothetically that these factors must support the clinical findings as evidenced in the postoperative results.

Some of these design variations originated from a wide experience in reconstructive surgery with use of the V–Y island flap (of which the Keystone represents a duplicated version) and earlier work on the **Limberg Flap** [8] and its designs on the flap integumentary surface.

The reliability of the Keystone is its main characteristic, and the main limitation of the technique is closure under tension but the use of supplementary grafting on appropriate bed overcomes this problem. Lack of adherence to such principles, as enunciated here, has led to necrosis, as I have observed with other operators. Presumably undermining and disturbing support from the suprafascial and infrafascial perforators. In all reconstructive techniques, venous drainage must be respected and microanastomosis and repair of any inadvertent venous damage can thus be repaired. The hairline vascular perforator supports are thus embedded in the fascia and the depths of the Keystone (Fig. 1.3).

In the original dermatome mark out published in 1900[23] using the virus infiltration by Herpes Zoster to establish the dermatomal mark outs and as viruses follow the nerve patterns. Extrapolating from this on an embryological basis if there is a nerve supply, there must be a blood supply and arterial flows create their own venous exit as they expand into the final developmental design. The vessels that grow with the nerves must have

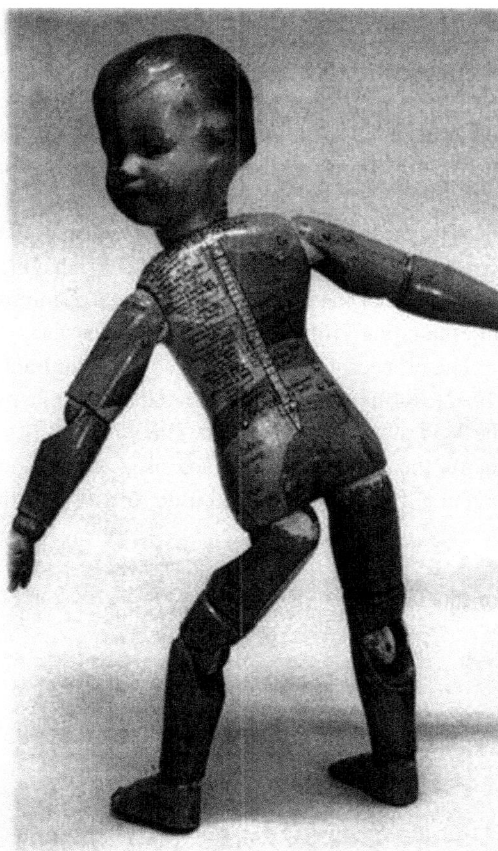

Fig. 1.3 The baby doll of the 1930s shows the dermatomes which were taken from Sir Henry Head's publication in 1900, "Brain. The Pathology of Herpes Zoster and its Bearing on Sensory Localisation". (Reproduced with permission from the 2016 autumn catalogue by antique book library Alain Brieux, Paris, and from Henry Head, A. W. Campbell, 1900, Macmillan and Company)

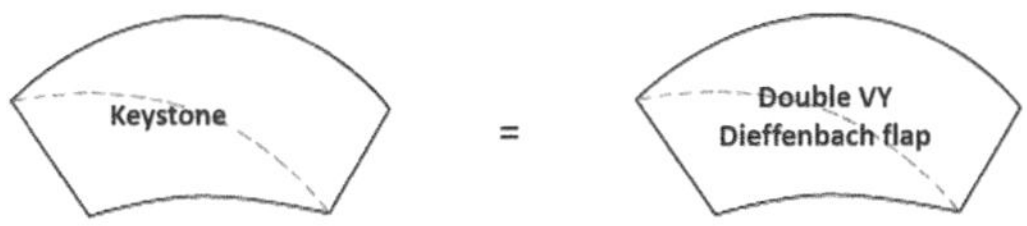

Fig. 1.4 The Keystone flap is a double V-Y Dieffenbach flap joining diagonally opposite points

autonomic supply to control their dilation as well and likewise a somatic input allows their tactile sensation to recover. Technically, a lesion pressing on the L1 root of the spinal cord creates an anaesthetic patch below the inguinal ligament on the anterior thigh (Fig. 1.4).

A demarcation of perforators with their angiographic definition has not been a pattern in this reconstructive series of Keystone uses in the thousands. However, the aide memoir in raising the flap within the dermatomes has been the basis of this clinical success because if there is a dermatomal blood supply embryologically, there must be an accompanying blood supply with these neural mark outs which are dragged in continuity as development continues. The Keystone is really an umbrella of tissue expanded to cover various surgical defects with V–Y points at their apices. The random pattern of the perforators is the source of vascular support ensuring advancement, rotation and transposition (ART) of Keystone island flaps as long as one third of deep attachment of the cutaneous island flap is maintained. I repeat, the gamut of vascular changes in the Keystone island flap come from observational findings not experimental investigations, and the usual restrictions one observes in closing large defects enable wound apposition. However, the Keystone principle, as these are fascial based, allows one to **close under tension**—breaking one of the mandated rules of plastic surgery. Why is this possible or to quote the late Sumner Millar 'Why is it so?' Again, observationally there are two aspects to this vascular perfusional increase we call **Reactive Hyperaemia** [9], it is the same as a lumbar sympathectomy effect, creating a pink foot in due course to assist healing in the elderly diabetic with distal perfusional restraints. This reactive hyperaemia takes 10–15 min to reveal itself when using the Keystone island flap repair. However, others have observed that the island principle creates a hydrostatic barrier to perfusion forcing the venous exit to the line of least resistance down the perforator stalks. These findings may be cyanotic from an observational point of view thus, if we have a combination of two hypotheses working out a combined outcome the hyperaemia causes the **Red Dot Sign**—the suture point site of exit through the Keystone is arterial red not cyanotic bluish which seems to convey there is an arterial factor in preference to a hydrostatic factor.

The Keystone experiences began in 1995.

The origin of the Keystone, being a double V-Y island, comes from my experience in using V–Y island flaps in many reconstructive options. As a preamble to the Bezier design, an ellipsoidal V–Y island flap—as illustrated in the diagrams, variations in the triangular design arise by joining the opposite extremes of the rhomboidal shape. The next stage in island flap design—the Keystone—is when this arc flap is a combination of two V–Y island flaps conjoined. In other words, this elliptical shape allows an easy apposition without tension in the closure of a surgical defect, one of the limitations of the straight V–Y flap (Figs. 1.5 and 1.6).

Any reconstruction based on a defined perforator may experience interference with their somatic, autonomic, lymphatic or humeral supply. The Keystone concept retains these neurovascular supports at the arterial, venous, somatic, autonomic and lymphatic support which has clinical applications in reviewing the postoperative effect of the Keystone.

1.2.1 The Science Behind the Keystone Flap: Based on Observational Findings and Recorded Clinical Findings Documented Digitally

Quoting Osler, Cheng Lo and Stecco.

William Osler (1849–1919), the influential Canadian physician said that *'observation is the basis of scientific advancement in medicine'*. My observations of the behaviour of various islanded

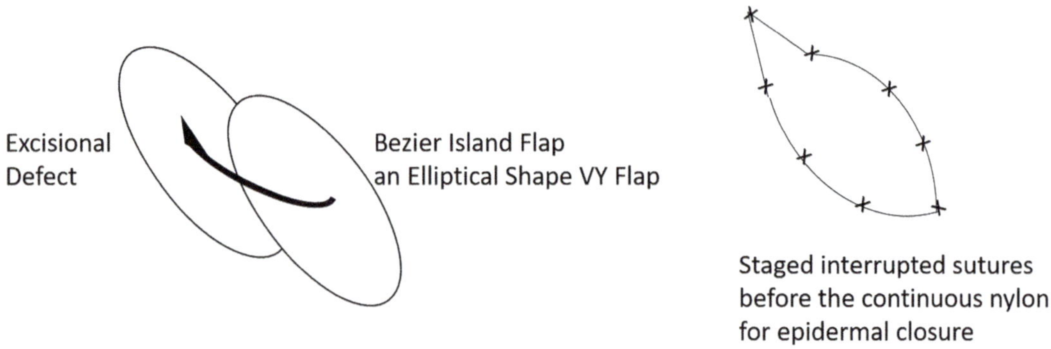

Fig. 1.5 Illustrations of the Bezier curvilinear V–Y island flap

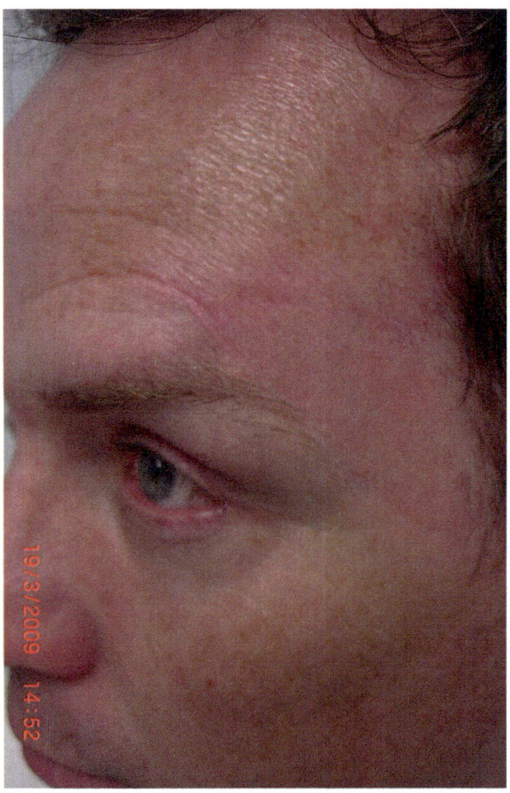

Fig. 1.6 A clinical example from my melanoma series using the Bezier curvilinear V–Y island flap with its subsequent applications applied in orthopaedic management—appearance at 6 months

local flaps led me on to search for the physiological basis for these findings using the digital images as a basis for comparison and control. This was inspired by other research published in the surgical literature on angiogenesis, the increased blood supply in tissue-expanded flaps, concepts in endothelial stress and facial nerve repair. These observations have not been the subject of pathology investigations to date but to quote Carl Sagan the Physicist who said 'The absence of evidence is not the evidence of absence' [10]. We have repetitive observational findings with the Keystone—all our observations are clinically recorded in digital format.

The challenge was how to come up with good **research projects** confirming the clinical findings which have been observational. The Cheng Lo [9] paper on vascularity of Keystones is the only one referenced about these tissue findings confirming the increased vascularity in island flaps.

However, a recent verbal communication thanks to Mr. Naveen Somia with Professor Carla Stecco, Orthopaedic Surgeon from Padua University and an expert on fascial innervation and vascularity has put the science factor into these clinical characteristics, besides observational findings. As evidenced by her 2022 publication [11, 12], she affirms that there are implications for the sympathetic nervous system as she has described in her communication. In a recent work, Stecco et al. revealed a huge innervation of the superficial fascia: the nervous structures were found above and around blood vessels and close to fatty tissue, adipocytes, but they penetrated also in the connective tissue itself and are found in the midst of fibro-adipose tissue. The diameter of the nerve fibres ranges from 2.5 to 35 μm, and the fibres are both sensitive and autonomic nerve fibres. The relative percentage of autonomic innervation of 33.82% in the superficial fascia was found in association with a huge vascular network forming a plexus. Additionally, it was possible to detect arteriovenous shunts, under the control of sympathetic innervation. In the light of these findings, it is evident that the superficial fascia can play a role in thermoregulation, proprioception and pain perception. The creation of the Keystone flap can alter the sympathetic innervation of the superficial fascia and consequently causes a vasodilation of the vessels inside the superficial fascia. This would explain the Red Dot Sign.

1.2.2 The Clinical Characteristics of the Keystone: More Observational Findings

The acronym P.A.C.E.S. becomes a natural application:

Pain: The **pain free** characteristic is a remarkable finding in the Keystone application in its postoperative phase. In simplistic terms, this may be explained that the cutaneous somatic supply divided around the arc of the Keystone creates an anaesthetic surface which recovers in some weeks as experienced in all linear surgical wounds. The only symptom the patient notices is a feeling of tightness which is one of the keynote features when wounds are closed under such tension.

Aesthetics: The Gillies principle of using **like-for-like** is standard reconstructive idea entrenched in history and producing outcomes which are most satisfying to the patient, particularly on exposed sites. The normal attractive appearance of the integument is lost when large defects are grafted or microvascular free flaps, without tissue match, fill the soft tissue defects as part of the orthopaedic repair.

Complications: Complications and adverse outcomes are not frequent. Wound breakdown when tension sutures are removed prematurely by an outside clinic may occur. Vascular complications are rare because the perforators are not individually skeletonised. Such technique may strip away the filamentous autonomic, somatic and lymphatic supports along the axial channels of such vascular perforator of the suprafascial and infrafascial perforators. Irradiated tissue is not a contraindication in the Keystone applications because of the hypervascularity principles established by this design concept. In the diabetic lower limb where the microcirculation is the centre of pathology, the elements of partial necrosis have occurred in type II diabetics and as a consequence closure must be done without tension and a generous use of skin grafting.

Expeditious in Execution: Time is money is a Benjamin Franklin quote from Fisher's book of 1748. If one can operate in a reduced timeframe, this has benefits for all modalities in the treatment and care of patients, particularly the elderly. It has also an economic factor and theatre throughput, whereas long reconstructive sagas may produce an adverse alternative. The implications for staff allocation need no elaboration in microsurgical team procedures. We need not repeat that the longer the operative procedure, particularly with microsurgical techniques, then pressure areas amplify the co-morbidities.

Somatic Recovery and **S**welling with the Resolution of Oedema: These final characteristics of the Keystone go hand in hand. As in any surgical wound, the division of the filamentous cutaneous branches creates a temporary anaesthetic field around the operative site. This may recover in the weeks that follow when the integument has healed and the scar is maturing. A final characteristic in observation is the resolution of swelling and oedema (cases 3.1.7 and 3.1.10) which goes hand in hand over this recovery period of up to 8 weeks.

A Synopsis of the Observational Findings Case by Case as Digitally Recorded:

A case example exemplifying the P.A.C.E.S. characteristics:

Mitotic lesion of the scalp Merkel cell (the appearance of an amelanotic lesion) follows biopsy clearance and repair using Keystone principles. The tumour defect on the vertex of the scalp produced an oncological clearance of a defect 8 × 8 cm (Figs. 1.7, 1.8, 1.9, 1.10, 1.11, 1.12, 1.13, 1.14, 1.15, and 1.16).

In summary her aesthetic result without complications is an acceptable outcome. All the P.A.C.E.S. characteristics were evident throughout.

The patient responses, recorded on video and including video supplement, puts a realistic perspective on the technique—it works and is pain free.

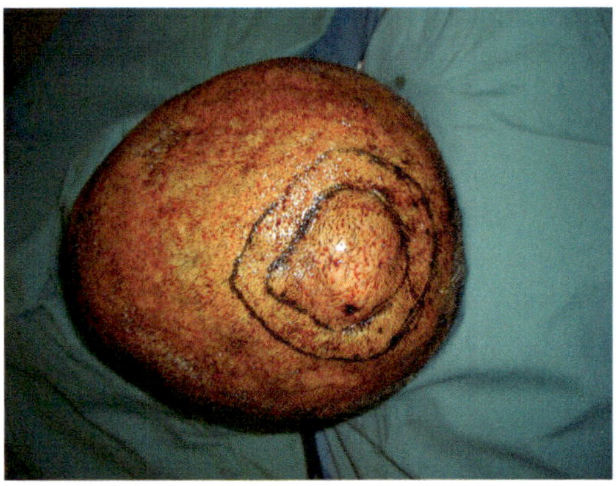

Fig. 1.7 The mark out of the tumour macroscopic and the 2 cm peripheral clearance of 1 cm into the outer table of the scalp

1.2.3 Dermatomal Precincts: A Link Back to Embryology When the Neural, Vascular, Autonomic and Lymphatic Links Are Part of the Developmental Process

The dermatomes are the aide memoire to define random perforators. This avoids the costly investigation of angiography, which has not been applied to any of these Keystone cases, which is standard in microsurgical procedures, another cost saving benefit. Intact nerve supply is consistent with an intact blood supply. The universal dermatome designs are the basis for Keystone orientation and then elevated with a fascial substrate. It is essential for undermined flaps when advancement, rotation and transposition are necessary but essentially one must leave, cautiously, one third of deep attachment is any undermining is deemed necessary however while the epidermal division ensures the island flap design which is just closed directly on completion as a single layer using locking mattress sutures and a continuous 3/0 nylon for epidermal seal. These dermatome precincts are illustrated in Fig. 1.17, and it is essential that the Keystone design lies within the dermatomal mark outs.

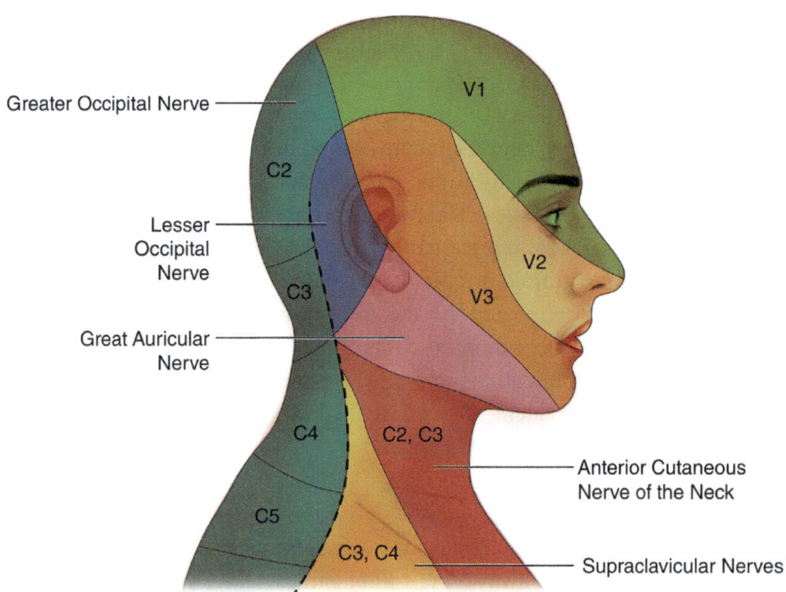

Fig. 1.8 The dermatomal mark out is the guide for the location of the random perforators coming through the fascia

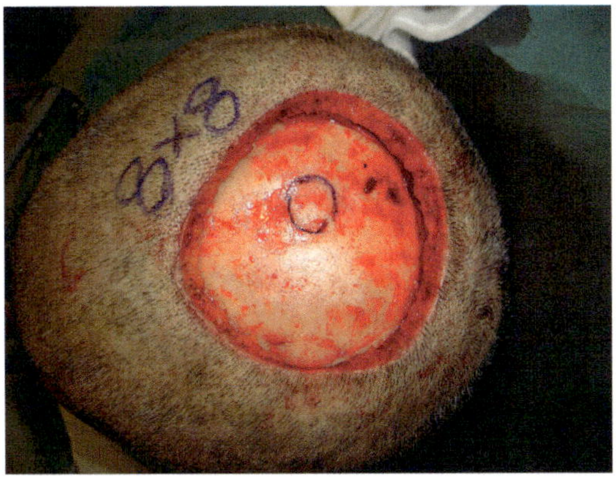

Fig. 1.9 The peripheral clearance before additional removal of the outer table of the scalp for clearance of the Merkel cell tumour producing a defect 8 × 8 cm

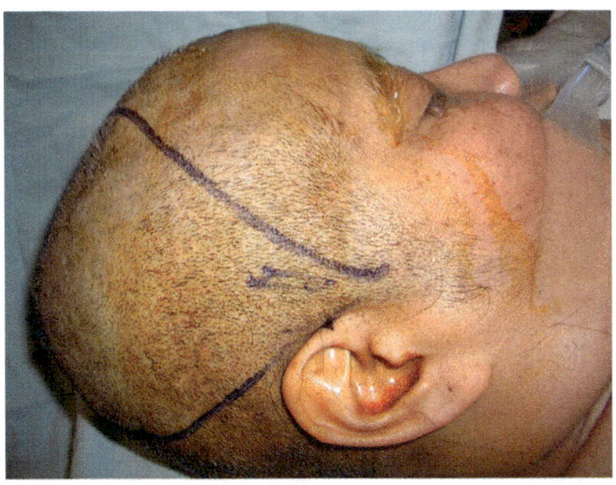

Fig. 1.10 Superficial temporal artery mark out. The flap is raised retaining and not skeletonising the axial neurovascular structures. This retains periadventitial tissue to ensure autonomic and somatic input

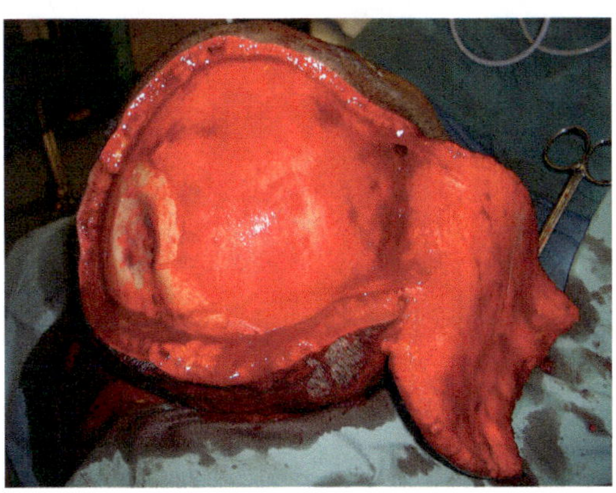

Fig. 1.11 Raising the flap using blunt dissection once the integument is divided around the periphery

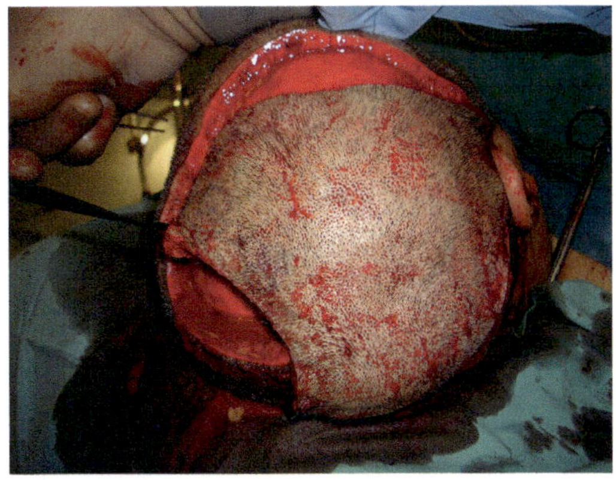

Fig. 1.12 Staged closure sequence

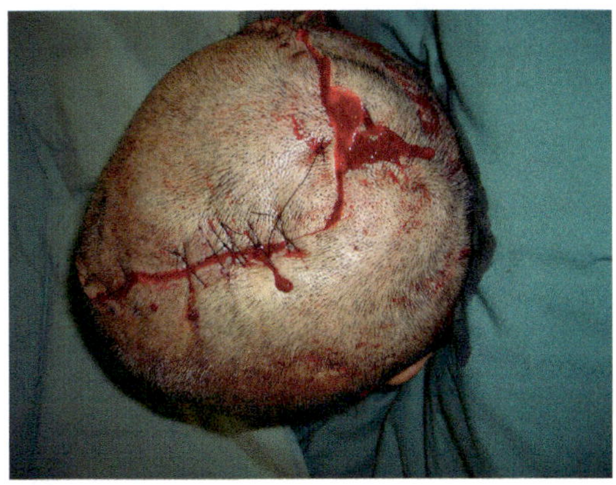

Fig. 1.13 The locking mattress sutures at the points of maximum tension to close the defect before ordinary mattress sutures produce wound closure

Synopsis of surgical principles for raising a keystone island flap

1. The dermatome alignment is an absolute prerequisite in the flap location.
2. The standard Keystone repair is a single unit straddling two surgical defects which are closed under tension.
3. With advancement, rotation and transposition of the fascial-based Keystone, it is raised in a distal to proximal direction, clipping any fascial perforators but leaves one third of proximal attachment in any therapeutic repair.
4. The flap consists of skin/fat/fascia and longitudinal anatomical structures in the vicinity, e.g. any venous line and neural are all retained in the initial dissection as deemed appropriate.

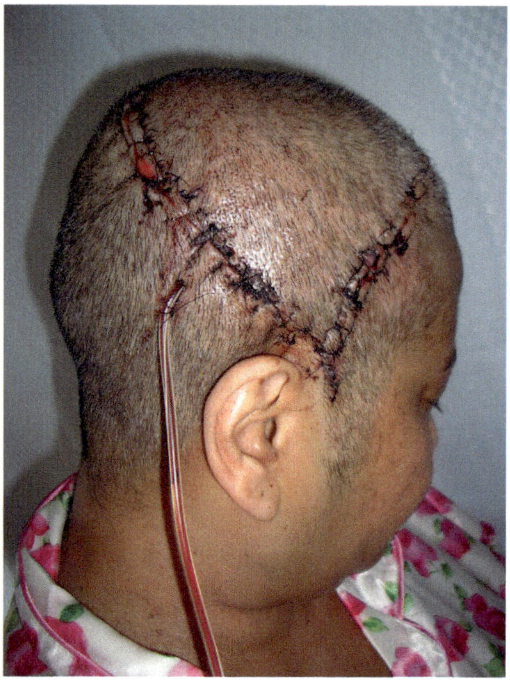

Fig. 1.14 On completion with Redi-vac drainage. Note the hyperaemic flare in the island flap compared with the image of the surrounding scalp. Hypothetically a sympathectomy effect

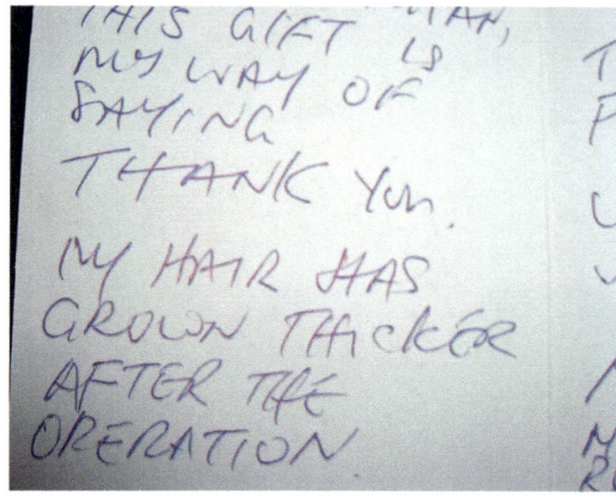

Fig. 1.16 Her Christmas card thanking me for the surgical procedure and stating that her hair is now growing thicker as a result of the Keystone reconstruction. Again, a reflection of hypervascularity of the sympathectomy effect

Fig. 1.15 The appearance 6 months later and I bring to your attention the patient's observation of the increased hair growth and thickness. Again, a clinical outcome of hypervascularity in the scalp as seen in Keystone reconstructions

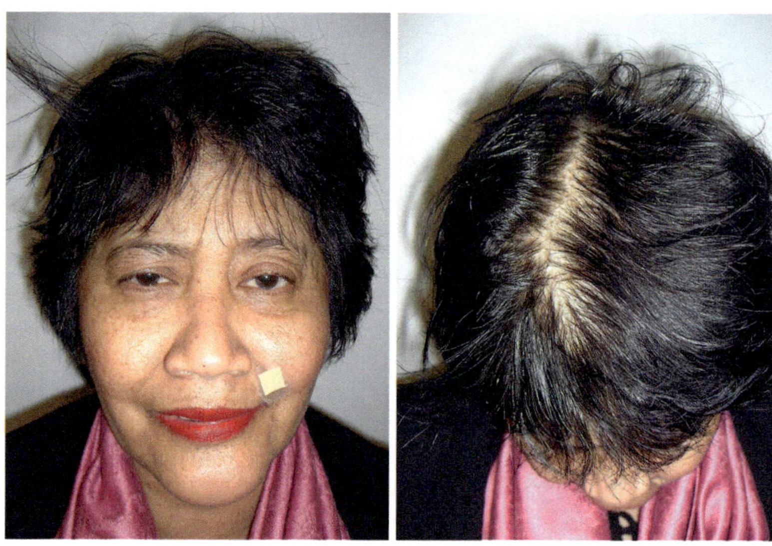

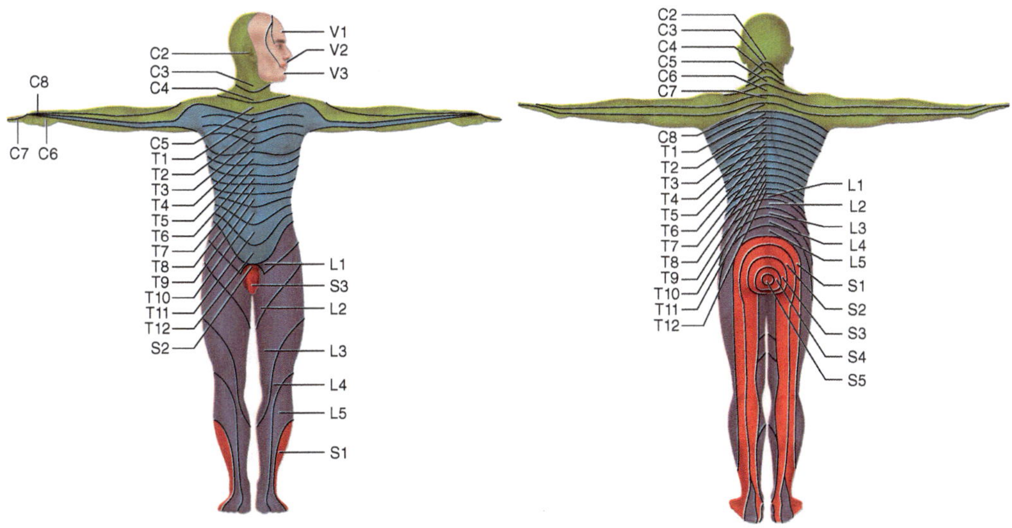

Fig. 1.17 The dermatome precincts

5. Two thirds undermining is a valid technical modification, with the remaining proximal one third attached for random perforator perfusional support allowing closure under tension where deemed necessary. The vascular perfusion may be slightly imperilled but a relocation of sutures on release helps to solve this temporary problem.
6. The cases and their digital images, some with time and date stamps, allow us to be specific about documented data.

The Keystone success in reconstructive surgery is based on the dermatomal outlines of the body which incorporates embryological principles in development. This implies the absolute necessity, when tissue is developing from its embryological phase, there must be some stimulus to make the organelle (the viscous or the limbs) develop in a certain way to match the final outcomes to create a human specimen when treated clinically or when researched in the anatomy museum. What goes to where to produce the ultimate outcome? But harking back to experimental or physiological outlines, such observational findings have been the stepping stone when one looks for an aetiological explanation. The history of the lumbar sympathectomy is worth recalling as an adjunct to my findings in clinical anatomy with the Keystone.

Thanks to Professor John Royle, a former Royal Australasian College of Surgeons dignitary and a former Vascular Surgeon could reveal the story of the development of a lumbar sympathectomy [13]. It was following the treatment of wounded soldiers after the Great War that the thought of spasticity in muscles with still ongoing intact motor and sensory innervation that could have been a contribution from the autonomic nervous system and its sympathetic overlay? This orthopaedic surgeon did anatomical investigations down the lumbar chain looking for elements of the sympathetic nervous system, all of which were operational, all from an anatomical point of view. Besides the sympathetic nervous system, the somatic nervous system had an important contribution for sensory protection and proprioceptive function. So, this combination of neural elements became the basis for the research before the clinical application in doing a lumbar sympathectomy became accepted.

It was the observational findings following such a procedure that the 'warm foot' observed in

24 h became the natural consequence following the operation of a lumbar sympathectomy. But as an additional finding, this hypervascularity had important implications in wound healing with the increased blood supply providing a solution to elements of trophic ulceration in those lower limbs that were still recovering from war injuries.

So, it was concluded that the division of the lumbar autonomic trunk had a collateral effect of vascular dilatation, increased vascular perfusion and a corollary of this was expediting healing for elements of trophic ulceration which is of a diabetic or pressure origin.

Could it be that making an island flap of the integument with a fascial base was similar in principle to a lumbar sympathectomy and its distal foot manifestations? When creating an island flap and the division through the integument removed the somatic sensory response and local changes, like the swearing response, in an area so demarcated.

Thus, when we raise a Keystone flap, we are dividing in fact filamentous branches of somatic or autonomic nerves, allowing the remaining networks, sourced from the lumbar origin, to function accordingly with their manifestations of hypervascularity. We have observed constantly with the Keystone the vascular flare where the flap, as an island, has the apparent appearance of increased vascular flow. But, more importantly, the suture point for surgical apposition bleeds more on the flap side than the receiving side or insertion site.

In the article by Professor Brendon Coventry and John Walsh ANZ Journal of Surgery 2003; 73:14–18. It is quite coincidental that my initial Keystone publication was in the same year in the same journal—*ANZ Journal of Surgery*.

The background to the Coventry article discusses the issue of ischemic rest pain and that lumbar sympathectomy had been used over the years, the mechanism by which improvements achieved as both sensory and vasomotor fibres travel in the lumbar sympathetic chain and the effects of a lumbar sympathectomy on these nerve types have been the basis of investigation. Normal and PVD controls had intact sensory and vasomotor nerves around dermal cutaneous blood vessels, but these were complete or virtually completely lost after lumbar sympathectomy, by either chemical or surgical means. To conclude: lumbar sympathectomy severed both vasomotor and sensory fibres suggesting the relief of rest pain may be explained, not only by increased cutaneous and muscle blood flow, but also by nociceptor sensory denervation.

Hence, by reverse thinking, when we have the vascular changes in a Keystone island flap, there must be a dominating sympathectomy effect to enunciate the characteristics of the Keystone with the acronym P.A.C.E.S.— they are Pain free, tissue match like-for-like in an Aesthetic manner with minimal vascular Complications and Economically feasible in time with cutaneous Sensory recovery – hence the acronym P.A.C.E.S.

1.2.4 Traditional Teaching

Keystone management has broken certain management rules in the reconstructive field allowing us to continue the Gillies dictum of like-for-like in any reconstructive saga. The microsurgical dominance now has to be revisited when one sees the advantages of the Keystone repair summarised by the P.A.C.E.S. acronym. Governed by the need for success, let alone aesthetic outcomes multiple descriptions of techniques plague the literature with various anatomical and architectural variations. The value of pedicle flaps, a follow on from microsurgical repair has been the vogue and the Blondeel perforator book [14] is the latest update summarising such applications in a universal way. And the Keystone technique is based on random perforators from the suprafascial and infrafascial layers sourced from deeper perforators often from a muscular orientation. This avoids the angiographic investigation and its cost saving implications.

1.2.5 How the Keystone Universalises the Clinical Outcome at Most Sites

As the possibility of long-term outcome and the patient's wish for an aesthetic outcome, this is where the Keystone seems to unify all the variables and as described above, the P.A.C.E.S. acronym is synoptic. Another advantage of this expeditious means of reconstruction is governed by the patient's co-morbidity status and the concerns with complications from mismanagement aggravate the morbidity factor in the elderly. Thus, if radical removal of groin mass or access to the neck of the femur for an ORIF can be done by a simplified technique, this is where the Keystone application becomes pre-eminently successful and the simplified closure using the L1 dermatome, moving upwards and inwards with division of the tensor fascia lata and the fascia down the medial side of the thigh. Distally, the island design is completed by creating a division in the epidermis across the suprapatellar region to ensure the hypervascularity factors of the Keystone are retained to ensure expeditious healing.

1.2.6 Arteriovenous and Lymphatic Communications in the Perforator Support Passing Through the Deep Fascia

The advantages of a non-complicated surgical repair need no elaboration, and the Keystone has one preeminent characteristic, i.e. neurodermatomally based within embryological mark outs. This has the accompanying arteriovenous, autonomic and somatic supply. All Keystones must be fascial lined for advancement, rotation and transposition and for more awkward loco-regional repairs along the anterior tibia and can be undermined two thirds along the peroneal L1 dermatome while preserving deep attachment to the remaining third over the neurovascular perforator supports, these must include lymphatic drainage. This embryological background has been the basis for the clinical characteristics synopsised by the acronym P.A.C.E.S. covering Pain, Aesthetics, vascular Complications, Expeditious in execution and the subsequent recovery of Sensation with the resolution of oedema, presumably dilating lymphatic channels after clinical healing. Again, these are all observational phenomena gleaned over the cases done to date in the thousands. The DRAPE [15] procedure (Delayed Reconstruction After Pathology Evaluation) while awaiting pathology clearance is a necessary prerequisite in good clinical management with cases of mitotic malignancy of the integument (Melanoma, SCC etc.).

1.2.7 Microvascular

We have all been victims of metamorphosis through the reconstructive perspective from Ian Jackson's work with Gwynn Morgan and the groin flap leading to Taylor, Daniels and Palmer of 1987 had a microsurgical perspective and the quote for success ranged from 95% but there can be adverse findings, particularly aesthetically. Aesthetics and function can be found wanting as that applies to many microsurgical applications as illustrated in Cases 3.1.7 and 3.1.10. None of the cases in this series needed microsurgical reconstructive input as a last port of call. Another plastic surgical edict that has been questioned is the use of the Keystone in irradiated tissue which happens frequently in head and neck cases and is the domain for microsurgical repair in most units—in Case 3.1.11 where 3 microsurgical procedures—lat dorsi, radial forearm and gracilis—all failed when basic surgical principles were ignored, and they were the victims where the dead space in the bone was not corrected with any filler.

The Lamberty [16] classification of vascular perfusion may need to be revamped because of these ongoing clinical experiences and not latex injection studies in cadavers. I repeat, the success of the Keystone reconstructive technique is based on ongoing clinical successes as revealed by the patient's personal responses on video. Perforator flaps need reassessment as the Keystone has proved its clinical value by not skeletonising perforators presumably stripping them of somatic, autonomic, lymphatic support. The Keystone preserves the integrity of all random perforators suprafascial and infrafascial. As I stated above, its success is based on fascial lining with a deep third attachment always retained if any release is necessary for advancement or rotation and the variations of the Keystone design, as discussed above, observes and respects the integrity of the random perforators.

1.2.8 Closing Under Tension: Another Edict of Plastic Surgery Called into Question

This basic dictum of general surgical principles applied universally is part of our surgical training because closure under tension produces epidermal necrosis. However, the Keystone has reorientated the thinking of this concept because of the redirection of vascular flow—the vertical infrafascial and suprafascial perforator support are hydrostatically superior to that of the horizontally orientated subdermal plexus. For example, dynamically one can compare fire hydrants and garden hoses, both have their specific uses. All the cases illustrating the hyperaemic effect in the text have all been closed under tension. Absolute white lines of tension are a warning to reinsert and realign the suture orientations but in the main the vascular flow on the fascial base to the microperforators eventually creates the dynamic effect of hyperaemia and the Red Dot Sign of the blood at the suture site of the flap confirms this dynamic, bleeding more on the flap side than the receiving side—under tensional closure we have increased flow. Variations on the design like Hatchet flaps completely miss the point of this dynamic perfusion concept and all gleaned from thousands of cases done over 30 years. It is mentioned here merely to dispel the clinical applications of such variations and this reflects erroneous thinking – however based on tradition from the times of Barron and Emmett [17] and island flap designs. From experience, the Keystone on lax tissue for example the Keystone in the lateral peroneal compartment will cover defects close toward the anterior tibial line but do not base Keystones on the resistant tissue of the underlying bone of the shin—doomed to failure because there is no muscle compartment to compress to facilitate these elements of closing under tension which happens when they have a peroneal compartment orientation. Discretion must always operate and when an area like the anterior tibial wall is needed for repair site, it is wiser to use a loco-regional Keystone to cover any bony defect from the lateral L5 dermatome, with or without grafting over muscle.

An overview of the Keystone concept can be read from this summary of my article in Surgical News [18]:

My Lightbulb Moments in Surgery—all Thanks to the Keystone

In the recent period of surgical development and the design and applications of the Keystone flap, certain physiological elements have surfaced by way of observational findings. It respects the Louis Pasteur statement on observation 'chance favours the prepared mind on observational findings' and it has remarkable clinical applications.

It was on the Feast of the Epiphany that I attended a church service in our local community in Parkville, when the homily focussed about the importance of the revelation of the baby Jesus when the three wise men from the East bringing their gold, frankincense and myrrh to the revelation of the spiritual event. The feature was the Almighty showing himself to the world by way of revelation. In colloquial terms, some describe it as a lightbulb moment—no matter what ethnic background would apply.

Revelation is a word used in the lay press when something is elucidated from an unknown source. It is worth recalling the Archimedes story and his 'eureka' expression after he had stepped into a bath and noticed that the water level rose, whereupon he suddenly understood that the volume of water displaced must be equal to the volume of the part of his body he had submerged. Volumetric measurement was an intractable problem and Archimedes solved the problem in a measurable way.

Such was his ecstasy and eagerness to share this discovery that he leapt out of his bathtub and ran naked through the streets of Syracuse (see images).

As a little cooking story when putting these lines together making fried rice, I my 'eureka' moment when dicing the onions. Tears did not surface as I did this under running water which prevented the sulfenic acids irritating my conjunctiva.

It made me think twice about the Einstein quote and his equation of nuclear energy $e = mc^2$ and his other adage eminently reflecting his brilliance that a straight line is the shortest distance between two points. If one goes conceptually into a circle enclosing the universe, how big is that circle? So large that the curvature resembles a straight line because of its miniscule circumference - billions of light years across.

But let us add a touch of humour quoting Mae West who once said 'a curve is the nicest line between two points'. I will leave this to your personal interpretation.

Now let us get back to clinical medicine and my lightbulb moments in clinical surgery in the development of the Keystone Flap—all observational findings with image photography.

Case 1 was a closure of a compound tibial fracture and I used a Keystone island flap designed along the L5 dermatome, compressing the muscles of the lateral calf to achieve closure under tension. Yes, it was fascial lined, there was no definition or skeletonisation of perforators, it was just an umbrella of tissue based on non-defined stalks, which allowed perfusional healing to occur in spite of tension, breaking one of the basic rules in surgery of not closing under tension. In other words, they hypothetical suggestion of a sympathectomy effect because of the island design caused vasodilatation, replacing free flap alternatives.

It was only at the completion of the procedure when I said to my registrar 'look it is bleeding more on the suture sites aligned along the island flap than along the margin where it was inserted' - was this Stephen Doig, Edward Ek or Fraser Gilmour? I cannot recall and I doubt if they can recall it either. So, I presumed I had done a sympathectomy by creating the fascial based island flap. No, I did not run down the theatre corridor in ecstasy going to change and not repeating the Archimedes story as above.

The wound healed perfectly and has been part of a publication of lower limb reconstruction1 with an orthopaedic bias and more cases came my way and more observational findings surfaced. Even the anaesthetic pain team could not understand why it was not pain free, offered Panadol which the patients rejected 'I have no pain, this is unnecessary'. The sequalae of the healing wound was pain free, in spite of closure under tension, aesthetic match side by side (like-for-like) is irreplaceable compared with free flap reconstructions. Vascular complications were not evident and in terms of economics of theatre time it is a welcome compromise to a busy workload and expeditiously completed compared with alternative methods, reducing staff and numbers for monitoring—a premium in other surgical procedures. It is strange it should happen in the postoperative phase that any postoperative distal oedema responded to elevation and compression stockings. Could it have been lymphatic channels recommunicated with the natural alignment of lymphatic drainage lines. Somatic sensation returned when the wound was healed.

Case 2: My second lightbulb moment relates to a chronic wound of the anterior tibial line which had been there for 14 years following a compound fracture and had been the subject of 21 procedures over this period to close this chronic wound. The patient was told nothing more could be done apart from an amputation. I just happened to walk by him in the outpatient department at the Western Hospital and said 'I can solve that for you' but his initial reluctance of accepting my advice reflected 14 years of complicated outcomes in surgery.

Yes, he finally let me get the ulcer covered using a Keystone of the peroneal compartment designed along the peroneal dermatome with its neurological, lymphatic, autonomic and somatic support intact. Again, this has been published [19].

In the postoperative consultation I have recorded his response that the leg was the best it had felt for 14 years. His initial reluctance reverted to admiration. But most importantly, the peripheral oedema of his lower limb resolved completely and he was no longer forced to buy two pairs of shoes because of the unilateral swelling. Long-term standing was no longer a problem and he even returned to work standing up all day at an industrial bench. Needless to say, he was grateful.

So, that made me conclude that with retained neurovascular support and the sensate and autonomic supply intact with somatic supply the associated lymphatic channels must have re-anastomosed. The academic verification of this is contained in the patient's response. I suspect it was the dermatome Keystone design retaining its somatic and endolymphatic supply, merely maintaining embryological factors – another somewhat speculative but another lightbulb moment—the patient's story is always accurate.

Case 3: The final case I must mention is the closure of large parotid defects of the face the size of one's palm. These can be closed using the loose neck tissue in the C2, C3 dermatomes, based on random perforators at the base of the sternomastoid perforators near the muscular attachment and the loose neck tissue is rotated to close these palmar sized defects easily and comfortably, particularly in the elderly. The tension closure of the neck wound of the secondary defect requires the help of locking mattress sutures, which stay in 3 weeks. I repeat the Keystone characteristics are evident throughout these procedures and we have coined the acronym P.A.C.E.S. which best describes the usual postoperative features—Pain free, Aesthetically matching, vascular Complications are rare, Economically responsible in terms of time and nursing staff monitoring, with Sensory recovery and resolution of oedema. We have followed in the late Sir Harold Gillies edict of using 'like for like' in the repair of tissue.

In all surgical wounds we all appreciated the anaesthetic margins are noted, taking some months for the reinnervation of the filamentous units that must realign to provide intact sensation.

Louis Pasteur is worth quoting 'Science knows no country, because knowledge belongs to humanity, and is the torch which illuminates the world.'

He also said 'chance observations favour the prepared mind'.

It was the chance observation through which he discovered that cultures of chicken cholera lost their pathogenicity but retained their antigenicity which became the basis of the vaccine. Pasteur was the father of immunity.

He was famous for making quotes based on his work on the germ theory of disease and he was prepared to grasp the key role of the microbe in the prevention of smallpox, something Jenner could never have known—the milking maids never got smallpox—a Jenner observation. He was world famous for the work on microbial disease and inventing the process of pasteurisation in preserving food.

Yes, he was a revolutionary and he introduced the concept that infectious diseases could be prevented by vaccination (let us not forget the French word for a cow 'vache' and the milkmaid story who never got smallpox). Hence, vaccination is a logical sequence in phoneticising the word and the origin of vaccination. He discovered that milk bacteria can be destroyed by heating and it helped in the development of cholera, anthrax, smallpox and rabies vaccinations. Some argue that he was not a doctor but he proved these antagonistic comments inaccurate and was right about the microbial background of disease. He obtained his Master of Science degree in 1845 before advancing to research commitments.

In a lecture presentation on his 70th birthday in a crowded amphitheatre in the Sorbonne, a university in Paris at the high end of town—all the university staff, state ambassadors and representatives from the Institute of France all attended, even including Joseph Lister of antiseptic fame, all full of admiring adulation as his intuitive research instincts produced.

Following his comment about chance favouring the prepared mind, he did note wine is the most healthful and hygienic of all beverages (my favourite Shiraz at 14% is superior to 13% Pinot Noir). He goes on to observe that a bottle of wine contains more philosophy than all the books in the world.

His pasteurisation process kills microbes and prevents ruination of our drinking favourites from beer, milk and iced coffee.

He also observed that microbes cannot arise from non-viable material.

However, coincidentally in association with Pasteur, the English surgeon Joseph Lister and the German physician Robert Koch have been given much of the credit for the development of the germ theory, which is really a focal point of Pasteur's scientific career.

So, his pioneering work in vaccination to produce a mild or attenuated form of the Rabies pathogen than the more harmful extended full-blown manifestation of the disease following a dog bite (the same principles are applied today in our COVID-19 vaccinations).

In the lay press today, the new version of COVID-19 JN1 has surfaced after the previous variants Omicron, Delta and Alpha and people should be aware that earlier preventative measures like crowd attendances and the wearing of masks should be mandatory. All work emanating from the eminent work of Professor Peter Doherty, whom I pass regularly perambulating through Parkville.

The Carl Sagan quote has always been at the forefront of my mind from the amassed observational findings, this clinical reconstructive flap has produced. I have documented the findings on the published material, made lists accordingly and hypothetically assumed that the hypervascularity phase was not dissimilar to **THE PINK FOOT** that was observed regularly after a lumbar sympathectomy to cure trophic foot ulcerations, thus, part of surgical history.

But my speculative hypothesis I have quoted regularly and if only one reverts to Carl Sagan's quote, it puts relevance into my findings:

The absence of evidence is not the evidence of absence

References

1. Behan F, et al. Island flaps, including the Bezier type in the treatment of malignant melanoma. ANZ J Surg. 1995;65:870–80.
2. Behrbohm H. History of facial plastic surgery in Europe. Lübeck: The European Academy of Facial Plastic Surgery; 2021.
3. Taylor I, Daniel R. The free flap: composite tissue transfer by vascular anastomosis. ANZ J Surg. 1973;43(1):1–3.
4. Behan FC. Atlas of keystone reconstructive technique in the management of melanoma. Cham: Springer; 2024.
5. Ockham W. Encyclopedia of philosophy. Stanford. Archived from the original on 7 October 2019. Retrieved 24 February 2016.
6. Behan FC, et al. Vascular basis of laterally based forehead island flaps and their clinical applications. Transactions of the 2nd Congress of the European Section of the International Confederation of Plastic and Reconstructive Surgery, Madrid, 1973.
7. Behan FC, Wilson JSP. The principle of the angiotome a system of linked axial pattern flaps. Transactions of the 6th International Congress on Plastic and Reconstructive Surgery, Paris, 1975.
8. Limberg AA. The planning of local plastic operations on the body surface. Toronto: The Collamore Press; 1984.
9. Lo C, Nottle T, Mills J. Keystone island flap: effects of islanding on vascularity. Plast Reconstr Surg Glob Open. 2016;4(2):e617.
10. "Absence of evidence is not evidence of absence". Quote Investigator. 2019.
11. Fede C, Petrelli L, Pirri C, Neuhuber W, Tiengo C, Biz C, De Caro R, Schleip R, Stecco C. Innervation of human superficial fascia. Front Neuroanat. 2022;16:981426. https://doi.org/10.3389/fnana.2022.981426.
12. Pirri C, Petrelli L, Fede C, Guidolin D, Tiengo C, De Caro R, Stecco C. Blood supply to the superficial fascia of the abdomen: an anatomical study. Clin Anat. 2023;36(4):570–80.
13. Royle JP. A history of sympathectomy. ANZ J Surg. 1999;69:302–7.
14. Blondeel P, et al. Perforator flaps: anatomy, technique and clinical applications. Missouri: Quality Medical Publishing; 2024.
15. Behan F, et al. Oncologic clearance with preservation of reconstructive options: literature review and the 'delayed reconstruction after pathology evaluation (DRAPE)' technique. ANZ J Surg. 2012;82(11):780–5.
16. Cormack GC, Lamberty BG. Cadaver studies of correlation between vessel size and anatomical territory of cutaneous supply. Br J Plast Surg. 1986;39(3):300–6.
17. Barron J, Emmett A. Subcutaneous pedicle flaps. Br J Plast Surg. 1965;18:51–78.
18. Behan F. My lightbulb moments in surgery. R Austral College Surg Surg News. 2024;25:1.
19. Behan FC. Keystone perforator island flap in lower limb reconstruction. Austral J Plast Surg. 2021;4(2):105–7. https://doi.org/10.34239/ajops.v4n2.341.
20. Behan F, et al. Fasciocutaneous island flaps for orthopaedic management in lower limb reconstruction using dermatomal precincts. ANZ J Surg. 1994;64(3):155–66.
21. Behan F. Evolution of the fascio-cutaneous island flap leading to the keystone flap principle in lower limb reconstruction. ANZ J Surg. 2008;78:116–7.

22. Behan FC, Lo CH, Ramin S. Perforator territory of the keystone flap – use of the dermatomal roadmap. J Plast Reconstr Aesthet Surg. 2008;62:427–562. https://doi.org/10.1016/j.bjps.2008.08.078.
23. Behan FC, Lo CH, Shayan R. Perforator territory of the keystone flap: use of the dermatomal roadmap. J Plast Reconstr Aesthet Surg. 2009;62:551–3.
24. Behan F, Sizeland A, Gilmour F, Hui A, Seel M, Lo CH. Use of the keystone island flap for advanced head and neck cancer in the elderly. J Plast Reconstr Aesthet Surg. 2010;63:739–45.
25. Behan FC, Rozen WM, Tan S. Yin-Yang flaps: the mathematics of two keystone island flaps for reconstructing increasingly large defects. ANZ J Surg. 2011;81:574–5.
26. Behan FC, Rozen WM, Lo CH, Findlay M. The omega-Ω-variant designs (types A and B) of the keystone perforator island flap. ANZ J Surg. 2011;81:650–2.
27. Behan F, Findlay M, Lo CH. The keystone perforator island flap concept. Sydney: Elsevier Textbook Churchill Livingstone; 2012.
28. Behan FC, Rozen WM, Azer S, Gran P. Perineal keystone design perforator island flap for perineal and vulval reconstruction. ANZ J Surg. 2012;82:381–2.
29. Behan FC, Paddle A, Rozen WM, et al. Quadriceps keystone island flap for radical inguinal lymphadenectomy. ANZ J Surg. 2013;83:942–7.
30. Behan F. Surgical tips and skills illustrating the keystone principle. Sydney: Elsevier; 2014.
31. Behan FC, Sizeland A. Keystone perforator island flaps in major head and neck surgery – the P.A.C.E. perspectives. World J Surg Surg Res. 2021;4(1):1293.
32. Rodriguez-Unda N, Abraham J, Saint-Cyr M. Keystone and perforator flaps in reconstruction. Clin Plast Surg. 2020;47(4):635–48.
33. Head H, Campbell AW. The pathology of herpes zoster and its bearing on sensory localisation. BRAIN Part III, 1900.

The Keystone Flap Technique to Reconstruct Palmar Defects Resulting from Dupuytren's Fasciectomy: The Province of Orthopaedic Hand Surgeons

2

Contents

Supplementary Information The online version contains supplementary material available at https://doi.org/10.1007/978-3-031-76702-9_2. The videos can be accessed individually by clicking the DOI link in the accompanying figure caption or by scanning this link with the SN More Media App.

F. Behan, *Keystone Flap for Complex Orthopaedic Problems*,
https://doi.org/10.1007/978-3-031-76702-9_2

2.1 Upper Limb: Soft Tissue Defects

The case range will encompass the following sites for expeditious soft tissue closure, all based on orthopaedic experiences:

Shoulder
Forearm
Elbow
Wrist

Hand and fingertips—palmar and metacarpal defects

This is usually managed with a fenestrated full thickness graft. However, the Keystone concept of flap reconstruction is a remarkably simple alternative to metacarpal island flaps [1]. The Keystone offers an alternative to microsurgical dissection defining metacarpal island flaps, and the time implications of this need no elaboration. The Keystone solves it expeditiously, and its characteristics referenced above are all evident when the reconstructive patterns are followed, i.e. using as a basis dermatological and embryological principles.

The acronym P.A.C.E.S. is a synoptic overview of the characteristics of the Keystone. The surgical delineation of the Keystone design divides temporarily sensory input to the integument which recovers. Aesthetically, it is a perfect match. Complications from a vascular strategy point of view are reasonably uncommon if the delineation techniques are followed. Economically, it is a timesaver from the point of view of surgical repair. Like the cutaneous supply across any surgical wound, sensory recovery returns in 2–3 weeks as the same timeframe as the resolution of oedema.

2.1.1 Case 1: Compound Forearm Fractures Involving Radius and Ulnar with the Usual Muscle Transfer Providing a Base for the Skin Grafting Cover After any ORIF

Traditionally, the standard practice is muscle transfer with grafting of the secondary defect. Again, repeat procedures take away the economic eficiency, whereas the Keystone solves it with one manoeuvre (Figs. 2.1, 2.2, 2.3, 2.4, 2.5, 2.6, 2.7, 2.8, 2.9, 2.10, 2.11, 2.12, 2.13, 2.14, and 2.15).

No other technique [2] around the world can close these forearm wounds so easily as the Keystone does based on dermatomal markings to define the orientation of the microperforators without multiple skin graft scar revision procedures to follow which may take years to complete. The PACES characteristics are quite relevant in this case of an ethnic background with pigmentation.

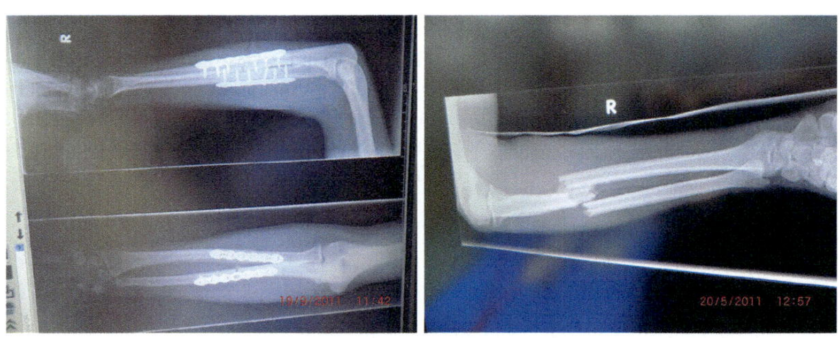

Fig. 2.1 X-ray images of the duplicated forearm fractures following ORIF reduction

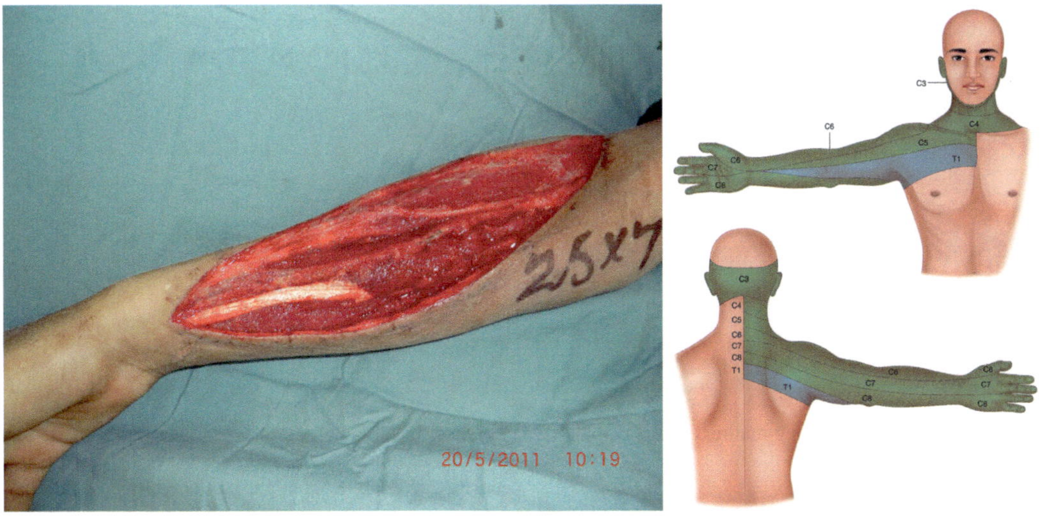

Fig. 2.2 The standard method of skin grafting the muscle bellies of the flexor/extensor compartments is thus obviated. This involves multiple repeat procedures to achieve healing before the patient eventually requests scar revisional surgery when the wounds are fully healed and the bones united. A routine appearance awaiting skin grafting

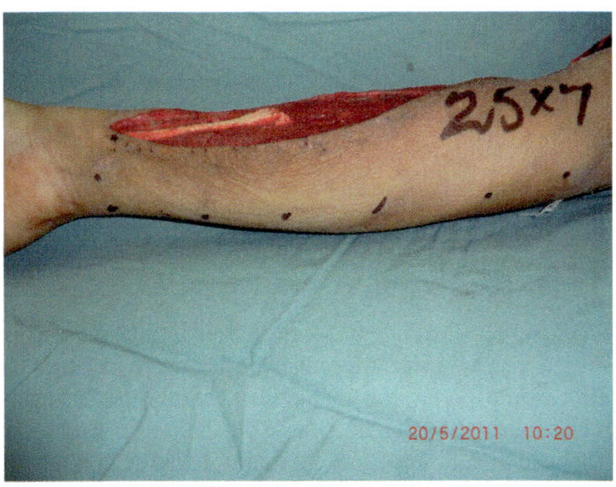

Fig. 2.3 Showing the Keystone mark out along the ulnar border of the forearm based on ulnar perforators to vascularise this unit at the fascial level, contributing to the suprafascial and infrafascial input (see operative sequence video)

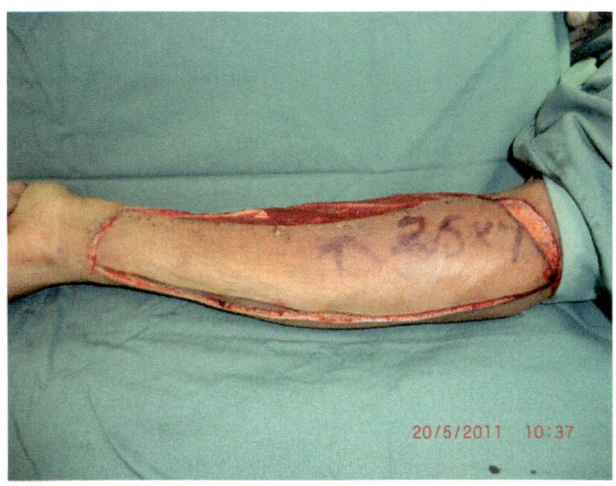

Fig. 2.4 The vascular flare is noted confirming its viability

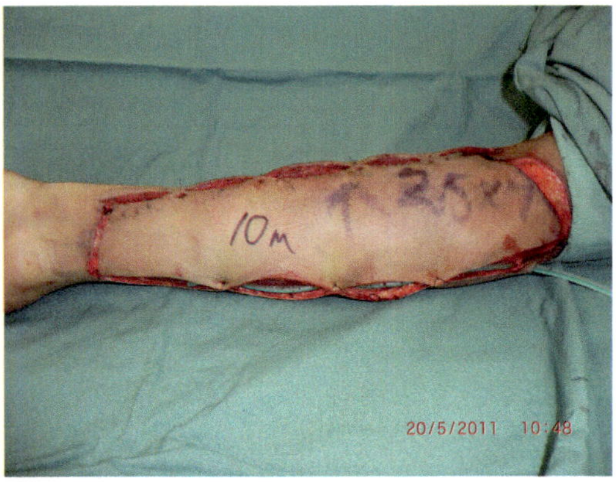

Fig. 2.5 Some staged locking mattress sutures along the radial and ulnar borders

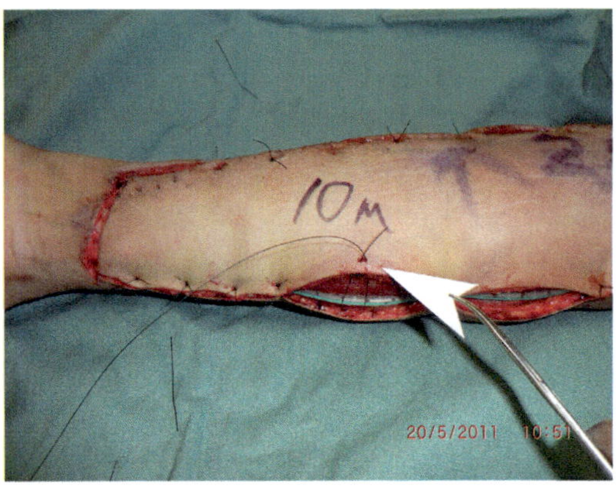

Fig. 2.6 The red dot sign characteristic of the Keystone

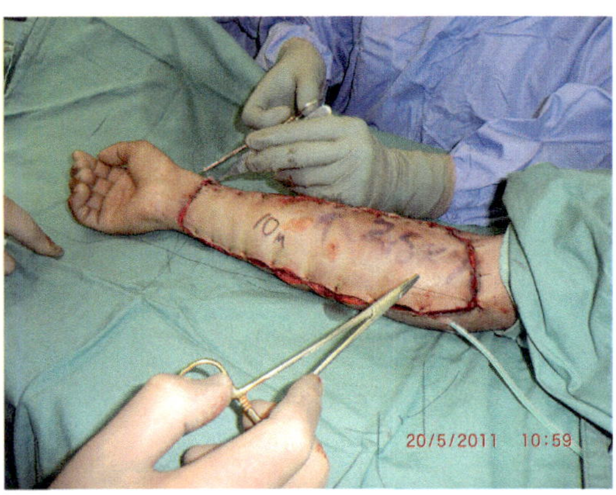

Fig. 2.7 The T3 dermatomal mark out aligns the random perforators in this fasciocutaneous island flap aligned along the T3 dermatome—there is no anatomical dissection defining perforators as this removes defined autonomic and somatic supply which accompany the vascular stalks. Thus, the retention of such anatomical normality allows sensory recovery and the sympathectomy effect creating hypervascularity is thus retained. This hypervascularity allows the wound to be closed under tension using mattress locking sutures

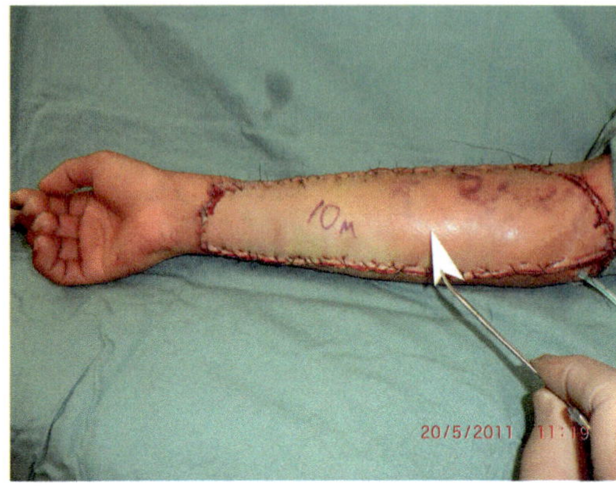

Fig. 2.8 On completion. No sign of any cyanotic demarcation and the proximal redness of the hyperaemia are more evident in the upper part of the flap

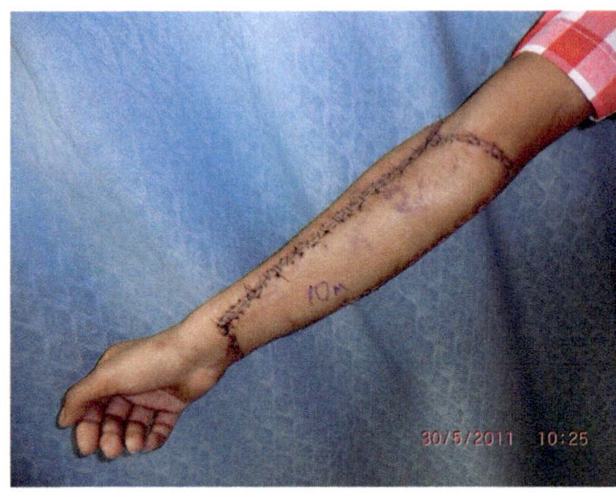

Fig. 2.9 The healing phase after 10 days. Note there is no evidence of vascular impedance or flap necrosis based on the random perforators (undefined) within the dermatomal precincts. Notice how the wounds have healed well. That trio of sutures of locking mattress, ordinary mattress and continuous nylon as a single layer gives perfect epidermal alignment, adding to its aesthetic appearance in this case with ethnic pigmentation the hypertrophic potential when using a skin graft is an important factor to be considered, both for the donor and recipient sites

Fig. 2.10 Full functional recovery, full range of movement and avoiding any scar revisional surgery

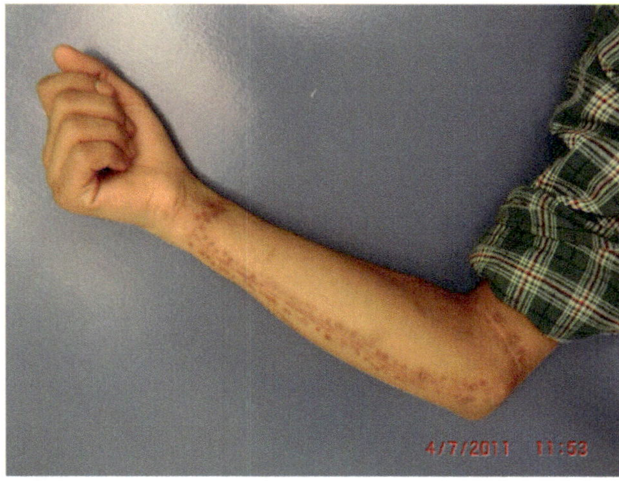

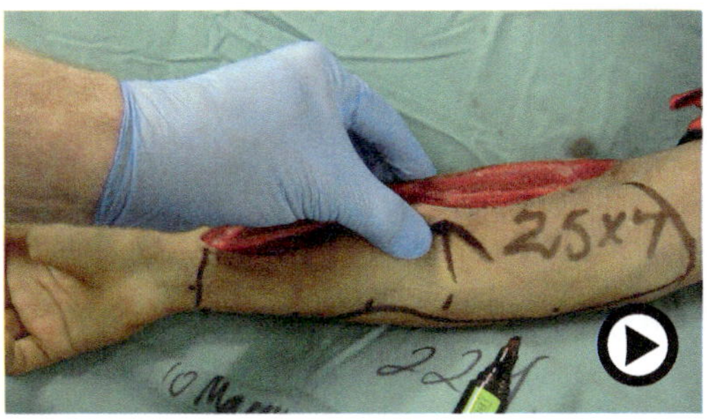

Fig. 2.11 Operative outline in detail (Video 2.1 Operative outline in detail) (▶ https://doi.org/10.1007/000-d4j)

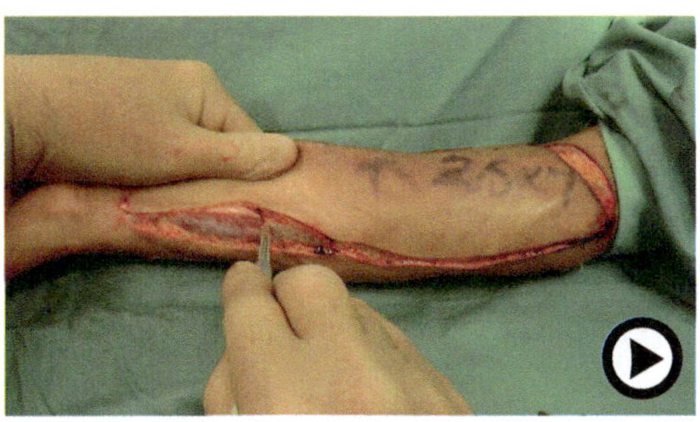

Fig. 2.12 Blunt dissection and dividing the fascia lining (Video 2.2 Blunt dissection and dividing the fascia lining) (▶ https://doi.org/10.1007/000-d4d)

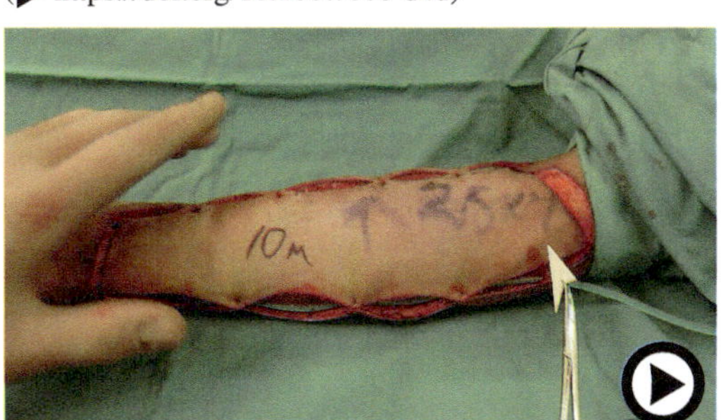

Fig. 2.13 Closing in stages (Video 2.3 Closing in stages) (▶ https://doi.org/10.1007/000-d4e)

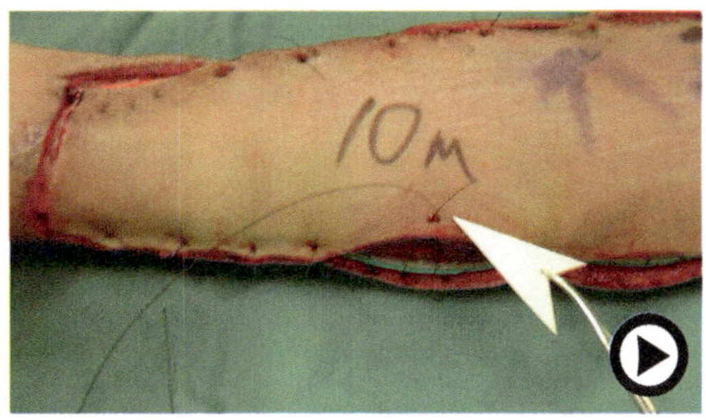

Fig. 2.14 The red dot sign (Video 2.4 The red dot sign) (▶ https://doi.org/10.1007/000-d4f)

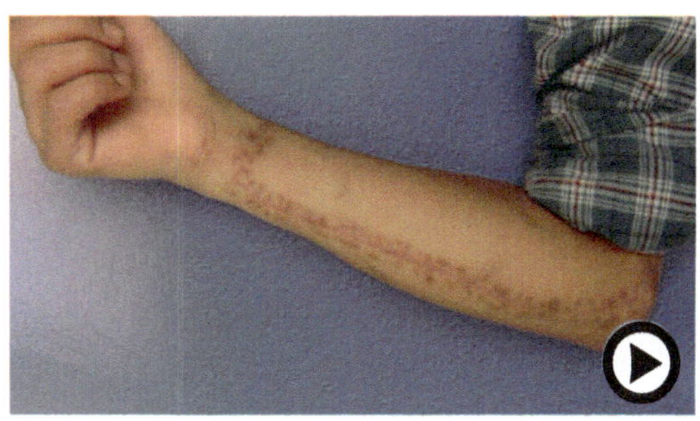

Fig. 2.15 Full range of movement recovery (Video 2.5 Full range of movement recovery) (▶ https://doi.org/10.1007/000-d4g)

2.1.2 Case 2: Gouty Tophi of the Olecranon of a Chronic Nature for this Complex Orthopaedic Closure

This was the site of recurrent suppurating gouty tophi of the olecranon. The Keystone mark out solved the problem (Figs. 2.16, 2.17, 2.18, 2.19, 2.20, 2.21, 2.22, 2.23, 2.24, 2.25, 2.26, and 2.27).

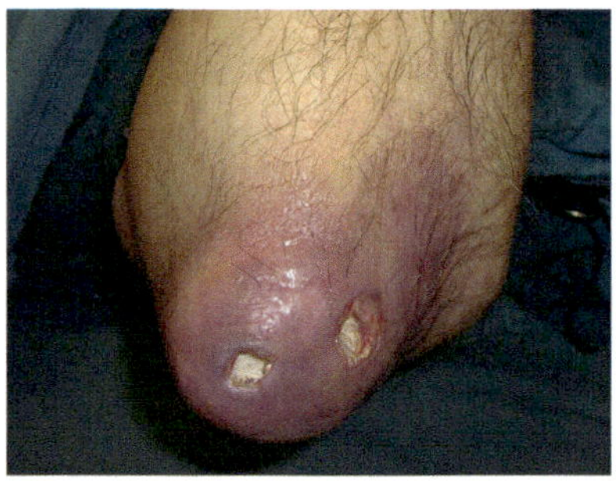

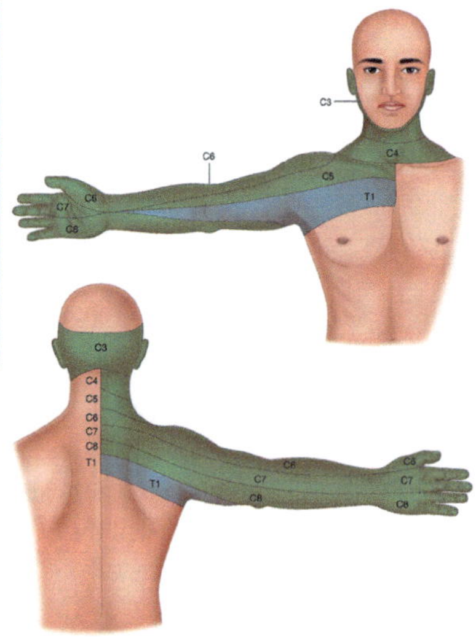

Fig. 2.16 Duplicated fasciocutaneous island flaps were necessary adopting the Yin Yang principle

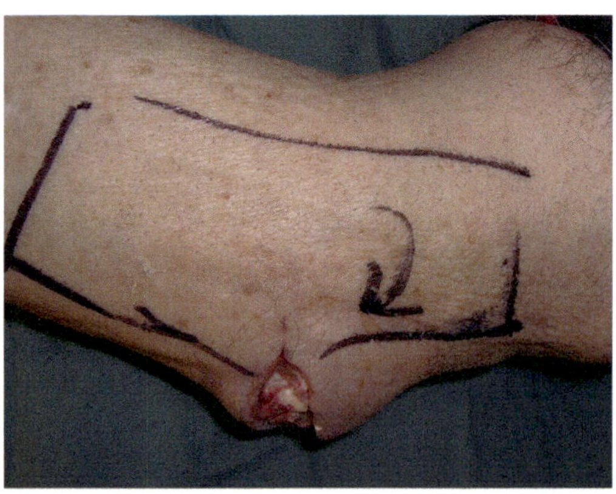

Fig. 2.17 The longitudinal alignment and mark out of the upper and lower flaps are so fashioned so they interdigitate. As long as a fascial base is released to allow cover over the bony defect

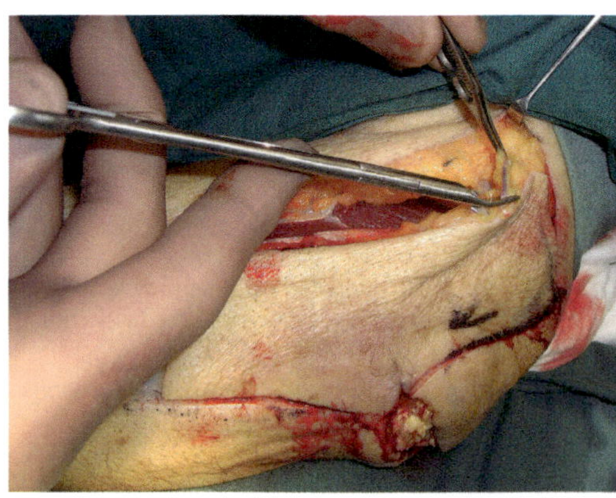

Fig. 2.18 Microvascular clips for haemostasis to avoid the use of diathermy and its potential for vascular necrosis, contributing to reliable perfusion

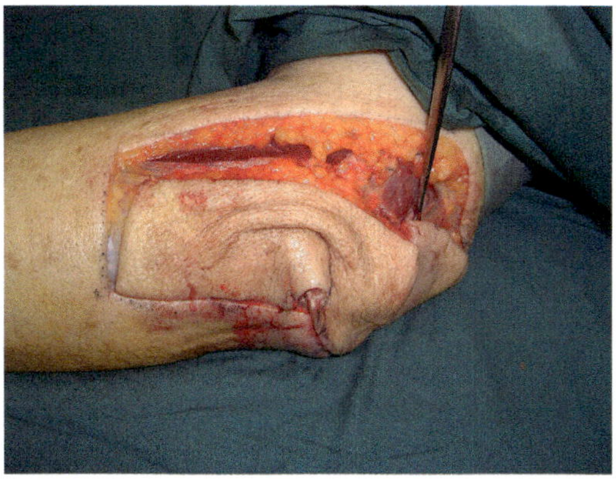

Fig. 2.19 The distal flap is islanded and released along the ulnar border which allows turn of the proximal 1/3 of the inferior Keystone

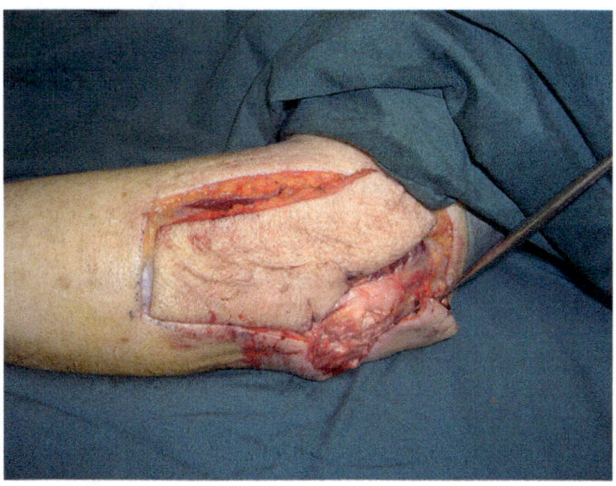

Fig. 2.20 Staged insertion of the flap reflecting the lines of tension

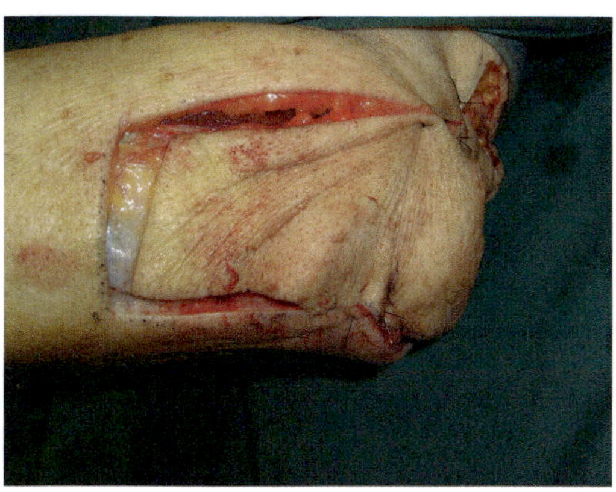

Fig. 2.21 Lines of tension are evident when the flaps are placed over the bony defect but the sympathectomy effect of the islands, exhibited by their hypervascularity phase, ensures sound healing if the 3-phase nylon suture technique is adopted

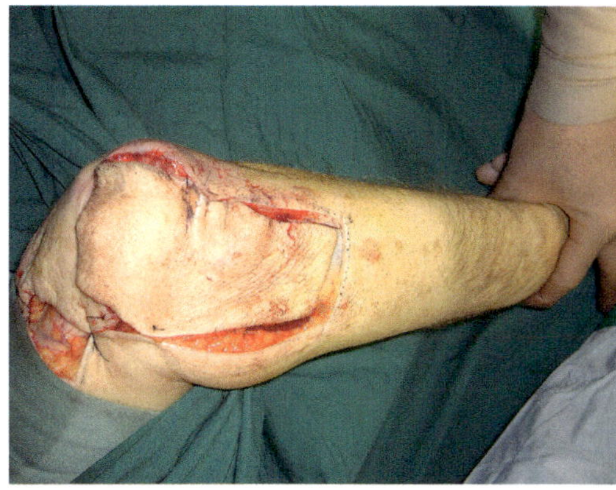

Fig. 2.22 Stages of the reconstruction

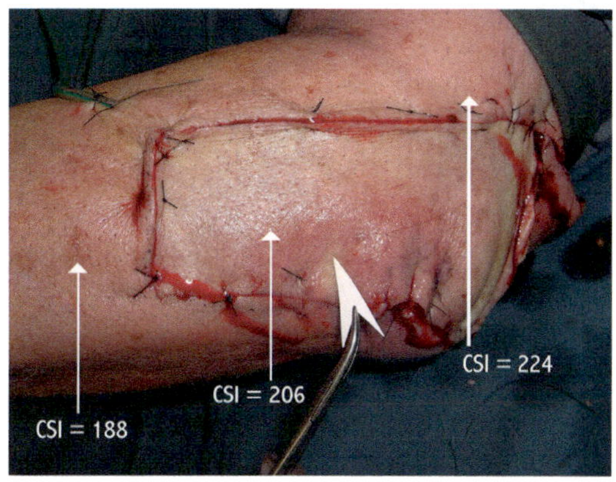

Fig. 2.23 Note the hyperaemia of the island flaps along the ulnar border, yet covering the olecranon, even with an element of tension which is not an impedance factor in closure. The alternative microvascular free flap closure with its limitations of donor site morbidity does not have the characteristics of being pain free in an economic time-frame with full recovery of somatic sensation

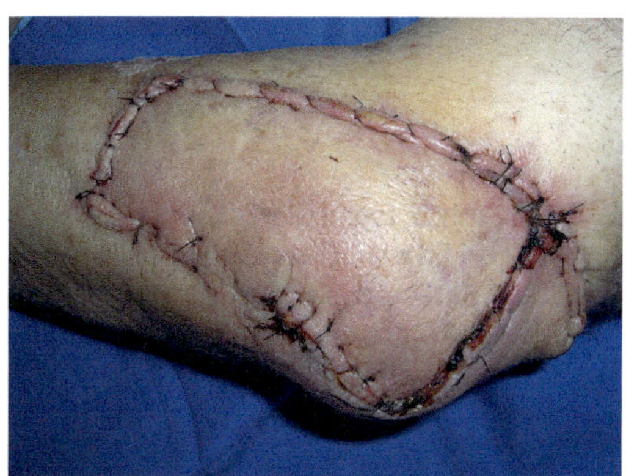

Fig. 2.24 The results are self-evident

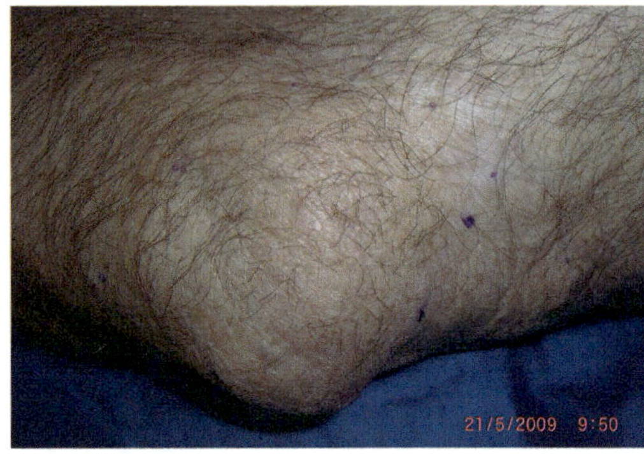

Fig. 2.25 Appearance at 3 months. The closure achieves an almost invisible scar line and they had to be dotted here to reveal their presence for those incredulous surgeons about this technique

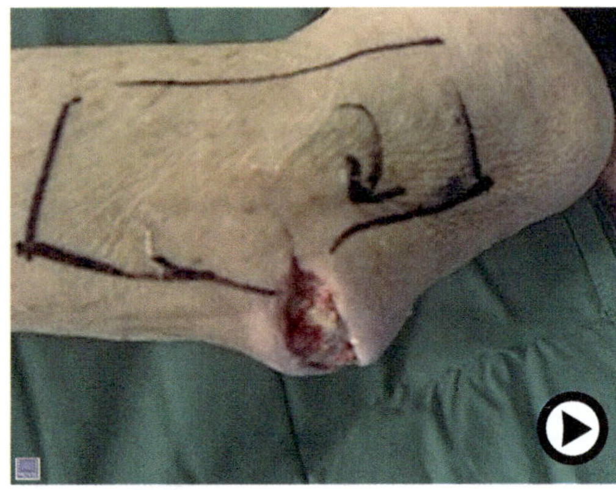

Fig. 2.26 Operative sequence (Video 2.6 Operative sequence) (▶ https://doi.org/10.1007/000-d4h)

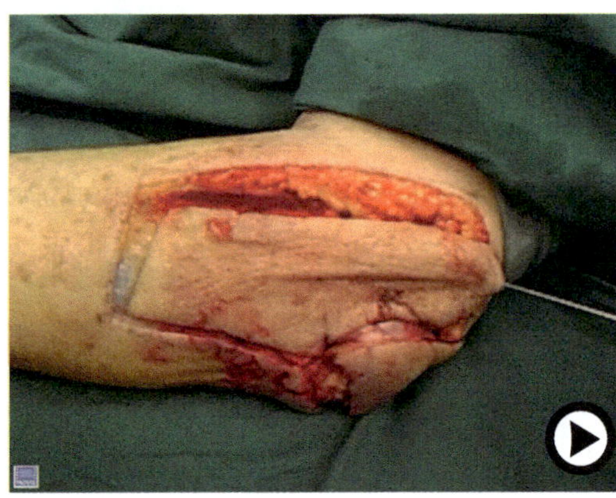

Fig. 2.27 Operative sequence (Video 2.7 Operative sequence) (▶ https://doi.org/10.1007/000-d4c)

2.1.3 Case 3: Exposed Bone at the Elbow (Olecranon) and Keystone Cover for Fractures and/or Coexisting Pathology

Using T1/T2 dermatome aligned fascial island flaps without skeletonising individual perforators to embrace the microperforators coming through the fascial lined Keystone design (Figs. 2.28, 2.29, 2.30, and 2.31).

Fig. 2.28 The 10 × 6 cm orthopaedic defect as marked and prior to flap elevation

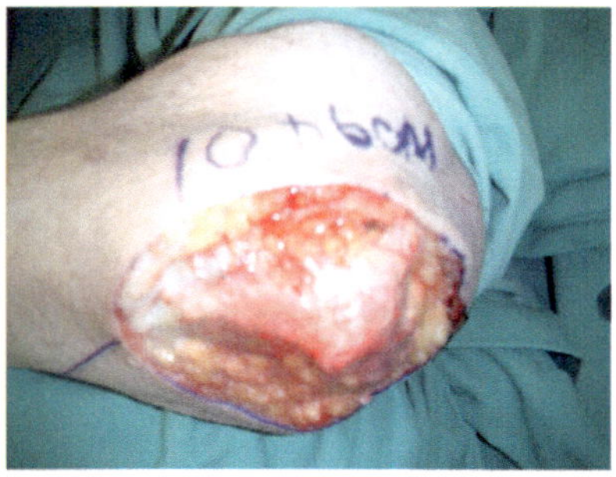

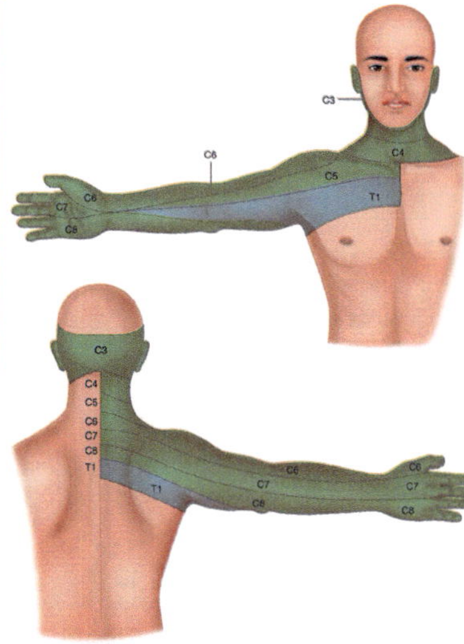

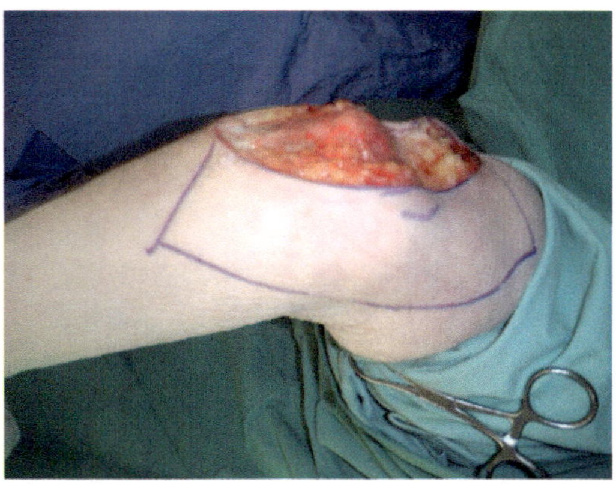

Fig. 2.29 The proposed Keystone flap mark out design for soft tissue cover over the olecranon to cover the exposed bone. Caution in the vicinity of the medial epicondyle and the cutaneous branches of ulnar nerve are to be handled with caution as they are often accompanied by microperforators

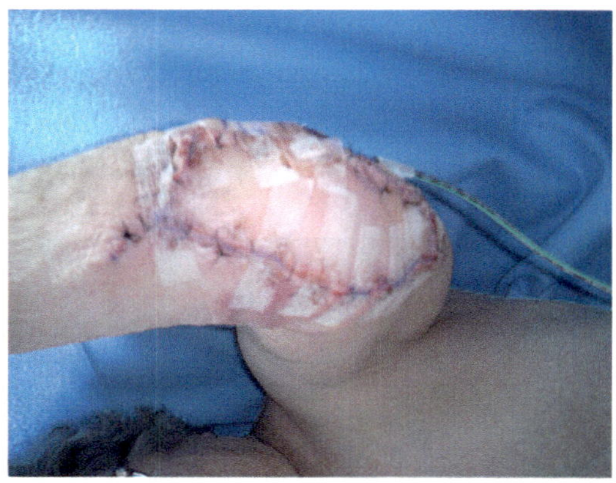

Fig. 2.31 Closure with the 3-phase single layer nylon locking mattress suture technique [3]. Elbow flexion and extension glide facilitate the closure to minimise points of tension which all settle. Redi-vac drainage is a prerequisite

Fig. 2.30 A progress image of flap elevation leaving the proximal 1/3 attached. This is orientated along the ulnar border of the forearm

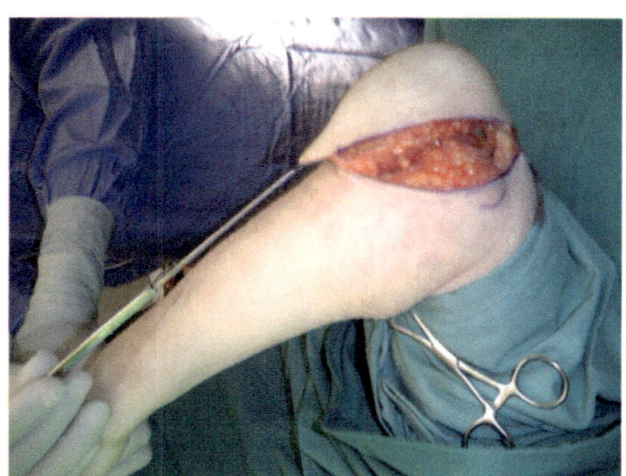

2.1.4 Case 4: Elbow Joint Cover Over the Olecranon (Figs. 2.32, 2.33, 2.34, 2.35, 2.36, 2.37, 2.38, and 2.39)

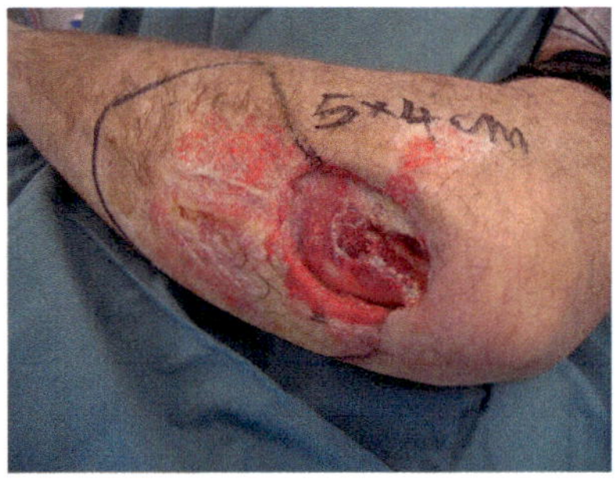

Fig. 2.32 The surgical defect following debridement with exposure of the olecranon area 5 × 4 cm with the mark out of the Keystone indicating planned closure

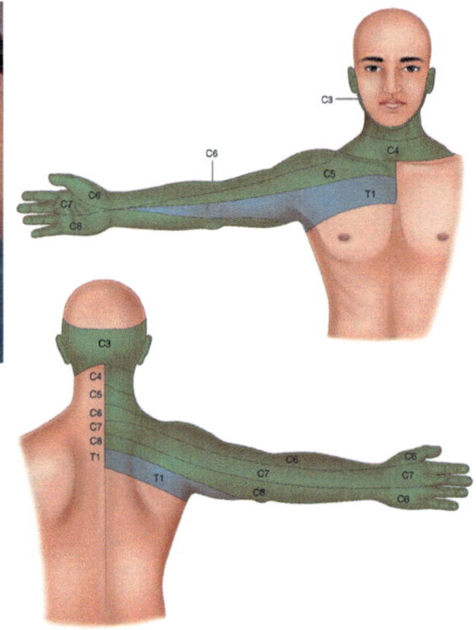

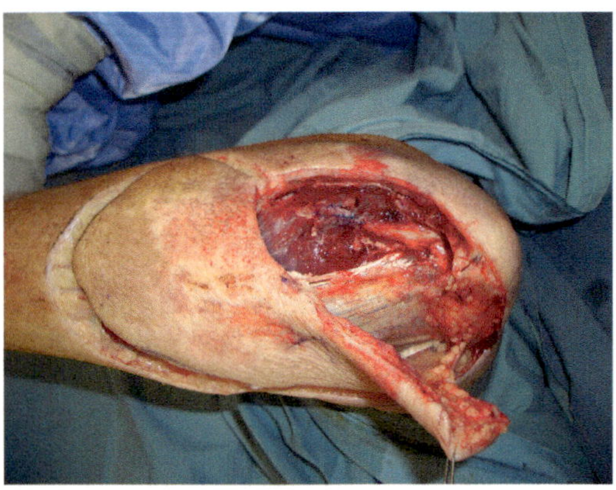

Fig. 2.33 Raising the fascial lined Keystone flap. The fascia is an absolute prerequisite to guarantee suprafascial and infrafascial circulation [4], and the outline of the Keystone is noted along the ulnar border before transposition of its proximal elevation

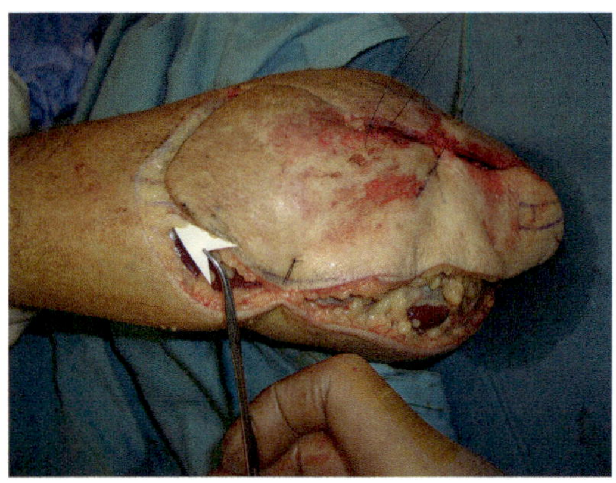

Fig. 2.34 Longitudinal neurovascular structures arrowed. These are retained at the perineural/perifascial level preserving their longitudinal alignment and integrity

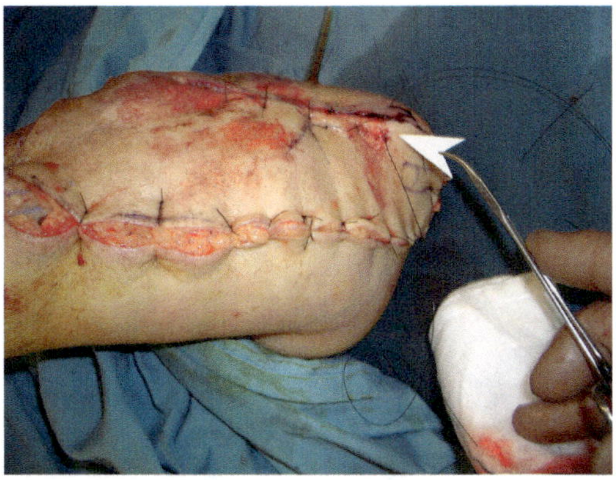

Fig. 2.35 Perfusional recovery after release of tourniquet, and the irregular distribution is consistent with flow up the suprafascial/infrafascial circulations

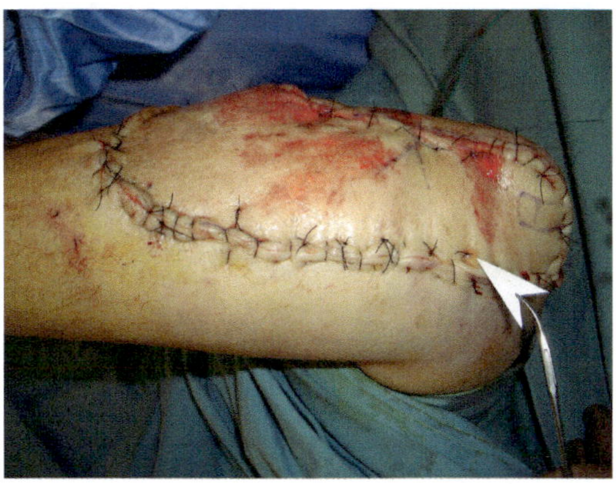

Fig. 2.36 Phase 3 of closure of a continuous epidermal nylon seal after the tension locking mattress sutures at key points to hold the flaps in alignment

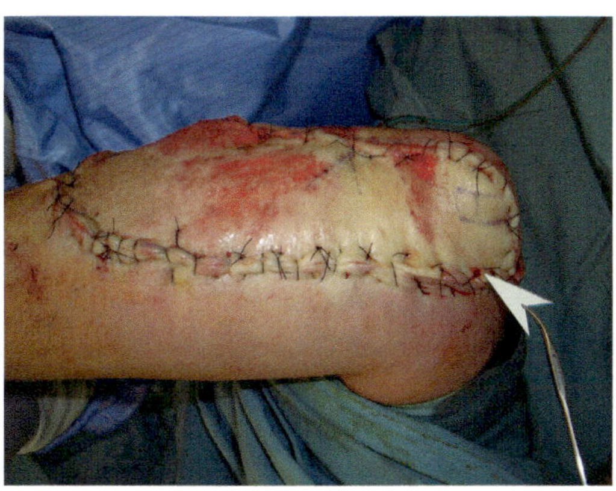

Fig. 2.37 The Red Dot Sign indicating vascular integrity and confirming the sympathectomy effect of increased vascular perfusion by way of the island design through the epidermis

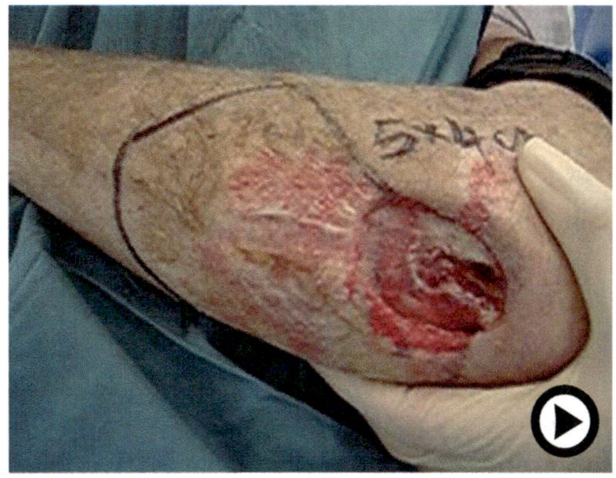

Fig. 2.38 Planned operative closure (Video 2.8 Planned operative closure) (▶ https://doi.org/10.1007/000-d4k)

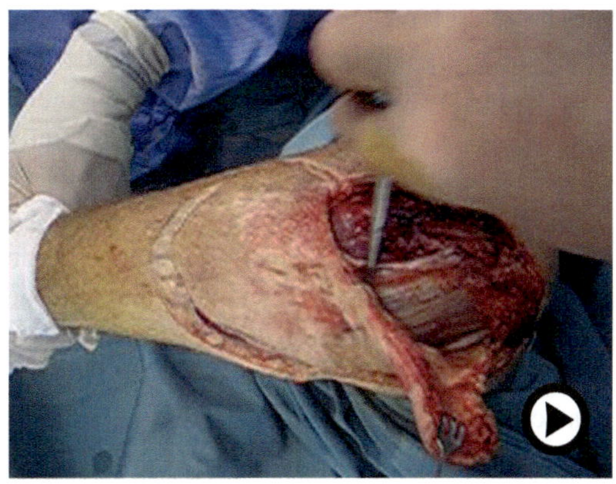

Fig. 2.39 Operative sequence (Video 2.9 Operative sequence) (▶ https://doi.org/10.1007/000-d4m)

2.1.5 Case 5: ORIF of Any Humeral Fractures Using the Keystone for an Access Technique

This melanoma excision and closure could well apply for design modification for ORIF closures along the humerous, sometimes a similar surgical defect is created following an ORIF for humeral fractures.

Reported relative indications for proximal humerus fracture ORIF include, but are not limited to, the following: displacement of tuberosities greater than 5 mm, marginal articular fracture with greater than 2 mm of displacement, greater than 100% displacement of the surgical neck, or a sufficiently large varus or valgus deformity [5, 6].

The Keystone repair orientated vertically along the biceps in the vicinity of the C3 dermatome is not disimilar to the flap used for melanoma closures over the upper limb in the vicinity of biceps, the original origin of this technique [4]. This nelanoma case helps to portray closure of a similary large surgical defect in the upper limb between the elbow and the shoulder and was the basis for this experience to give a flap repair in spite of closure under tension. Yet, the P.A.C.E.S. characteristics of the Keystone are all exemplified.

Any melanoma with a longitudinal biopsy orientation is well managed with the Keystone concept reconstruction vertically orientated. The soft muscle bellies of the biceps and triceps areas facilitate closure under tension based on random myocutaneous microperforators. In this case, the oncolological defect was 7 × 4 cm (Figs. 2.40, 2.41, 2.42, 2.43, 2.44, 2.45, and 2.46).

In summary, an aesthetically acceptable outcome for a young lady wearing summer clothing and the P.A.C.E.S. characteristics were all exemplified.

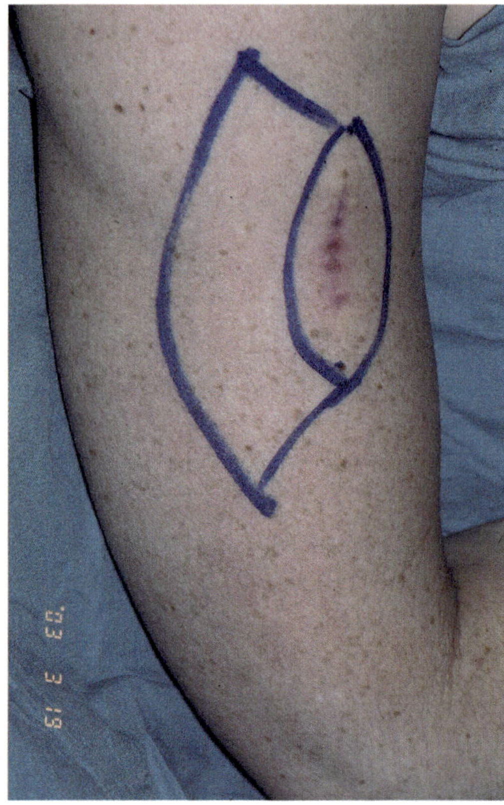

Fig. 2.40 In a well-presented young lady, fully aware of the problems of scarring deformity in her upper limb and the controversy such scarring produces mentally and physically is partially overcome with the Keystone technique. The alternative 'melon slice' scar deformity always raises questions over its lack of aesthetic appeal and resultant outcome. The standard technique of using a skin graft to close surgical/melanoma defects leave a lot to be desired from an aesthetic point of view. The patient regularly uses the words 'shark bite appearance' for their deformity, to the patient's embarrassment and dissatisfaction as well when wearing summer gear. The biopsy site and the Keystone flap mark out are illustrated between deltoid, and the lower third of the arm is evident where a single flap closes two defects where the Keystone flap really closes two defects, the surgical site and the design of the Keystone itself

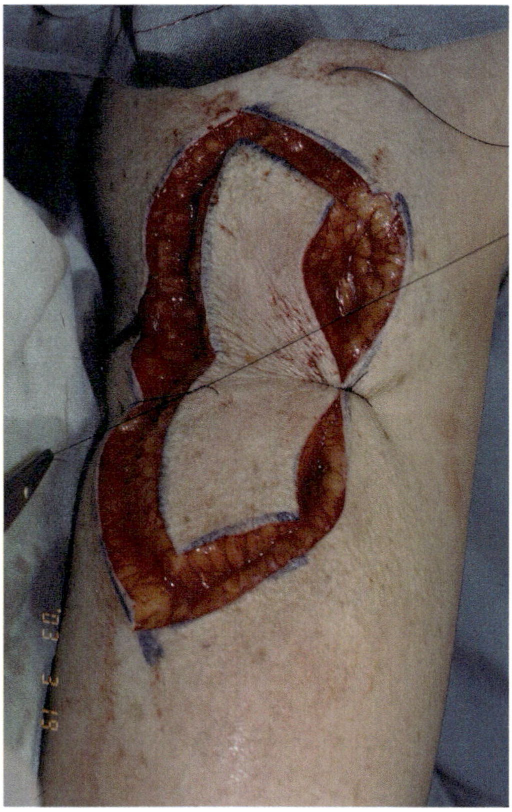

Fig. 2.41 The initial lines of maximum tension in this fascial lined island flap occur when the convex and concave sides are aligned. Note the pink flare reflecting hyperaemia, a confirmation of hypervascularity and attributed to a sympathectomy effect at the epidermal level because of the island design. Random perforators in the suprafascial and infrafascial compartments contribute to this vascular support. There is no skeletonisation of any defined perforator axes and no undermining of the Keystone flap should this detract from the neural basis at the autonomic and somatic levels

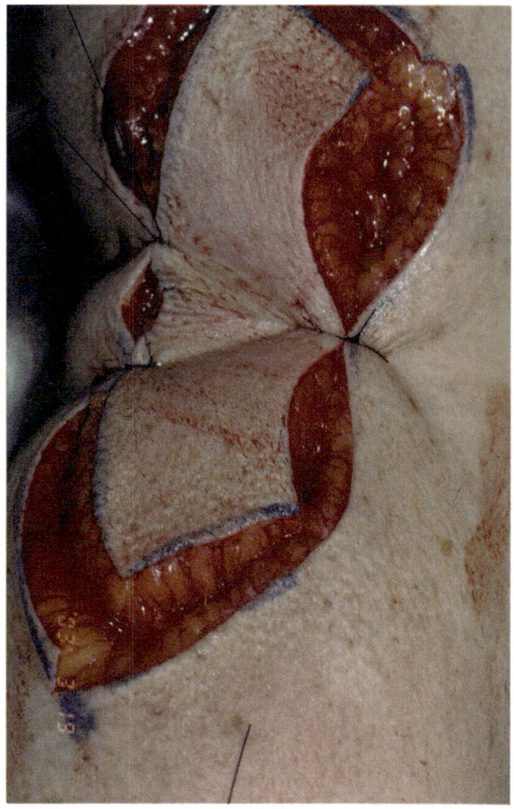

Fig. 2.42 Note the lines of tension—a contraindication in surgical wound closure as part of our teaching and unacceptable to some minds until they start using Keystone reconstruction—a point of contention - but these are not significant when adopting Keystone principles. Having broken this rule of surgery and used repetitively—it is because the circulation in the subdermal plexus is supported by the vertical fascial perforators from the laxity of the muscle bellies which facilitates the closure, achieved by compressing the biceps muscle volume

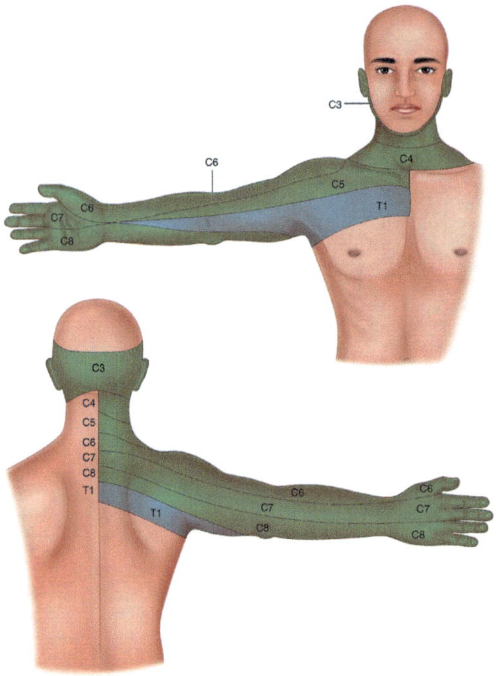

Fig. 2.43 The dermatomal mark out is a superficial guide to the location and orientiation of suprafascial and infrafascial random perforators coming through the deep fascia and part of the neurovascular embryological development

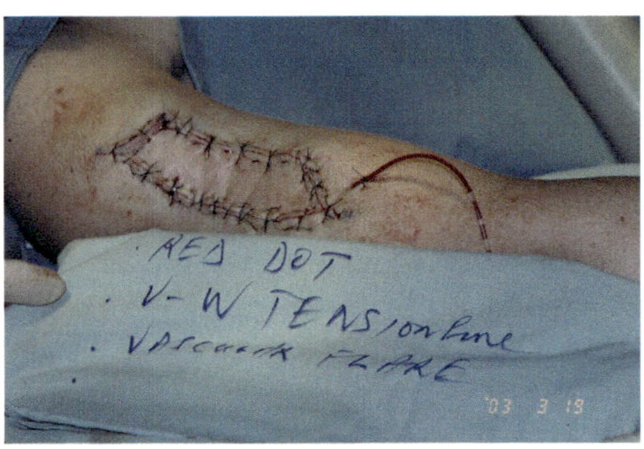

Fig. 2.44 Note the vascular flare, the lines of tension creases are disappearing usually in 10–15 min and the Redi-vac drainage is with the tubing folded in a U-shaped manner draining both surgical site and flap defect. The definitive closure—the simple 3-phase single layer locking mattress suture technique is applied where tension locking sutures in the epidermis in the centre of both arcs align the closure. There are no fascial deep layered sutures which may embarrass the circulation. The locking mattress suture provides a simple layered closure alternative. Further locking mattress sutures may be deemed appropriate before epidermal seal is achieved to achieve an aesthetic outcome

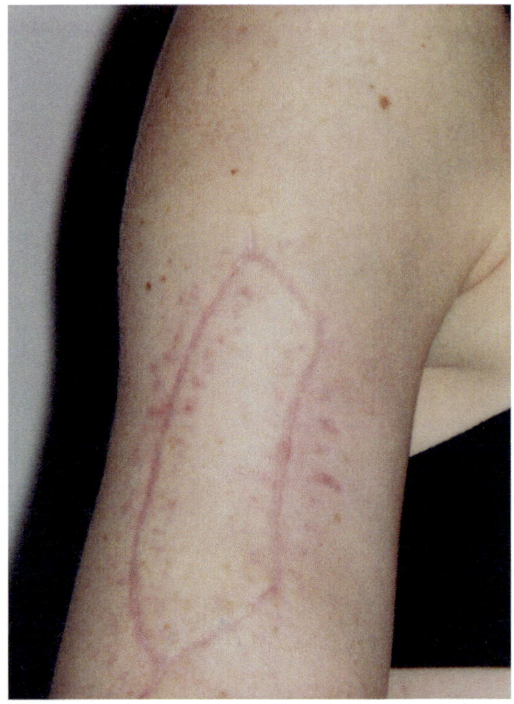

Fig. 2.45 The postoperative acceptable appearance after 3 years without any 'shark bite' appearance allowing her to wear full summer attire after a melanoma excision

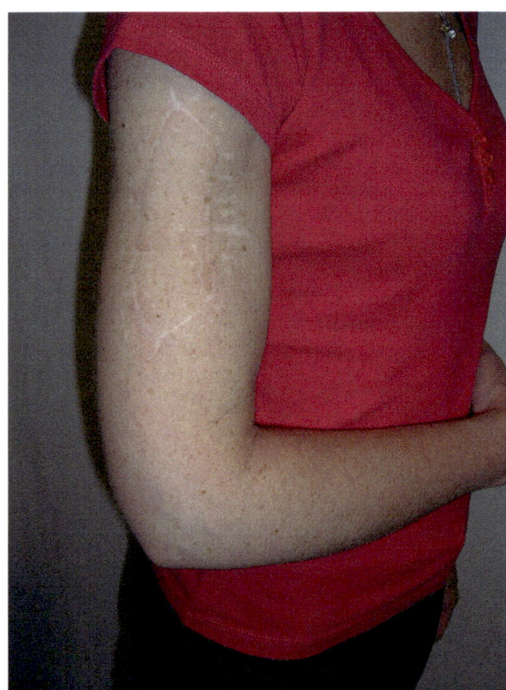

Fig. 2.46 An aesthetic outcome wearing summer gear

2.1.6 Case 6: Supracondylar ORIF of the Humerus with an Encircling Keystone to Achieve Cover Above the Olecranon

Case origin: Melanoma R elbow complicated reconstruction as the Clark Level II 0.6 mm biopsy was done in a circumferential manner. Hence, the Keystone had to be circumferential in the supracondylar region but equally pertinent for orthopaedic applications (Figs. 2.47, 2.48, 2.49, 2.50, 2.51, 2.52, 2.53, and 2.54).

In summary, the reliability of the Keystone allows closure of tissue when the biopsy orientation is circumferential and not longitudinal in this melanoma case used as a baseline for orthopaedic applications. Its hyperaemia and slow sequential suture removal ensures wound integrity.

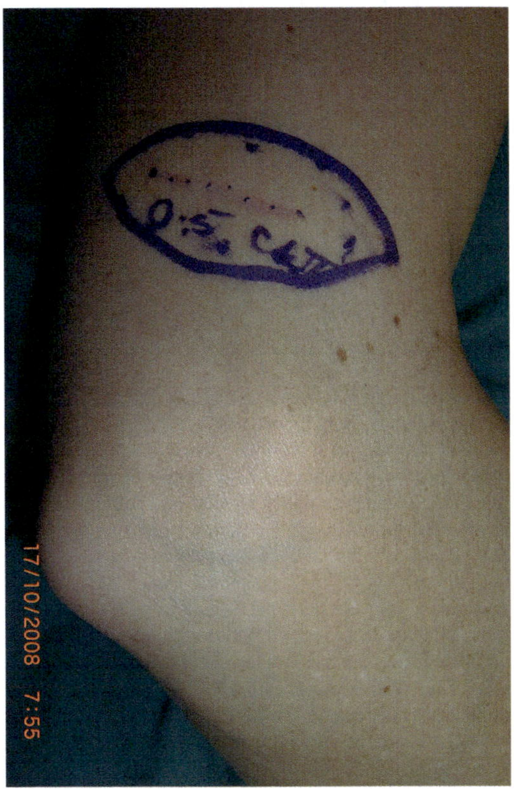

Fig. 2.47 Melanoma Clark level II 0.6 mm, bad circumferential biopsy, representing a poor orientation technique from an outside source. Such a defect and closure is also applicable to orthopaedic reconstruction when the traumatic injury and/or the ORIF repair need a soft tissue cover which is the basis for inclusion of this technique with such an orthopaedic necessity

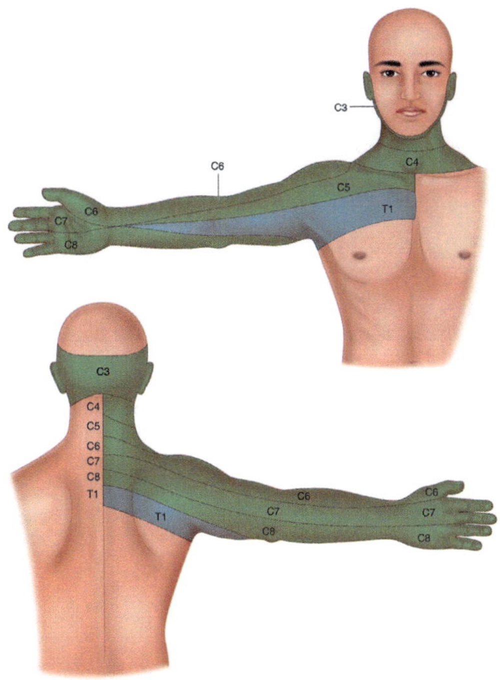

Fig. 2.48 The dermatomal mark out is the guide for the location of the random perforators coming through the fascia and they follow the neurovascular axes

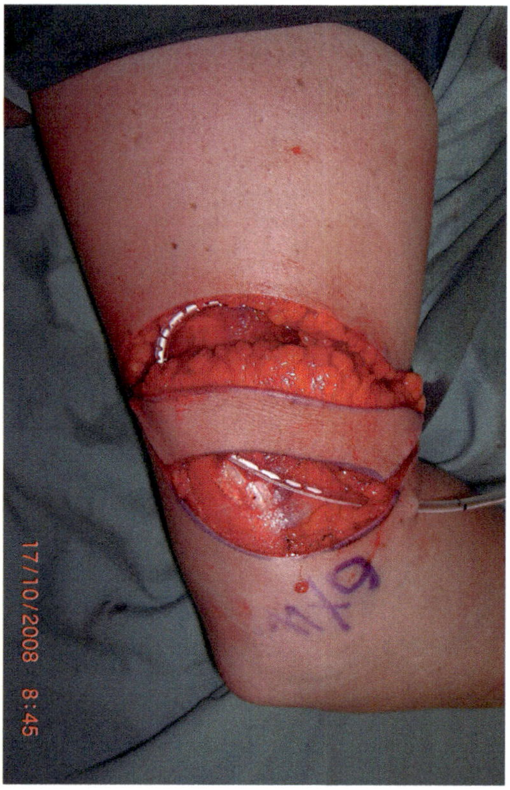

Fig. 2.49 A 6 × 4 cm excisional defect with a thinner 2 cm Keystone in the supracondylar region with a single Redi-vac tubing in a U-shaped design draining two surgical sites—oncological and Keystone sites

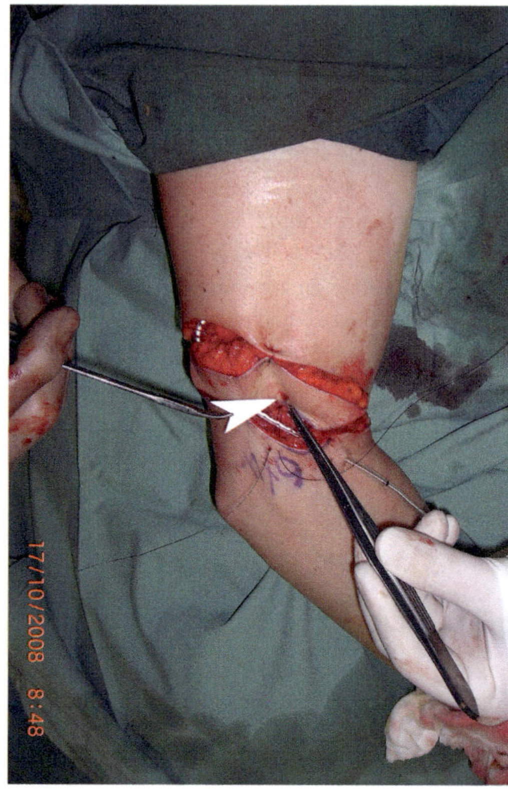

Fig. 2.50 Tensional closure is obvious with partial extension of R elbow. Note the red dot sign (arrowed) confirms vascular integrity in spite of the restrictions of direct closure under tension. This technique breaks the obvious surgical rule of closure under tension but because there is random perforator unaffected circulatory support suprafascial and infrafascial avoiding dependence on the subdermal plexus. This maintains vascular integrity minimising necrosis potential. Thankfully the sympathectomy effect with the island flap design ensures generous circulatory perfusion. Elbow extension facilitates the closure. Thus, this design location has not only oncological applications but can be associated with orthopaedic metal exposure where it warrants soft tissue closure replacing microsurgical techniques

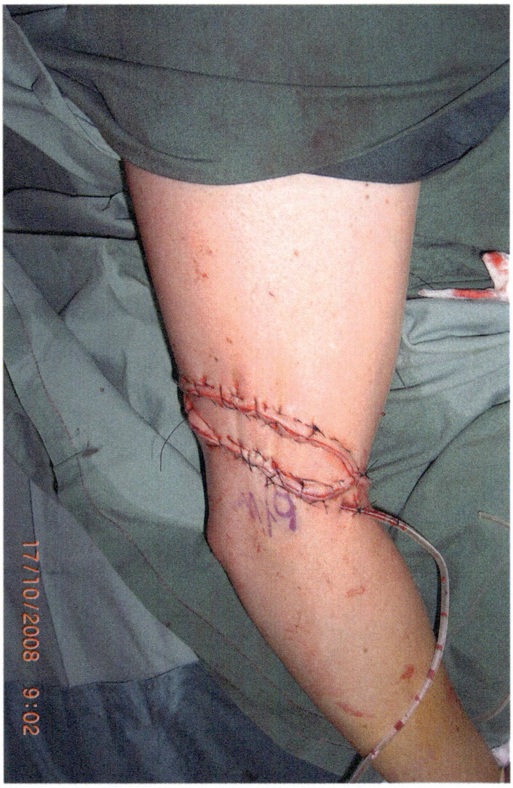

Fig. 2.51 The elbow had to be fully extended to achieve closure intraoperatively and gradually brought into flexion as healing became stabilised over the ensuing days. The 3-phase suture technique applies with these wounds closed under tension—locking mattress sutures along the convex and concave sides of the Keystone and further mattress ensures tissue apposition for wound closure and then a continuous nylon for epidermal seal. The 7, 14 and 21 day sequence is the wound dressing technique for suture removal

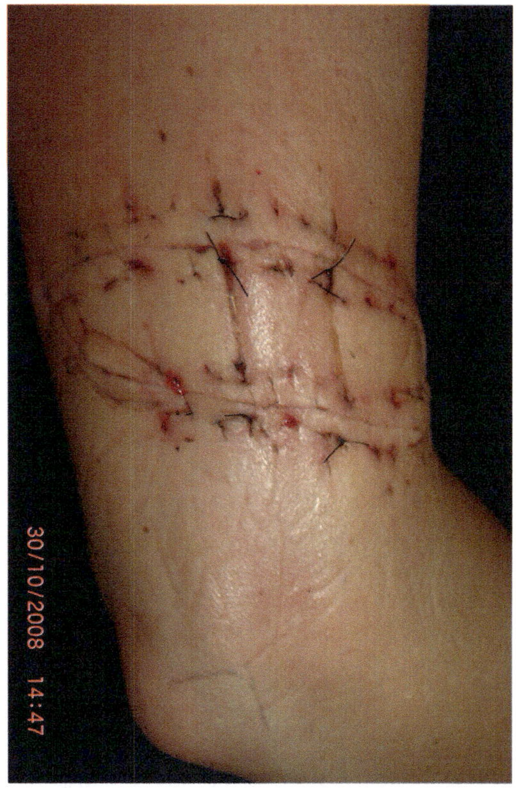

Fig. 2.52 The appearance at 2 weeks and the lines of tension are still evident because of the disorientation of the biopsy specimen. No necrosis evident

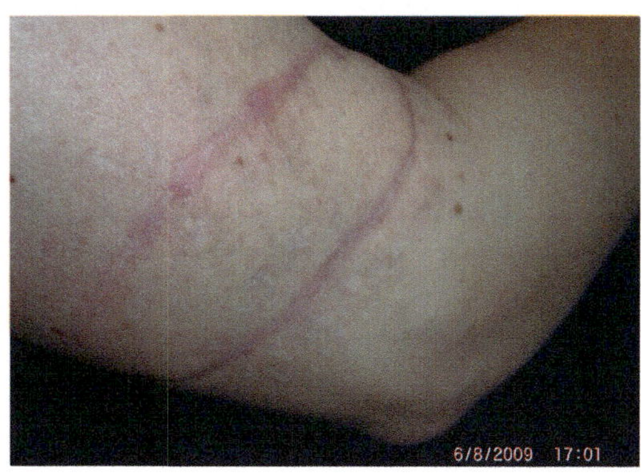

Fig. 2.53 Appearance at 10 months. The mildly hypertrophic scar reflects the closure under tension but acceptable to the patient and I repeat the P.A.C.E.S. acronym were all evident. Such wound dressings should be done at the major clinic rather than left to an outside source should premature removal of sutures lead to wound rupture

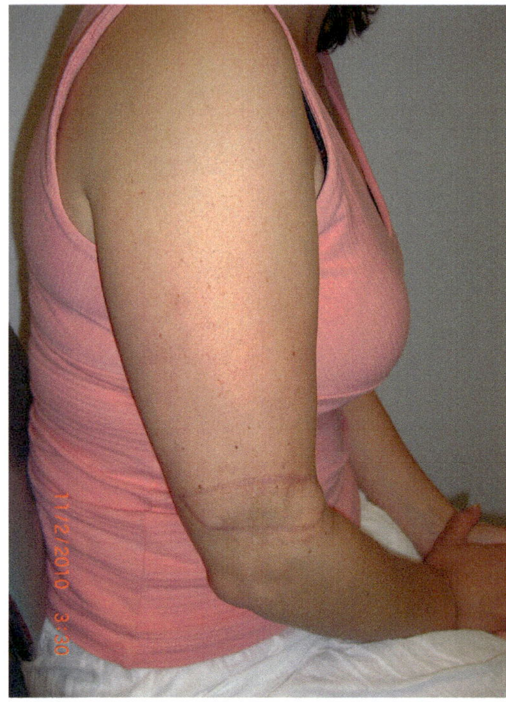

Fig. 2.54 Tumour free interval 16 months and an aesthetic outcome is evident allowing the patient to wear summer gear

2.1.7 Case 7: Fractures of the Spine of the Scapular and/or Acromium If and When an ORIF is Appropriate. The Keystone Flap Technique Provides Access and Facilitates Closure of the Shoulder Joint

I have included this case over the posterior deltoid region because even though the Keystone application is ideal for reconstruction, the movement of the shoulder girdle is a definate contraindication if the patient is non-compliant. In other words, a firm shoulder splintage girdle using an orthoapaedic appliance holds the joint relatively immobile while healing continues over this 3 week period. This may help prevent any wound breakbown with premature removal of sutures (Figs. 2.55, 2.56, 2.57, 2.58, 2.59, 2.60, and 2.61).

In summary, stabilising shoulder movement goes some way to ensure wound healing with the arced Keystone over the supeior deltoid region but the pain free recovery was the keynote of the repair and the P.A.C.E.S. characteristics were all exemplified.

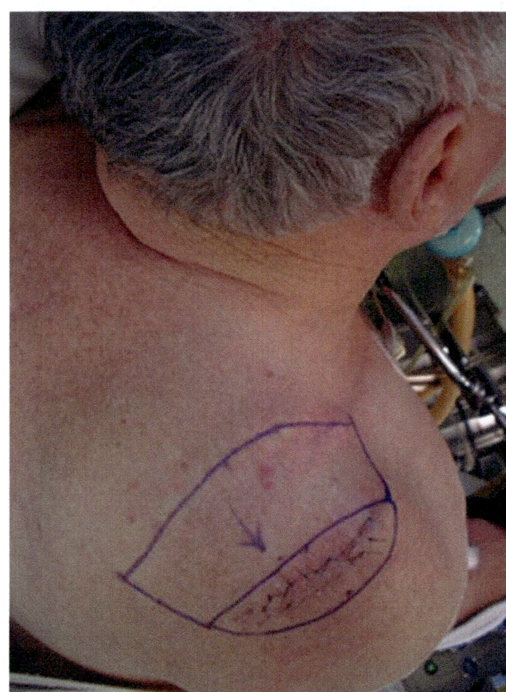

Fig. 2.55 Melanoma of the shoulder/deltoid region Level III—>1 mm and the closure of the surgical defect with the Keystone flap mark out as indicated. The size is larger in transverse depth compared with the marked excisional defect

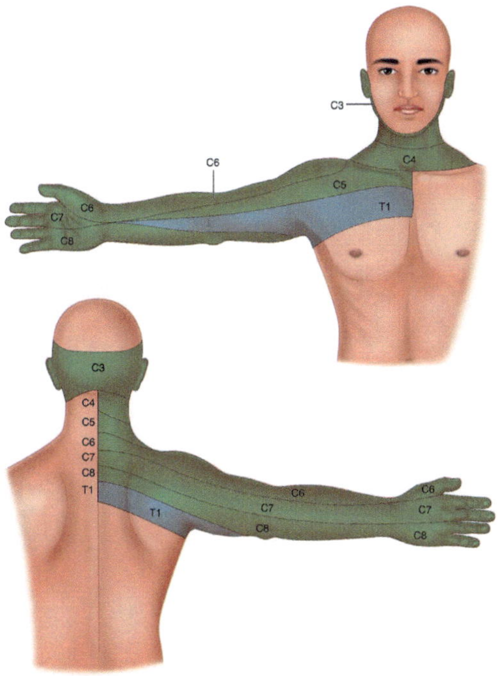

Fig. 2.56 The dermatomal mark outs have been the aide memoir to help orientation of any Keystone design and is the guide for the location of the random perforators coming through the fascia

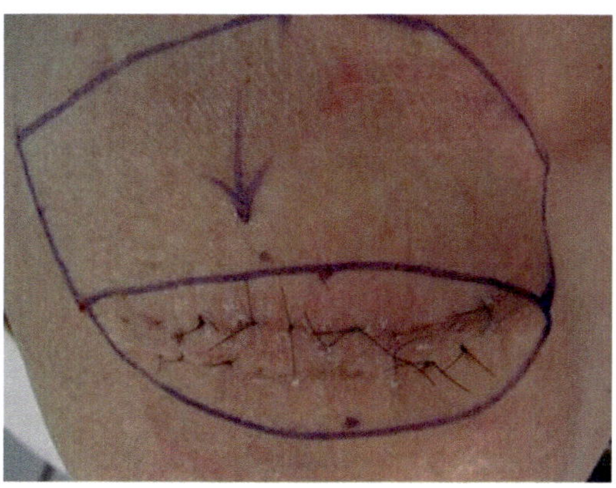

Fig. 2.57 The biopsy site and the subsequent re-excisional defect mark out

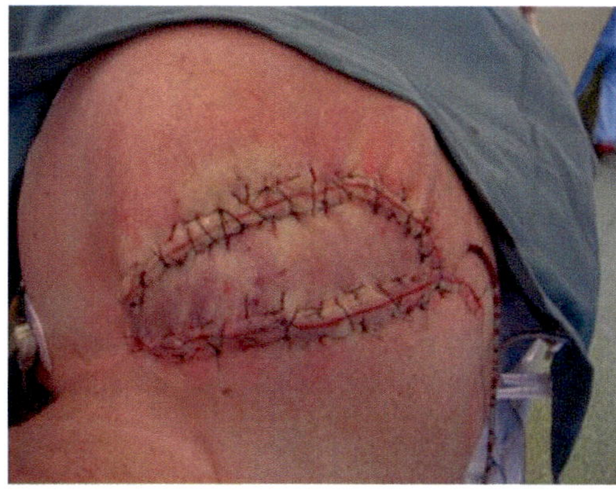

Fig. 2.58 The completed procedure. Note the area of hyperaemia throughout the flap displacing white lines of tension. This reflects the subdermal hypervascularity reflecting what is proposed as a sympathectomy effect as a hypothetical suggestion to explain the increased vascular flow [7]

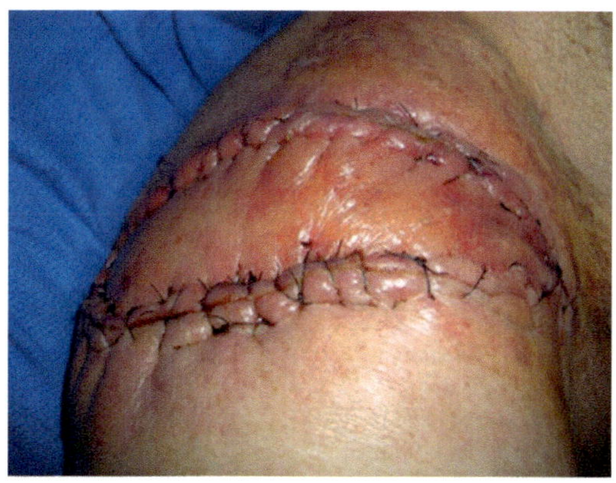

Fig. 2.59 Seven-day appearance. A note of caution, the patient must be splinted in an abducted position of the shoulder joint using a splint to obviate potential wound rupture complications which may occur with premature removal of sutures, i.e. cut the continuous loops at 7 days and the locking mattress sutures are removed sequentially over the next 14 days. Note the wound oedema around the direct closure using the Keystone and a warning sign to be cautious in the wound dressing and suture removal technique when delegated to an outside clinic

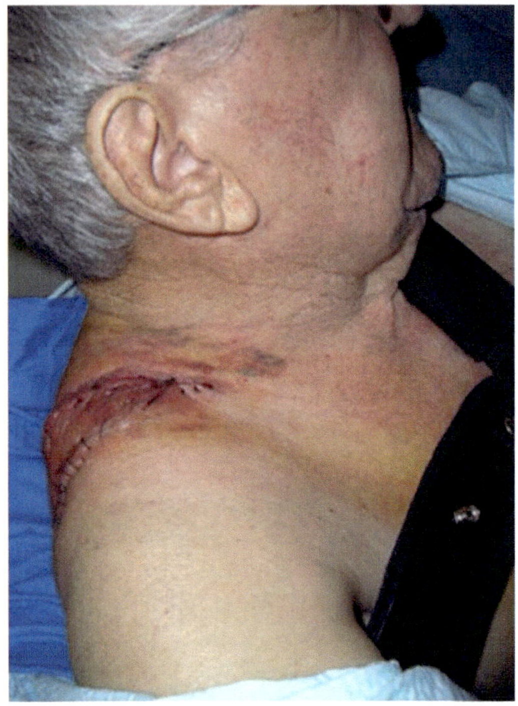

Fig. 2.60 The pain-free surgery and the P.A.C.E.S. characteristics were all exemplified in this sequence of images and in spite of having an oncological background the orthopaedic cases are all treated similarly when bone cover and/or ORIF metal procedures need soft tissue cover

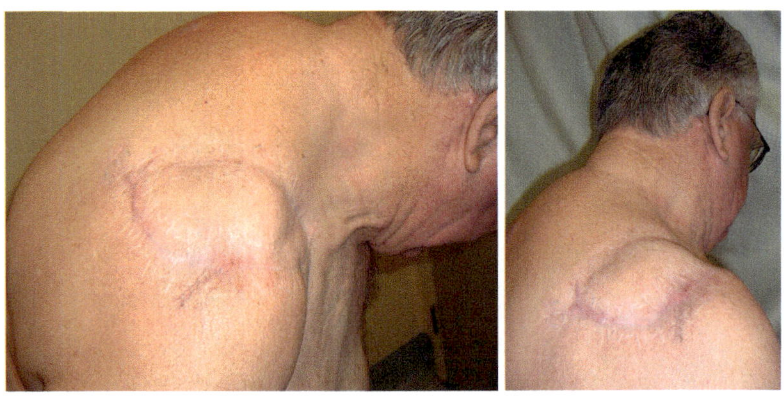

Fig. 2.61 Postoperative outcome and full range of movement and recovery of functional activity have all been achieved under the physiotherapy supervision for shoulder girdle splint is an absolute prerequisite to minimise wound rupture

2.1.7.1 Soft Tissue Palmar Defect

Soft tissue cover of the hand is well suited to the use of the Keystone application, and these cases will show that the design of the Keystone flaps can be used after surgical correction of Dupuytren's fasciectomy, particularly in the McCash version where the MCP 5 needs soft tissue cover.

2.1.8 Case 8: The Keystone Technique for Closing Palmar Defects—An Alternative to the McCash Skin Grafting Technique for Palmar Defects Over the 5th Metacarpal Utilising the Bruner's Exposure

This case was presented internationally at the Dupuytren's Meeting in Paris in 2015, and the use of the Keystone to close the palmar defect avoids skin grafting procedures and their slow recovery phase with hand therapy. Keystones are pain free—part of the Keystone acronym of P.A.C.E.S (Figs. 2.62, 2.63, 2.64, 2.65, 2.66, 2.67, 2.68, 2.69, 2.70, 2.71, 2.72, and 2.73).

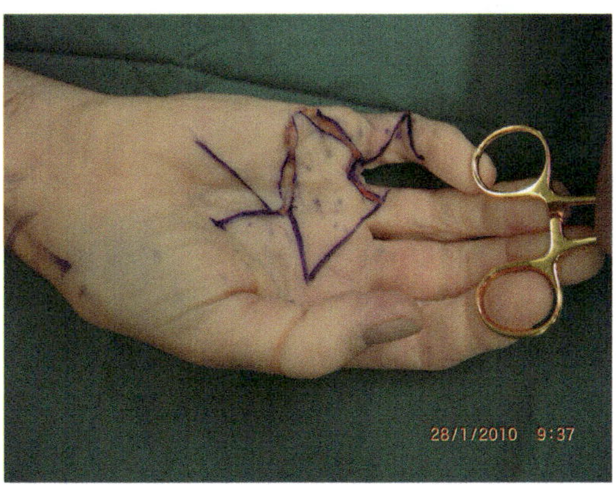

Fig. 2.62 The delineation of the Dupuytren's mass over MCP 4 and 5. The Bruner's [8] exposure excision—triangulate Zs facilitate delivery of the neurovascular bundles into the wound

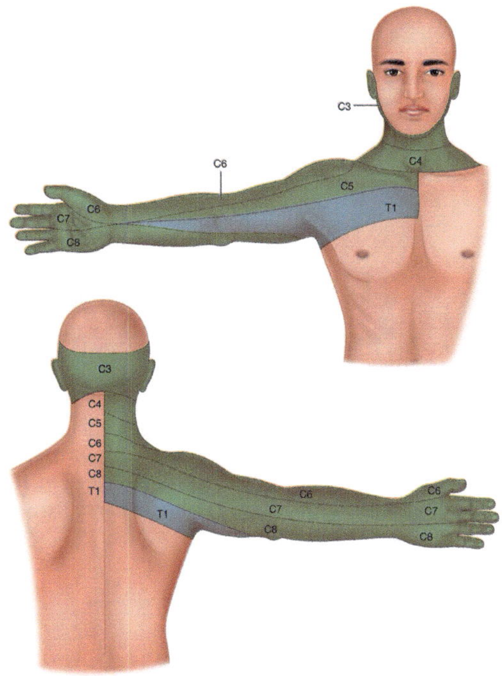

Fig. 2.63 Dermatomal mark out

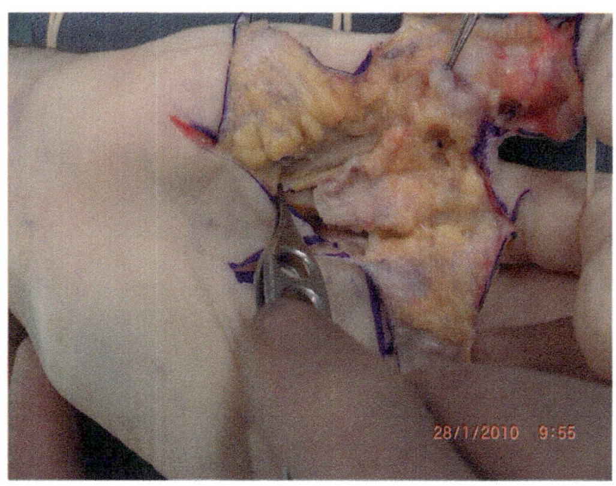

Fig. 2.64 The blue dots on the nerve is a safeguard trick to help in their delineation where with a slight tug they can be delineated from the Dupuytren's effect

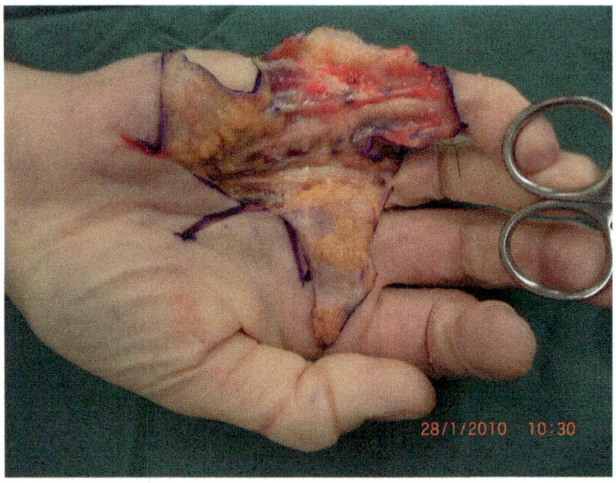

Fig. 2.65 The Z exposure facilitates exploration of the digits, clearing the neurovascular bundles. The triangles of tissue are folded back as though hinged as long as 1/3 or deep attachment is maintained to ensure microperforator support to the flaps

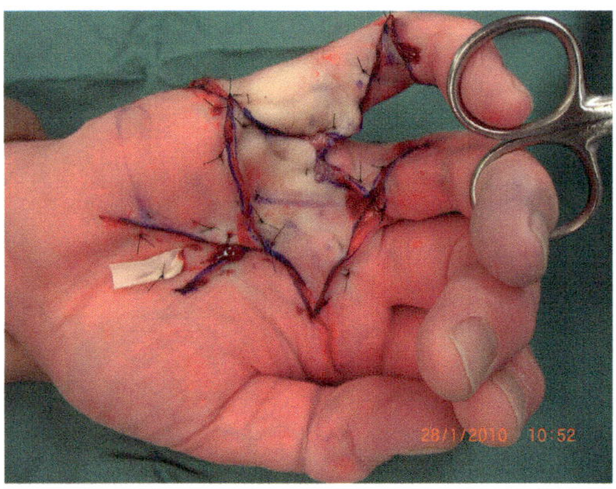

Fig. 2.66 Perfusion after the tourinquet release and the gradual recovery from the hinged margins of the triangulate margins of the Brunner's exposure

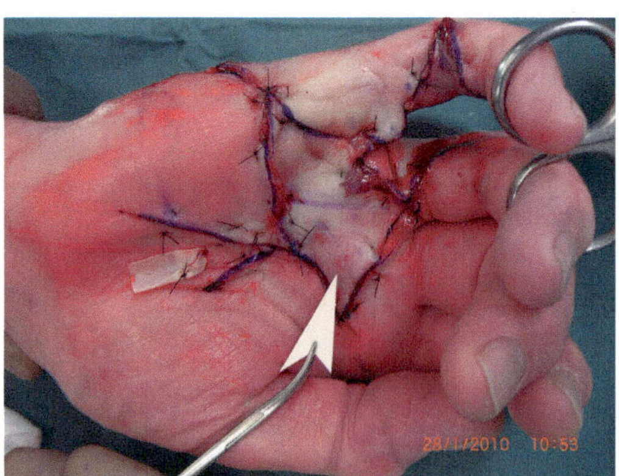

Fig. 2.67 Perfusion to the limits of the flap at the detached margin sourced from the attached side

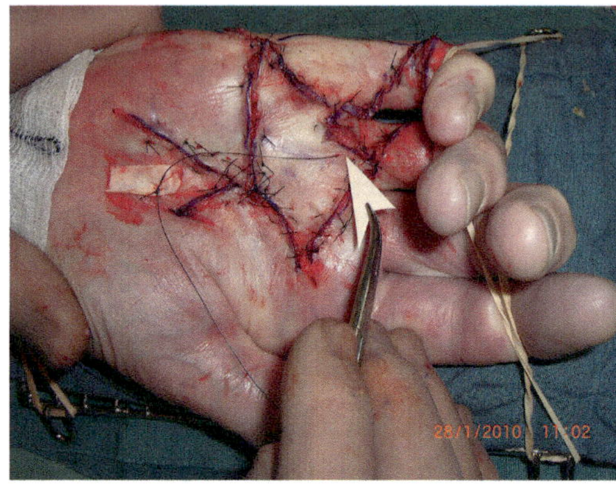

Fig. 2.68 Staged closure after 9 min from the date stamped image

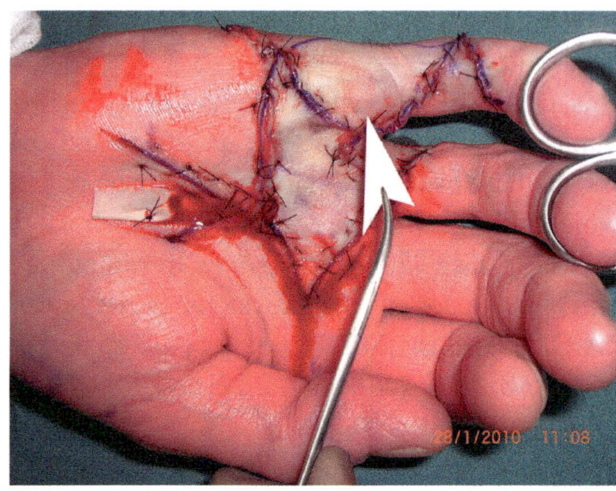

Fig. 2.69 Red dot signs indicating satisfactory perfusion following haemostasis and penrose drainage

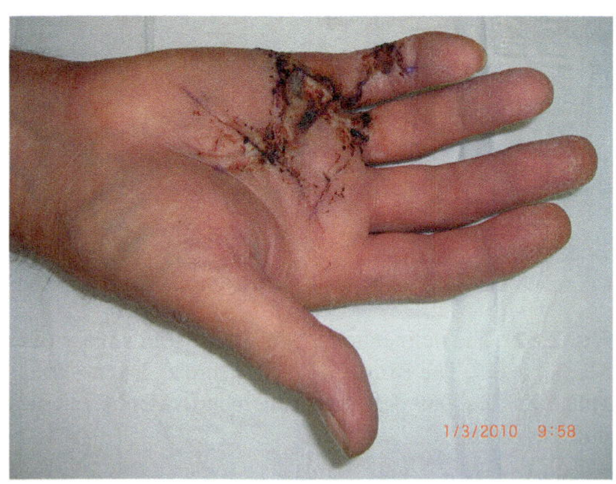

Fig. 2.70 Four weeks postoperative appearance with no evidence of any necrotic flap because of the hypervascularity developed from the Keystone principle

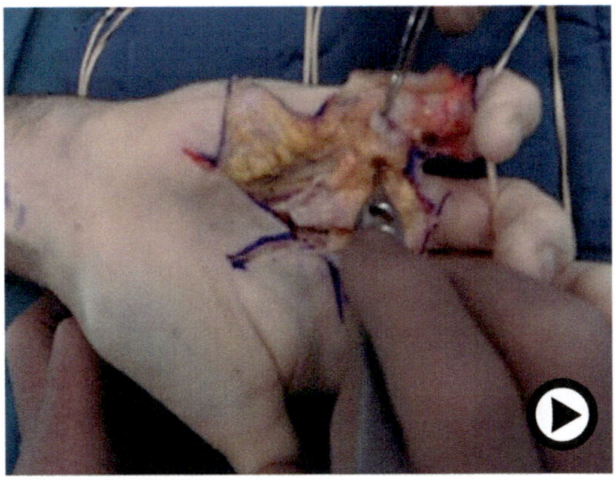

Fig. 2.71 The tug test to appraise the alignment of the nerve before dissection and operative release (Video 2.10 The tug test to appraise the alignment of the nerve before dissection and operative release) (▶ https://doi.org/10.1007/000-d4n)

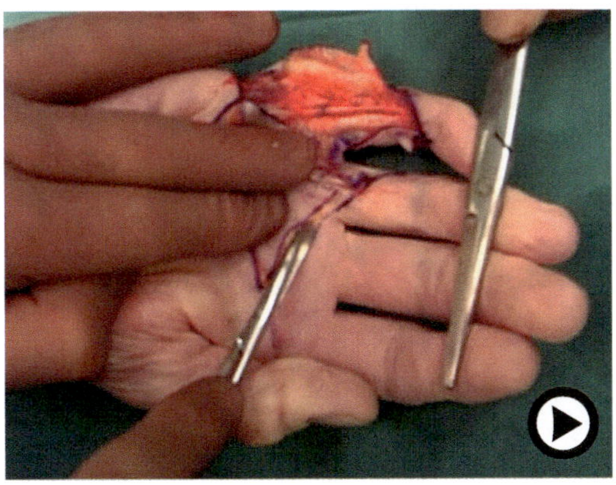

Fig. 2.72 Delivering the nerve with blunt dissection (Video 2.11 Delivering the nerve with blunt dissection) (▶ https://doi.org/10.1007/000-d4p)

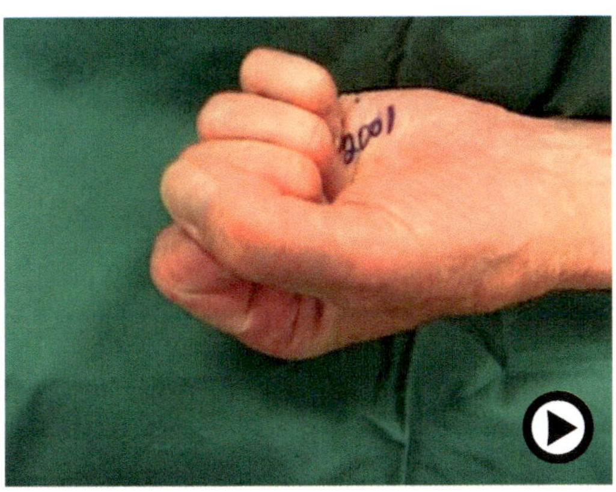

Fig. 2.73 Postoperative full range of movement achieved (Video 2.12 Postoperative full range of movement achieved) (▶ https://doi.org/10.1007/000-d4q)

2.1.9 Case 9: Orthopaedic Closures for Bony Defects Around the Anatomical Snuffbox

This melanoma case and closure with Keystone applications are equally applicable in the stages of repair of the reconstruction and its applications in orthopaedics apply the same principles. The 10 × 4 cm melanoma defect can be easlity closed with a variety of Keystone applications as illustrated should an ORIF of the metacarpal of a similar size needing soft tissue cover can be repaired using a similar flap technique adopting Keystone principles. The melanoma management follwowed a **biopsy Clark Level IV—3 mm thick in a farmer's wife.** The transverse orientation of the biopsy creates difficulties in Keystone reconstruction. Hence, the design along the limits of the anatomical snuffbox becomes the requirement. The same flap can be used for compound fractures of the metacarpal needing cover should orthopaedic soft tissue cover be necessary (Figs. 2.74, 2.75, 2.76, 2.77, 2.78, 2.79, and 2.80).

Again, in summary, this melanoma case which is circumferentially aligned at the wrist crease has been resolved by ensuring the integrity of loco-regional perforators, but more importantly in watching the cutaneous input from the radial cutaneous nerve which must not be disturbed in case any filamentous damage can produce a subsequent sympathetic distrophy and always a source of chronic regional pain syndrome. Thus there are orthopaedic applications for ORIF procedures over the anatomical snuffbox.

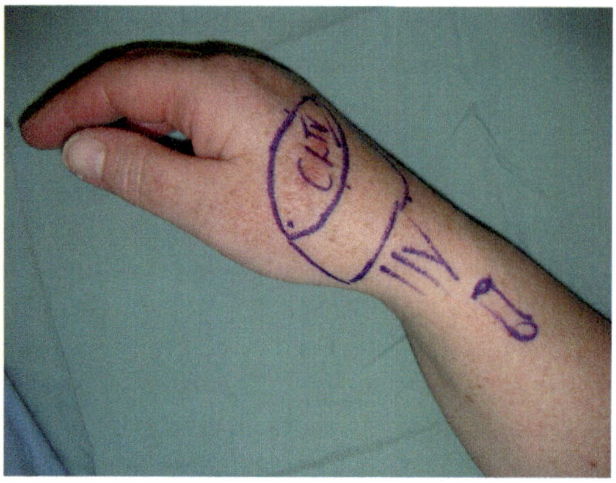

Fig. 2.74 The use of the circumferential Keystone designed from the anatomical snuff box and radially orientated towards the direction of the ulnar styloid. This circumferential Keystone is a very easy procedure while the integrity of the neurovascular channels, filamentous in nature, is defined and preserved across the wrist. The arrow indicates the direction in which the flap is raised based on ulnar border microcirculation. The neurovascular support of the radial cutaneous nerve and perforators through the anatomical snuff box are all visualised. As one raises the flap circumferentially, it is the ulnar styloid site which is the basis for the microvascular perforator support. A basic surgical requirement of surgical caution around the radial cutaneous nerves will help obviate any postoperative post traumatic neuritic symptoms leading to possible sympathetic dystrophy. The implications of hypersensitised pain are a well-recognised problem when focused on the radial cutaneous nerves

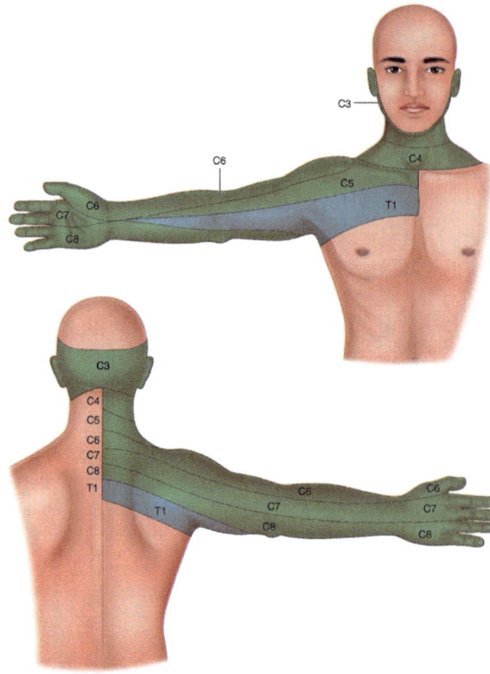

Fig. 2.75 Dermatomal mark out

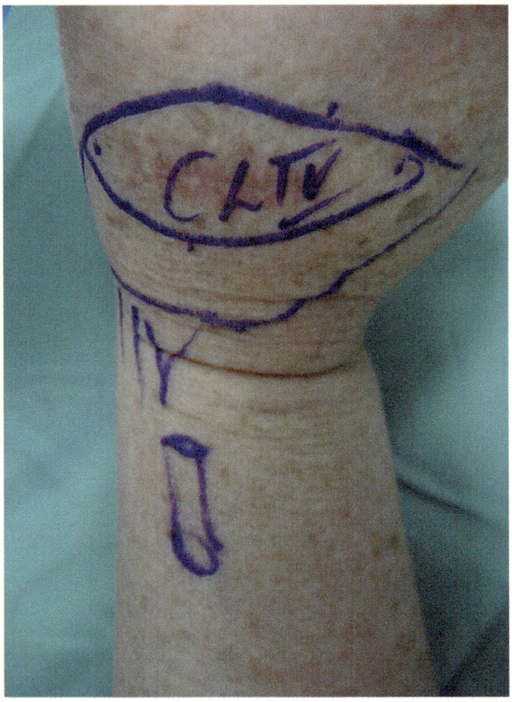

Fig. 2.76 The design of the circumferential Keystone is governed by the biopsy orientation in this melanoma case but the same closure sequence using Keystone applied. The wrist in extreme extension facilitates wound closure. The radial cutaneous nerve and the cephalic vein are part of the neurovascular support, and the integrity of these structures must be maintained to avoid any chronic regional pain syndrome. The dermatomal mark out is the guide for the location of the random perforators coming through the deep fascia. It is the dermatome that is the aide memoir in the design of the circulatory pattern with its deep attachment overlying the ulnar styloid

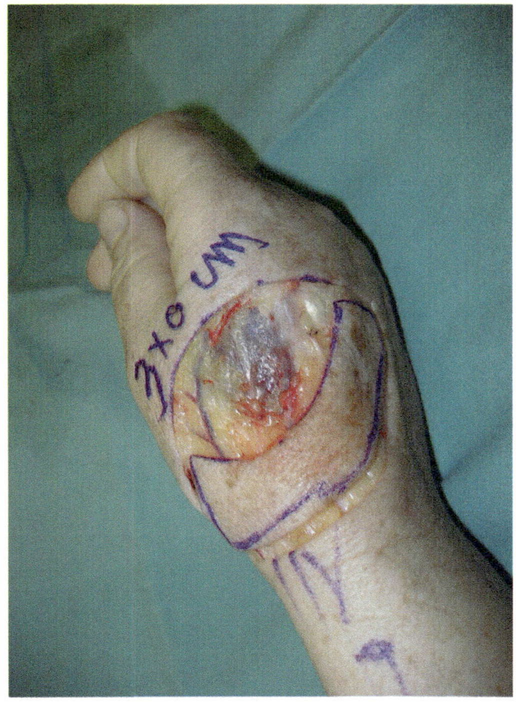

Fig. 2.77 The oncological defect 3 × 6 cm (as marked on the image) and the mark out of the proximal circumferential Keystone design to close the defect exposing the branches of the radial cutaneous nerve which must be preserved with discrete dissection. Avoidance of neural damage is an absolute prerequisite in this closure under tension to avoid any potential chronic regional pain syndrome. The wrist is held in extension with some radial deviation to facilitate wound closure. Again, this applies in any orthopaedic reconstruction

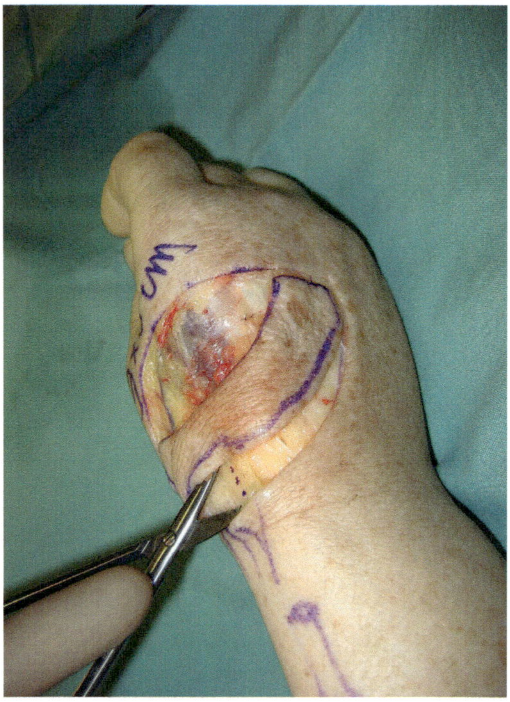

Fig. 2.78 The blunt dissection technique to help mobilisation of the Keystone, again avoiding neural damage associated with maintaining the integrity of microperforators, the anatomical snuffbox. This technique frees us the subcutaneous adhesions using blunt dissection (as illustrated) facilitating flap mobilisation avoiding undermining using the open scissors to free the flap from the underlying structures longitudinally while not damaging them anatomically and this facilitates closure. There is no undermining of the flap

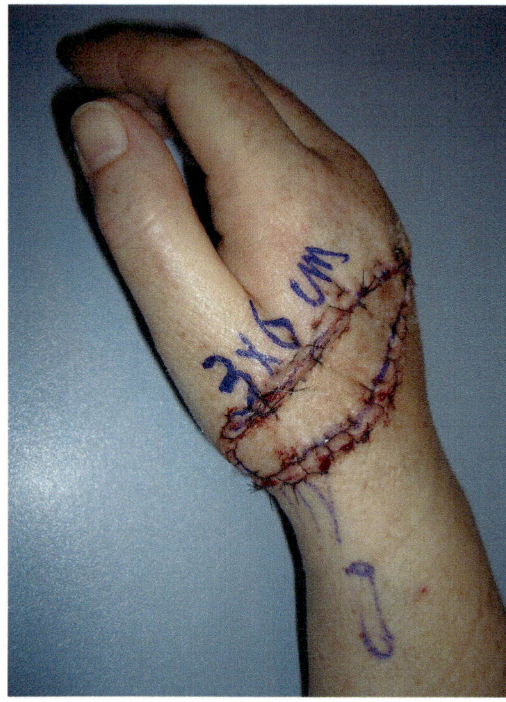

Fig. 2.79 The appearance at 7 days with the wrist in radial deviation facilitating closure. The hyperaemic flare is evident and settling consistent with vascular integrity without dissecting any particular perforators. The temporary swelling of the thumb and hand continues to resolve, and the patient is totally pain free consistent with the Keystone P.A.C.E.S. characteristics

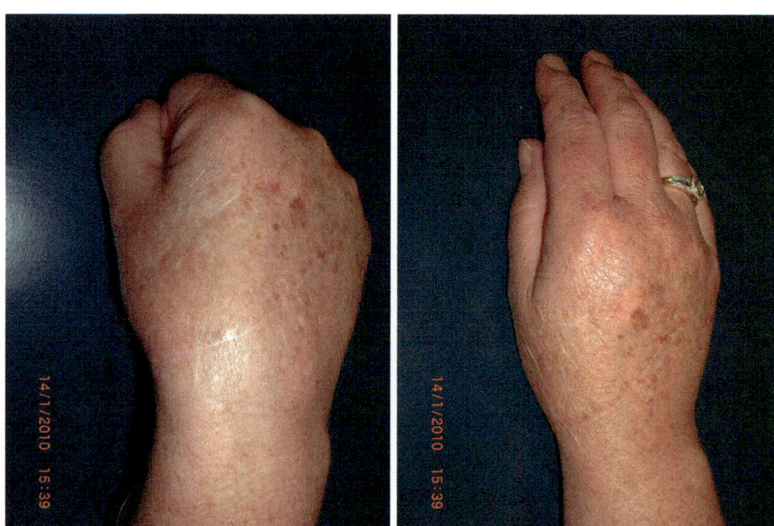

Fig. 2.80 The scarring is indiscernible and arrowed to visualise the margin of the flap in this aesthetic outcome after 3.5 years at the time of this image for a lady's hand. There is a full range of normal pain free movement of the R wrist in this farmer's wife who was still milking cows. The P.A.C.E.S. characteristics were all exemplified

2.1.10 Case 10: Thumb Reconstruction and a Littler Flap [9] Avoiding Terminalisation Procedure

The soft tissue flap can be divided in sequence optimising the extension of the island flap suspended on the neurovasular bundles with microvascular support not disimilar to clothes on a clothesline. The island flap in this variation repeats the vascular sequence one sees in the Keystone principles and its characteristic acronym P.A.C.E.S (Figs. 2.81, 2.82, 2.83, 2.84, 2.85, and 2.86).

A simple technique to get bone cover and avoid terminilisation procedures which shorten the thumb (40% of the function of the hand). All P.A.C.E.S. characteristics were exemplified, and the fenestrated full thickness graft in the gaps in the island flap ensured integrity in the wound closure.

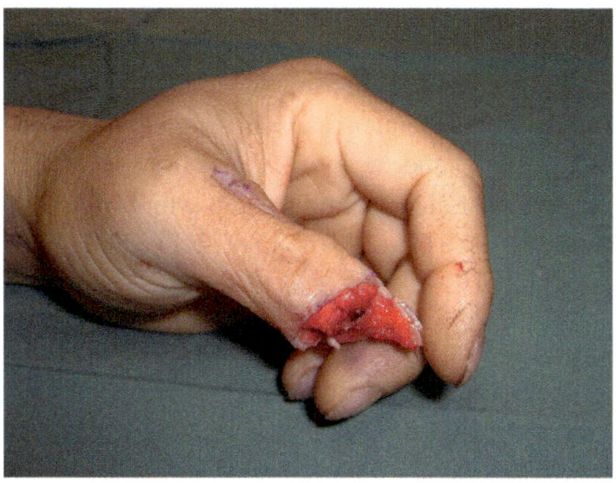

Fig. 2.81 The traumatic defect of the base of the terminal phalanx of the thumb in the C6 dermatome

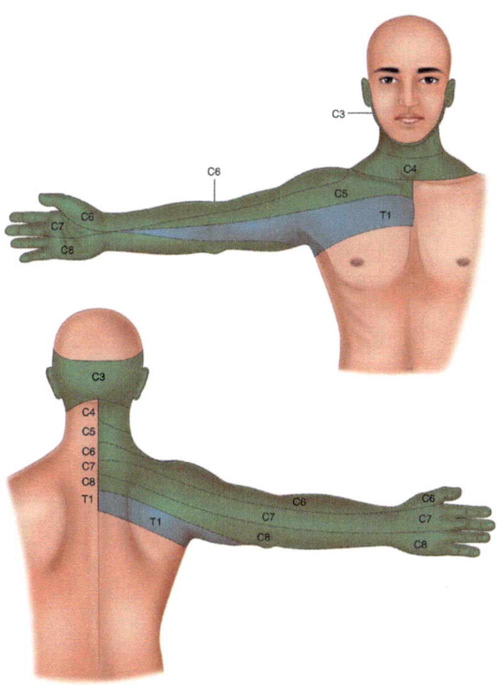

Fig. 2.82 Dermatomal mark out

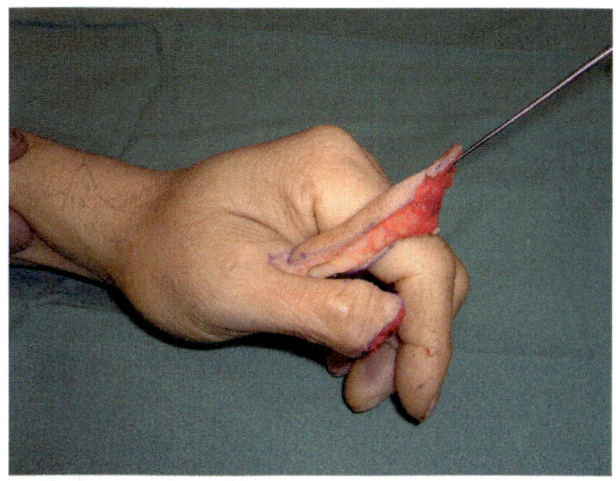

Fig. 2.83 Tailoring the flap proximally to cover the defect including exposed bone. The Littler island flap based on the neurovascular axes, in this case up the ulnar side of the thumb, is raised down the cleft side of the thumb maintaining vascular integrity. A second phase entails division of dermal continuity to allow stretch to cover the bony exposure optimising length.

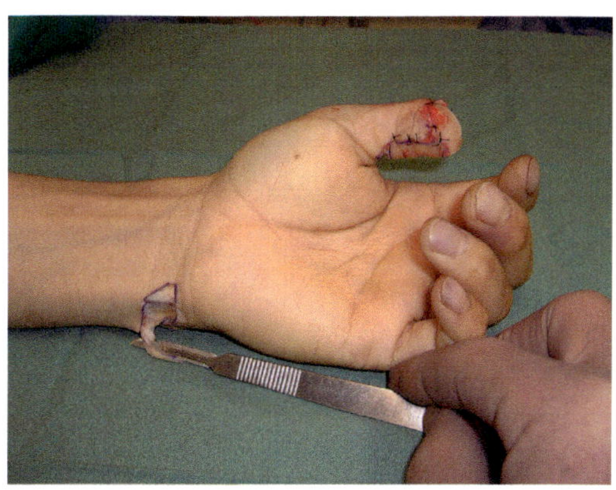

Fig. 2.84 Fenestrated graft technique: the harvesting of redundant tissue at the ulnar styloid crease is an ample source of donor skin which is pre-fenestrated before insertion over the divisions of the dermal flap-on-flap technique illustrated

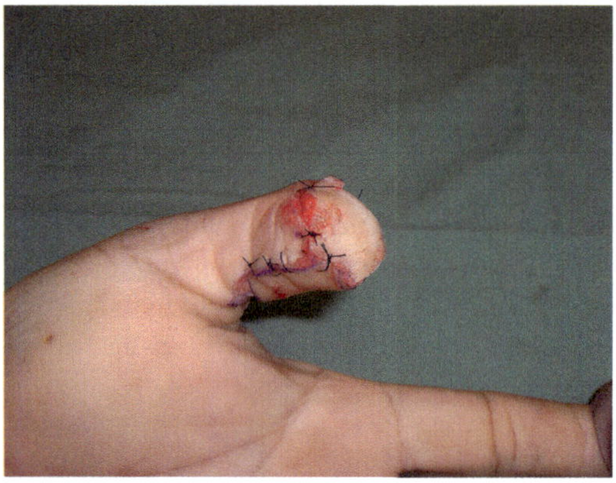

Fig. 2.85 The outcome achieved with full vascular integrity and the use of the full thickness graft contributes to this tension free closure of the thumb tip—this digit constitutes 40% function of the hand

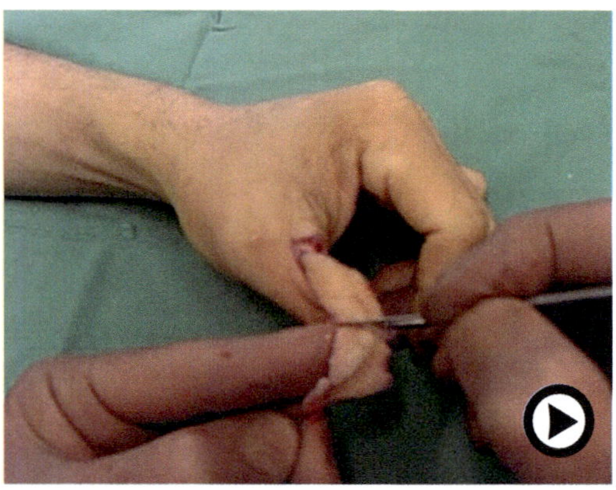

Fig. 2.86 Operative sequence dividing the island flap suspended on neurovascular structures for length increase (Video 2.13 Operative sequence dividing the island flap suspended on neurovascular structures for length increase) (▶ https://doi.org/10.1007/000-d4r)

2.1.11 Case 11: Digital Tip Reconstruction Using the Flap-on-Flap Technique—a Simple Method Optimising Length When the Double Flaps Are Suspended from the Neurovascular Axes by Blunt Dissection Stretch Achieving 1 cm of Extra Length with a Fenestrated Full Thickness Graft to any Exposed Area Created

Illustrated above. This simple technique of dividing the flap in sequence visualising the neurovascular axes, and a blunt dissection technique optimises stretch creating a gap which is closed with a graft (Figs. 2.87, 2.88, 2.89, 2.90, 2.91, and 2.92).

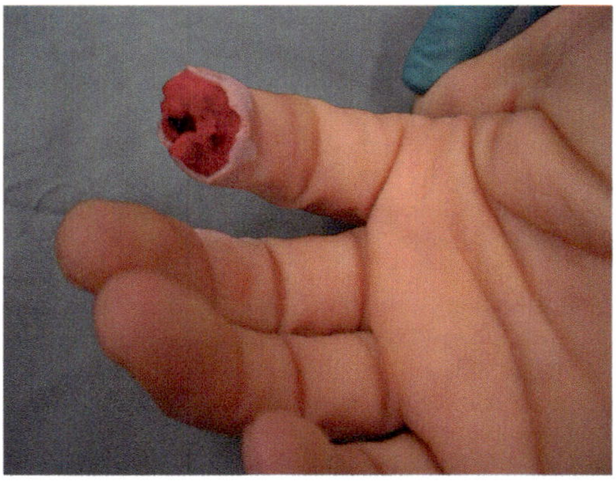

Fig. 2.87 Bony defect amputation at the base of the terminal phalanx of the index finger

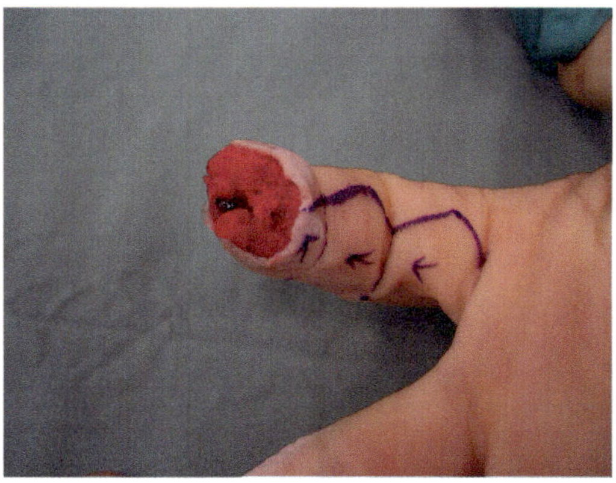

Fig. 2.88 The Littler flap is raised with a Bruner's exposure down the ulnar side of the digit, and these dermal divisions over the middle and proximal phalanges facilitate the stretch needed to cover the bony defect of the base of the terminal phalanx. Fenestrated full thickness graft helps bridge these dermal divisions

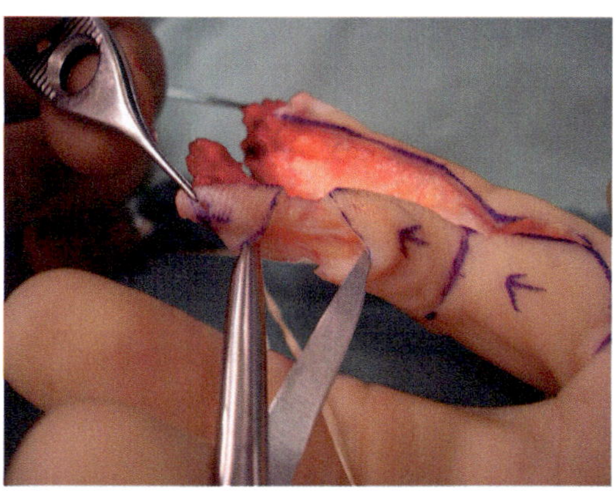

Fig. 2.89 The blunt dissection stretch technique showing the integrity of the neurovascular system, increasing the sensate cover for the bony tip, the site for future grafting

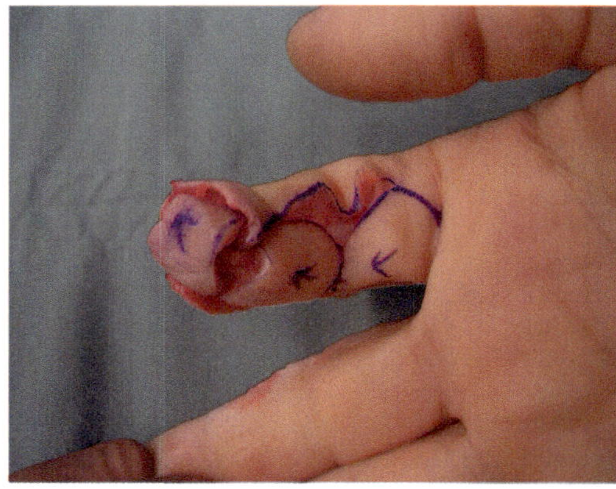

Fig. 2.90 Again, further grafting between the dermal bridges

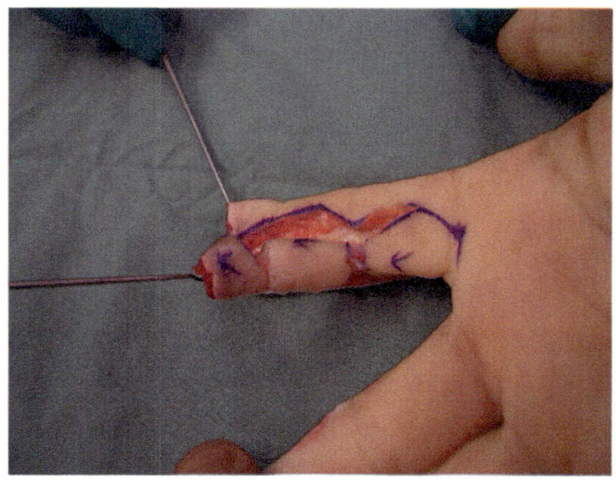

Fig. 2.91 The arrows indicate the lines of stretch facilitating the flap-on-flap lengthening covering the bony base of the terminal phalanx. The bridging between the tissue flaps is closed with a fenestrated full thickness graft which is just tacked into position without any pressure or tie over closure

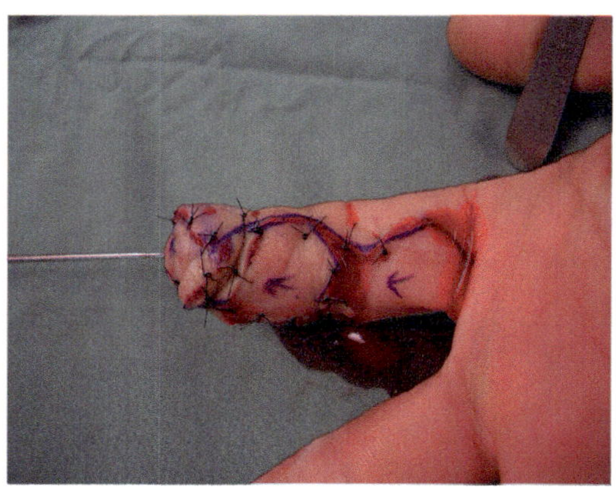

Fig. 2.92 The grafts in situ and the bony defect covered—a simple way of stretching the Littler flap. Note the viability of vascular flow without any vascular impedance contributing to the healing sequence without flap necrosis

References

1. Pelissier P, et al. Reverse dorsal digital and metacarpal flaps: a review of 27 cases. Plast Reconstr Surg. 1999;103(1):159–65.
2. Wong TM, Lau TW, Li X, Fang C, Yeung K, Leung F. Masquelet technique for treatment of posttraumatic bone defects. Sci World J. 2014;710302. https://doi.org/10.1155/2014/710302. PMCID: PMC3933034, PMID: 24688420.
3. Behan FC. Atlas of keystone reconstructive technique in the management of melanoma. Cham: Springer; 2024.
4. Rodriguez-Unda N, Abraham J, Saint-Cyr M. Keystone and perforator flaps in reconstruction. Clin Plast Surg. 2020;47(4):635–48.
5. Guy P, Slobogean GP, McCormack RG. Treatment preferences for displaced three- and four-part proximal humerus fractures. J Orthop Trauma. 2010;24(4):250–4.
6. Robinson CM, Amin AK, Godley KC, et al. Modern perspectives of open reduction and plate fixation of proximal humerus fractures. J Orthop Trauma. 2011;25(10):618–29.
7. Lo C, Nottle T, Mills J. Keystone island flap: effects of islanding on vascularity. Plast Reconstr Surg Glob Open. 2016;4(2):e617.
8. Bruner JM. The zig-zag volar-digital incision for flexor-tendon surgery. Plast Reconstr Surg. 1967;40(6):571–4.
9. Littler J. The neurovascular pedicle method of digital transposition for reconstruction of the thumb. Plast Reconstr Surg. 1953;12(5):303–19.

The Keystone Flap Technique to Solve Orthopaedic Defects of the Lower Limb from the Inguinal Region to the Dorsum of the Foot

3

Contents

Supplementary Information The online version contains supplementary material available at https://doi.org/10.1007/978-3-031-76702-9_3. The videos can be accessed individually by clicking the DOI link in the accompanying figure caption or by scanning this link with the SN More Media App.

F. Behan, *Keystone Flap for Complex Orthopaedic Problems*,
https://doi.org/10.1007/978-3-031-76702-9_3

3.1 Case Presentations

3.1.1 Case 12: Surgical Inguinal Closures Based on Integumentary Management of Melanoma of the Groin Which Has Orthopaedic Relevance for Wound Closure Application

In this oncological [1] illustration, a defect 10 × 15 cm is closed by a keystone of the anterior thigh, islanded throughout down the collatoral margins along tensor fascia lata incising medially up to the groin, having incised the tissue over the suprapatellar region to maximise mobility and faciliate closure over any femoral neck defects that may have to be covered. Thus, it has orthopaedic applications for wound closures around the upper femoral region, whatever the pathology but it is beneficial to know there is a flap available for application—the keystone (Figs. 3.1, 3.2, 3.3, 3.4, 3.5, and 3.6).

In summary, the P.A.C.E.S. characteristics of the keystone were all exemplified contributing to the patient's wellbeing including a pain free postoperative phase with good aesthetic presentation,

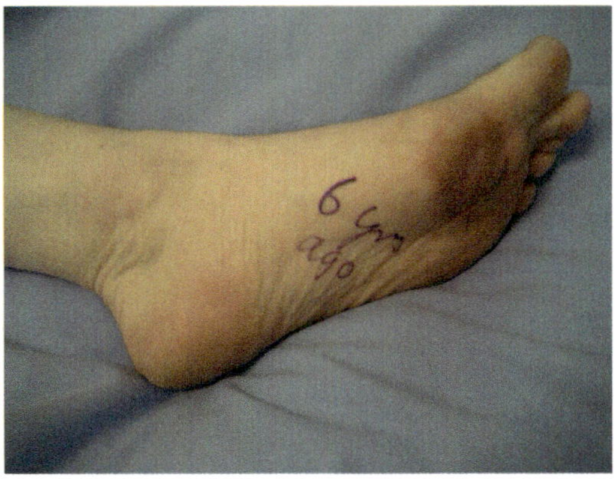

Fig. 3.1 Original presentation. No sign of local recurrence of the ALM of the plantar surface of the L foot over the 1st metatarsophalangeal joint

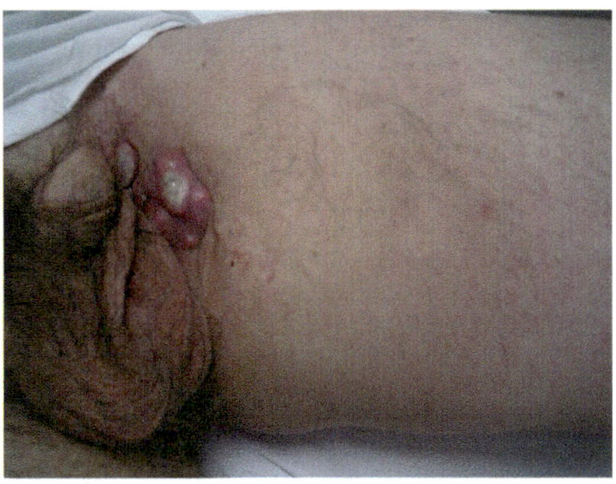

Fig. 3.2 More illustrations of the oncological case with secondary deposits in the groin to help define the outline for surgical removal and closure of the subsequent defect which is linked to the orthopaedic management of similar groin defects

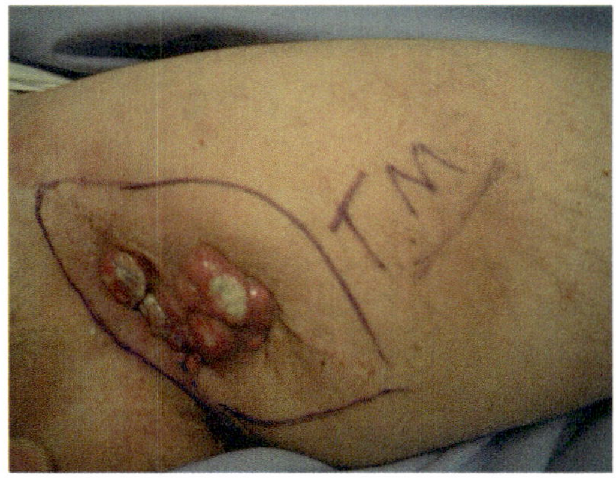

Fig. 3.3 L groin dissection including cutaneous clearance of the L inguinal tumour mass approximately 10 × 15 cm

no evidence of any vascular necrosis as a complication and the economics of operating time were well defined. There was recovery of somatic sensation and lymphatic channels presumably prevent any residual postoperative oedema.

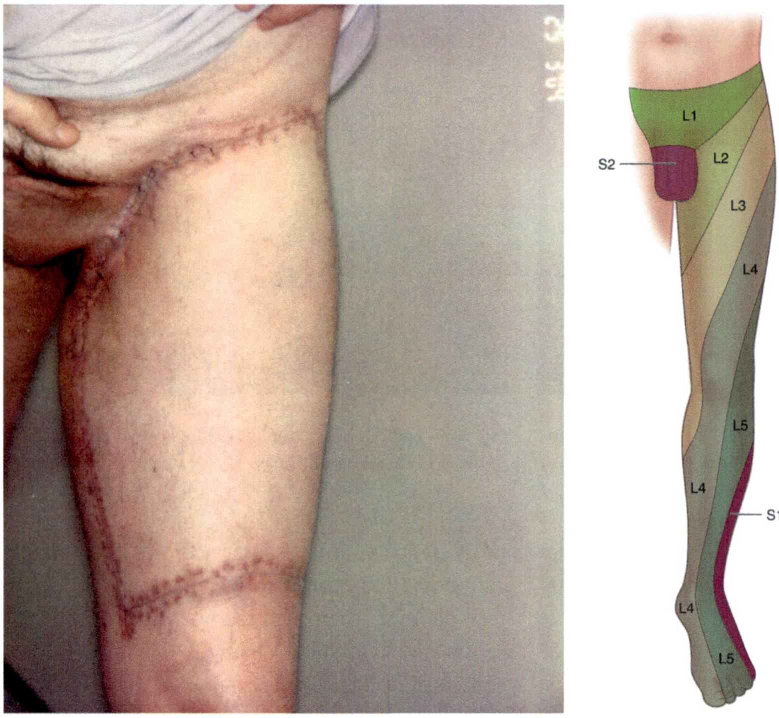

Fig. 3.4 The suture lines in the vicinity of the lateral thigh from inguinal level down to the suprapatellar bursa level. The tensor fascia lata along this lateral margin must be divided, so the other 3 incisions medially and inferiorly allow the tissues to be mobilised with ease closing defects of the groin 10 × 15 cm. This should be ample mobilisation to cover any ORIF defect of the femoral neck as orthopedically appropriate. Appearance of the healed wound of the L2, L3, L4 groin dermatome for this keystone groin flap technique (Reproduced with permission from [2]). Technique: The keystone, almost quadrangular in design, extends from the line of the inguinal excision at the upper level of L2 and is outlined. The operative technique consists of a lateral incision along and ascending the tensor fascia lata laterally, transversely across the suprapatellar region and ascending medially up the inner thigh still dividing the deep fascia. This creates an umbrella of tissue based on random perforators straddling L2, L3, L4 dermatomes and based on microperforators from the quadricep muscle group. These are not individually dissected because the random perforators are sufficient to maintain viability as evidenced on the healed wound. The filamentous contributions to neurovascular support up these perforators including lymphatic channels goes towards a simplified method of closure of groin defects or an orthopaedic origin up to 10 × 15 cm

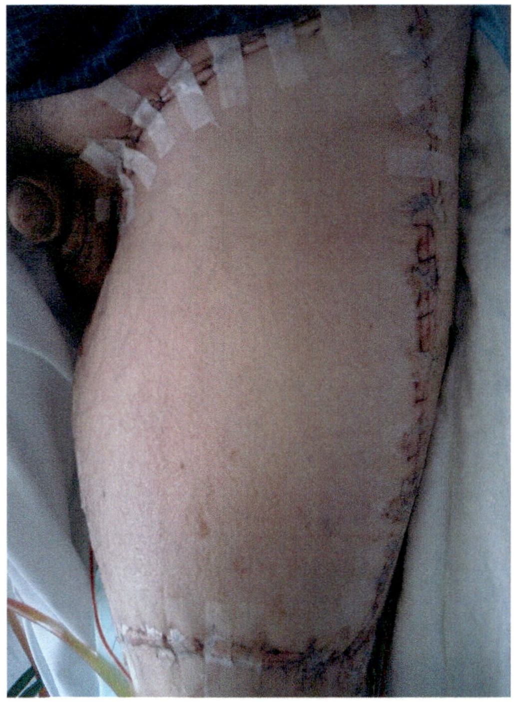

Fig. 3.5 The inferior wound of skin and epidermis is just closed directly and the rest of the wound is closed by the 3-phase nylon suture technique. An essential prerequisite is to have a large drain tube along tensor fascia lata for obvious reasons which can extend up into the groin. A medial drainage of a large bore drain tube is also an essential requirement. This immediate postoperative appearance shows the reactive hyperaemia, an important background for sound healing

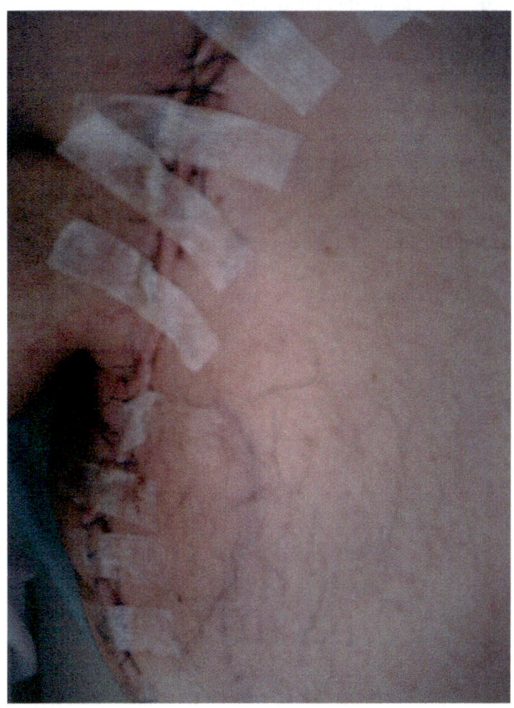

Fig. 3.6 A closeup of the groin defect without any evidence of vascular impedance or potential necrosis. The mild inflammatory reaction along the suture line settled with antibiotic cover reflecting its earlier inflammatory phase

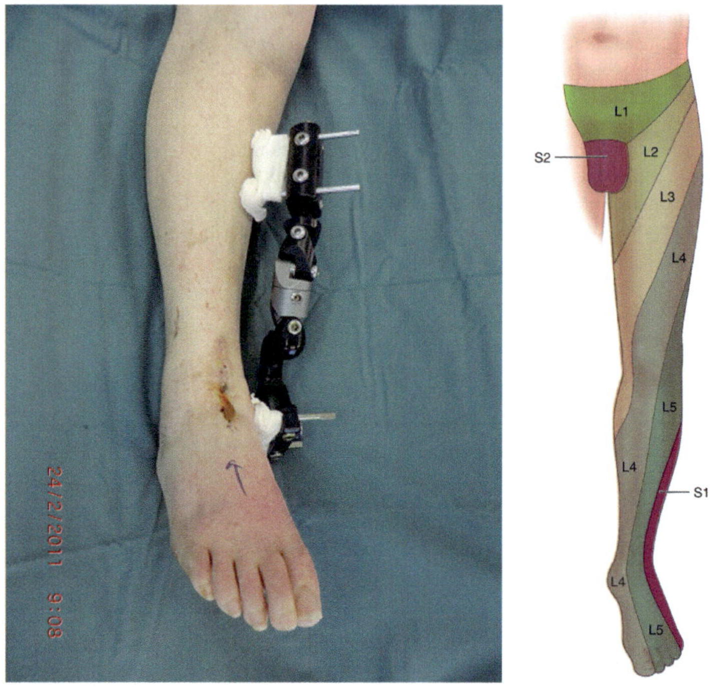

Fig. 3.7 Images of the healing phase with potential wound breakdown over the fracture site before referral

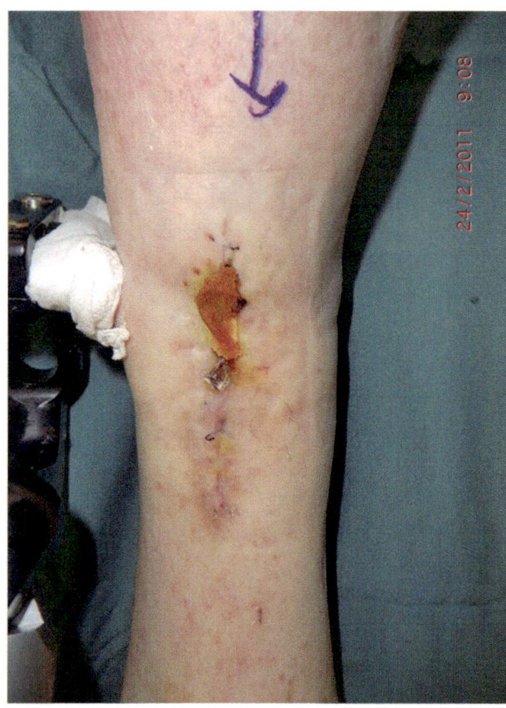

Fig. 3.8 The wound breakdown of a compound tibial fracture lower 1/3 of some weeks duration and closure under tension could have been avoided with the application of a keystone island flap technique. The surgeon in this case here was obviously trying to close the wound to avoid microsurgical reconstruction and its basic impedance in quick wound healing. The keystone used to solve such problems illustrated the expeditious nature of the repair, and all the keystone characteristics P.A.C.E.S. subsequently became exemplified

3.1.2 Case 13: Compound Fracture Lower 1/3 Tibia

This referral was for wound closure with a chronic infection of the ankle following joint replacement and fusion. The keystone provides a simple solution. Best viewed on video for the clinical summary of a fracture of the ankle followed by fusion and infection (Figs. 3.7, 3.8, 3.9, 3.10, 3.11, 3.12, 3.13, 3.14, 3.15, 3.16, 3.17, 3.18, 3.19, 3.20, 3.21, 3.22, 3.23, 3.24, 3.25, 3.26, 3.27, 3.28, 3.29, 3.30, 3.31, 3.32, 3.33, 3.34).

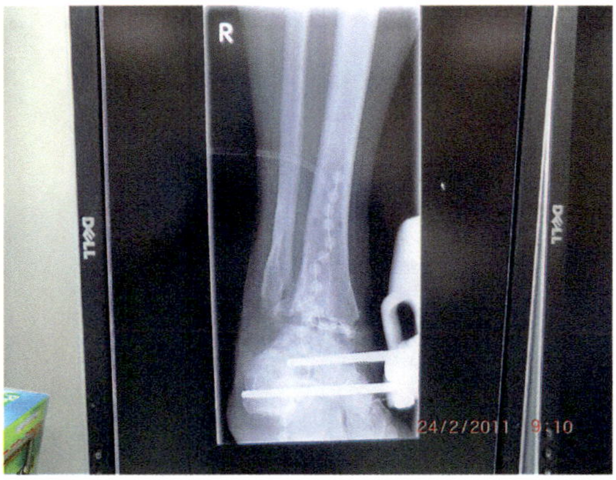

Fig. 3.9 ORIF R tibia with the transverse metal pins in situ. The joint alignment showing the incongruity of the articular lining—an orthopaedic issue and possible need for later fusion

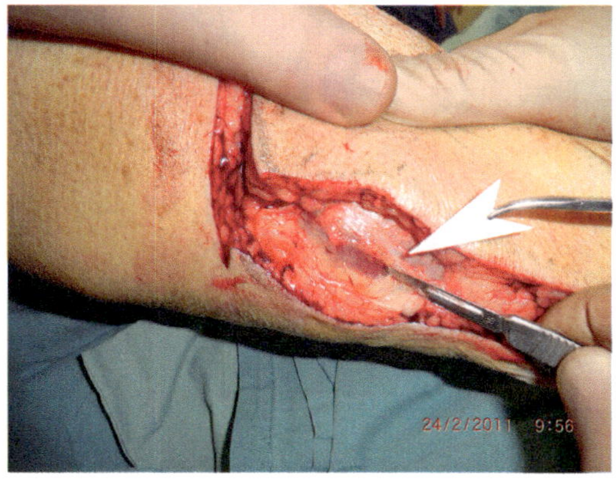

Fig. 3.12 Staged elevation of the flap cutting the deep fascia to facilitate transfer

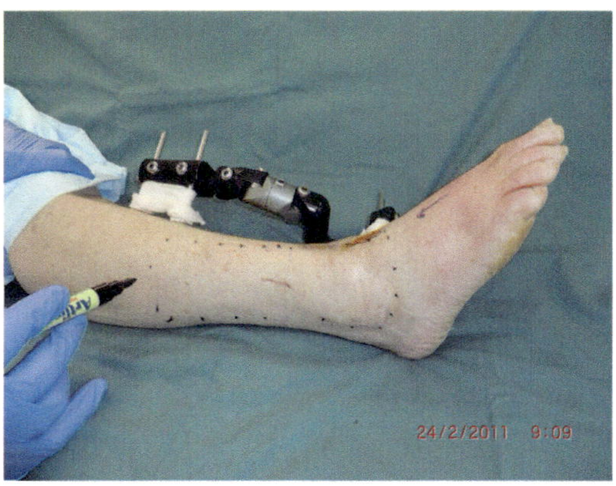

Fig. 3.10 Potential mark out sites of perforators of the superficial peroneal nerve region around the lateral compartment of L4 and L5

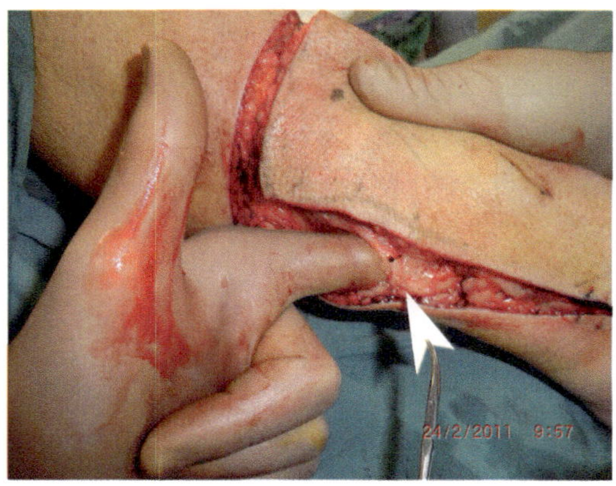

Fig. 3.13 Digital dissection of the fascia—with elevation under direct view to preserve any perforators

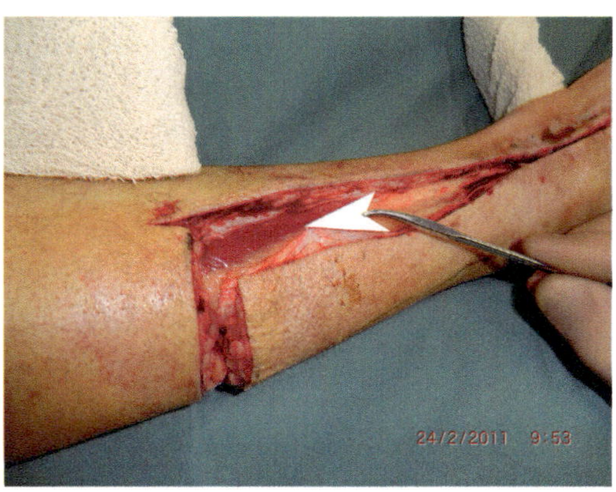

Fig. 3.11 The FCIF along the peroneal compartment from the mid-lateral point down to the lower limit of the R lateral malleolus

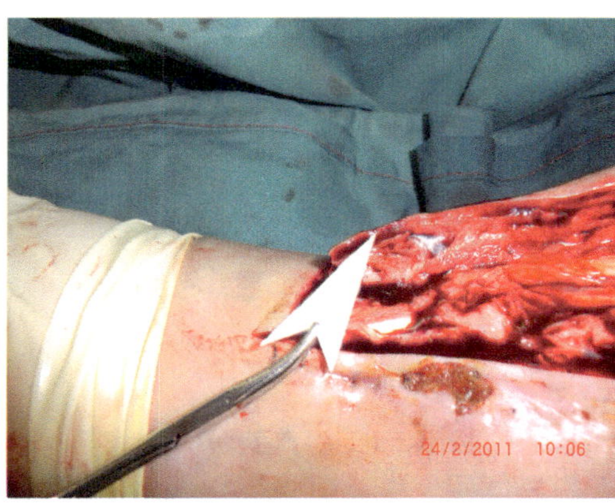

Fig. 3.14 Suprafascial circulation indicated with the arrow along the line of the subdermal plexus

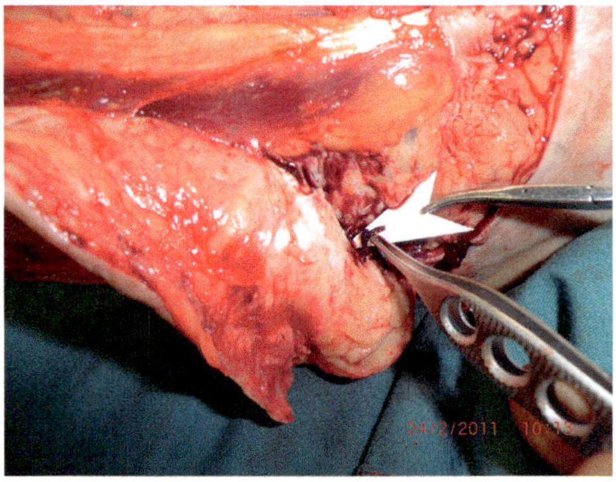

Fig. 3.15 The arrow is overlying the sural nerve which must be protected at all levels when the flap is raised along the peroneal lining

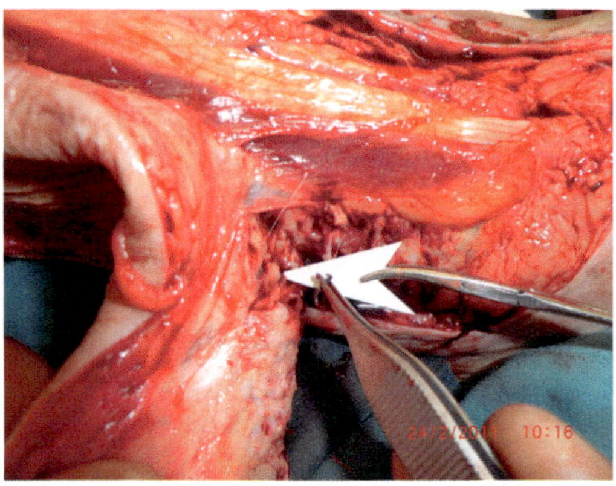

Fig. 3.16 Illustrating points of microvascular perforator circulation aligned along the suprafascial and infrafascial mark out of the flap which has to be sealed with micro clips as an alternative to the use of diathermy to control any tissue necrosis, thus impeding the peripheral flow

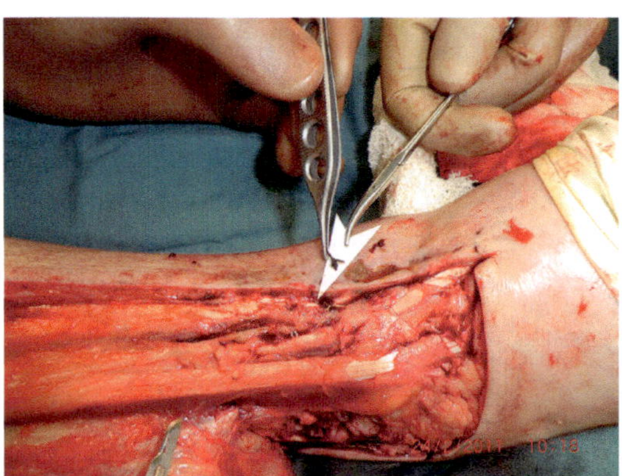

Fig. 3.17 Medial branch of the sural nerve confirming the fascial base of the flap is raised to preserve the integrity of the sural nerve and sensory innervation distally is preserved

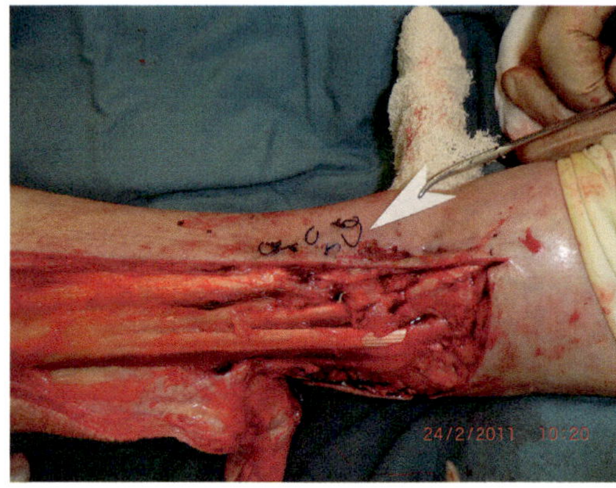

Fig. 3.18 The debridement of the wound is completed once the transposed flap alignment is finalised. In other words, place the flap over the defect to create the line for marginal debridement

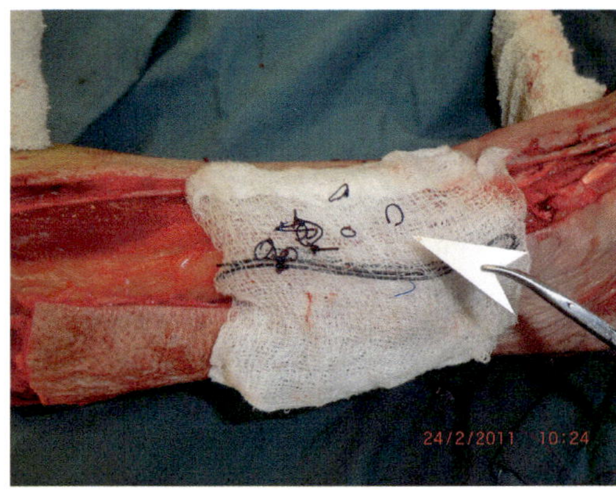

Fig. 3.19 The debridement has been removed along the line of the flap margin as a 'ruler' to fit exactly to avoid tension

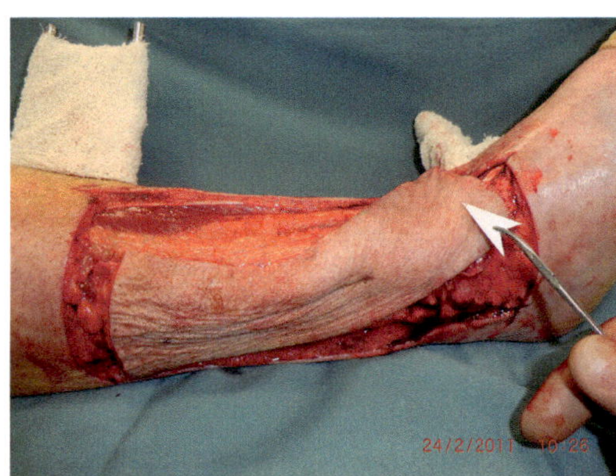

Fig. 3.20 The hyperaemic flare, one of the keystone characteristics, is evident after 6 min (see time stamped image)

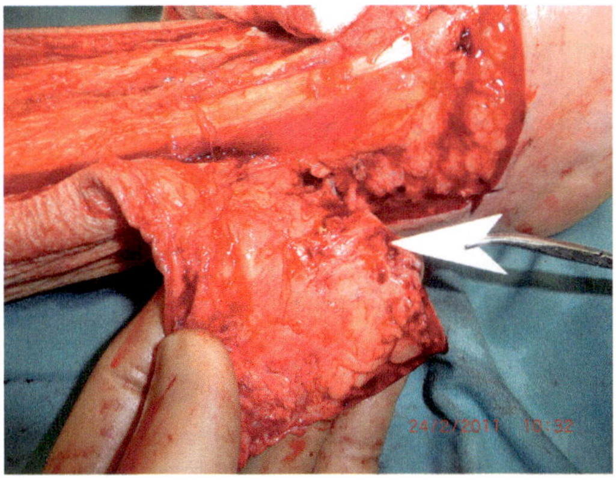

Fig. 3.21 The suprafascial and infrafascial circulation points are indicated with the white arrow before clip diathermy

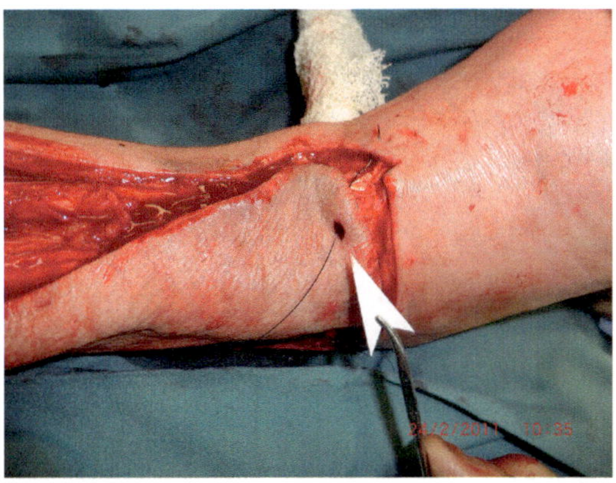

Fig. 3.22 The red dot sign sits on the flap at the entry point of the suture confirming intact vascular integrity with a pink flare and it lies on the flap side rather than the receiving side

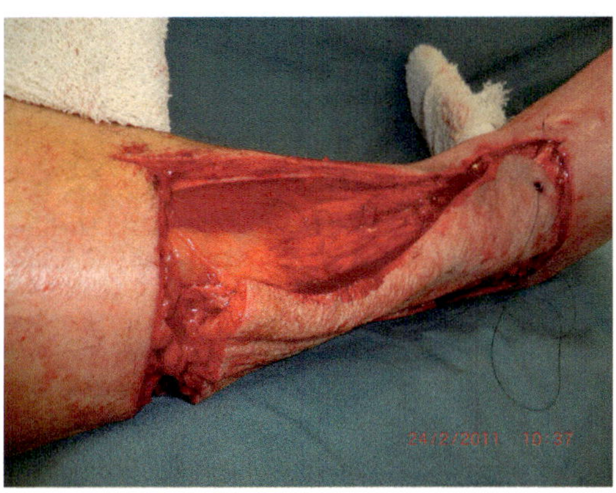

Fig. 3.23 Staged closure before employing the 3 phase locking mattress suture technique to close the defect before skin grafting the secondary defect

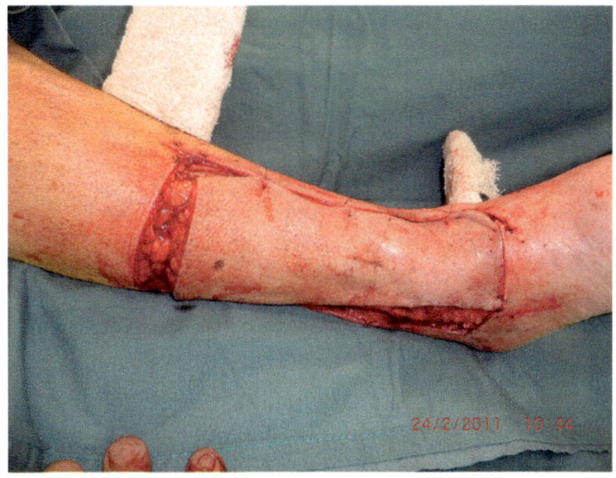

Fig. 3.24 Single layer staged closure with the 3 phase locking mattress sutures with intact circulation confirmed by the pink flare

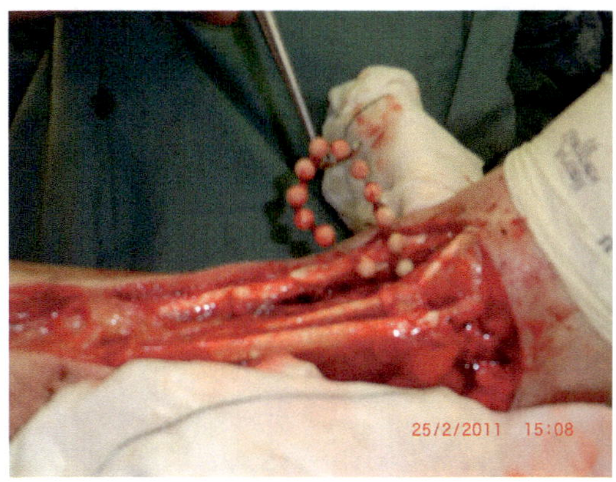

Fig. 3.25 The removal of the gentamicin beads, protective antibiotic cover for the wound showing delayed healing without cover, now solved with a keystone flap

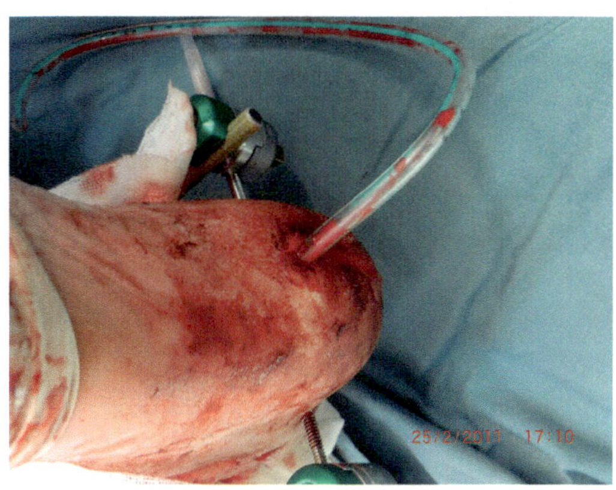

Fig. 3.26 The value of Redi-vac drainage to prevent any pooling in the dead space vacated by the gentamicin beads

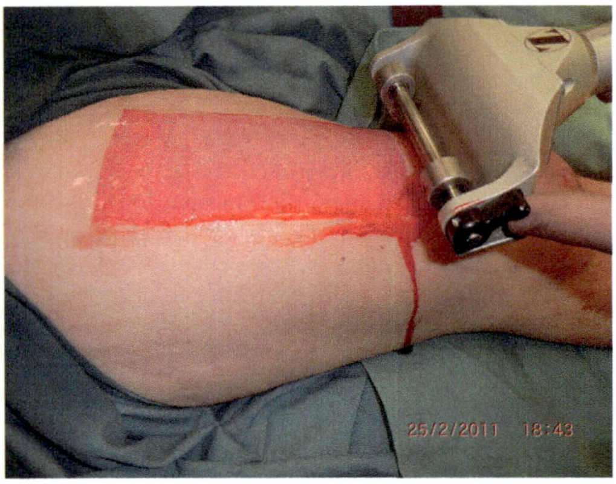

Fig. 3.27 A simple technique of harvesting skin with a powered dermatome is to raise the tissue at the appropriate level for a split skin graft (0.3–0.45 mm)

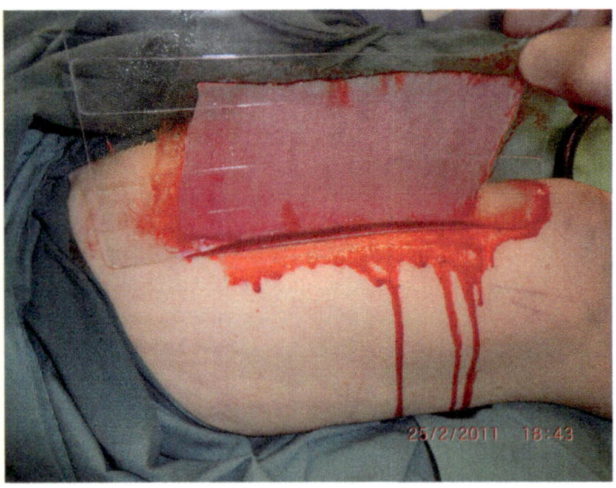

Fig. 3.28 If the blade adjustment is fully open and the roller blade is retracted, it can relay the skin evenly over the very dimensions of its harvest site. Once detached, it lies evenly over the meshing plate to give a symmetrical piece of split skin graft 0.4 mm prior to its meshing

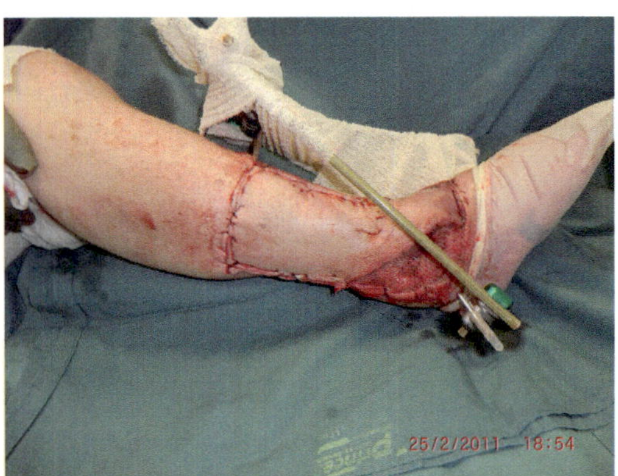

Fig. 3.29 A fenestrated split skin graft completes the reconstruction

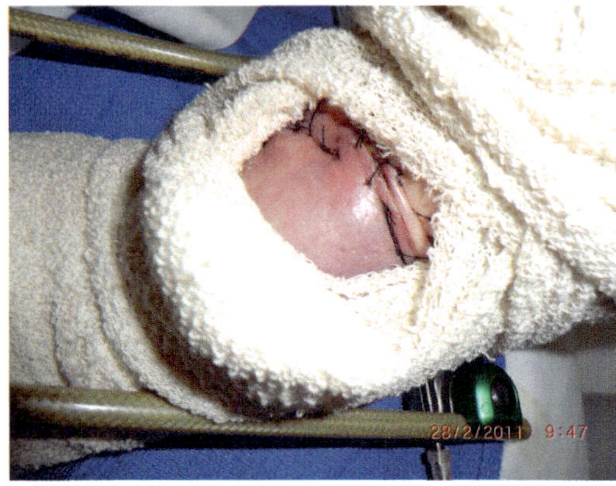

Fig. 3.30 This patient shows the integrity of the keystone on wound closure and absence of any vascular impedance or necrosis—intact vascular viability to accompany the island design and an exponent of the keystone characteristic

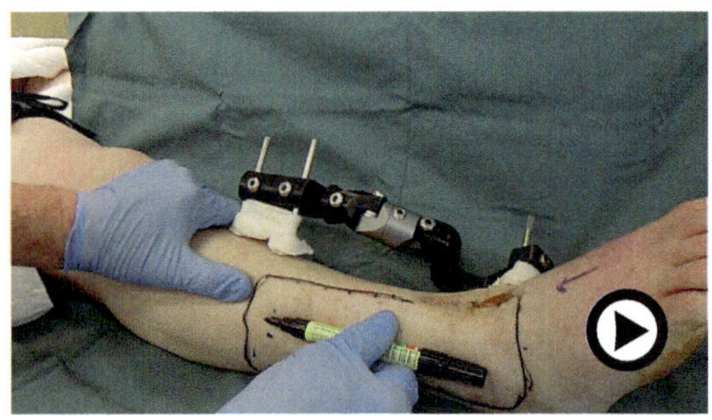

Fig. 3.31 Clinical summary (Video 3.1 Clinical summary) (▶ https://doi.org/10.1007/000-d6k)

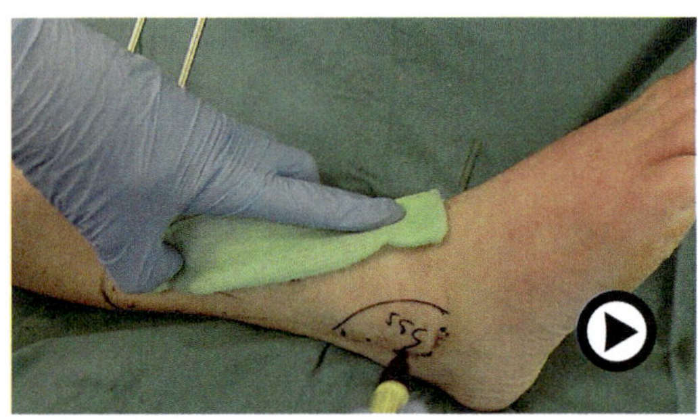

Fig. 3.32 Operative plan marking out the keystone and the SSG for secondary defect (Video 3.2 Operative plan marking out the keystone and the SSG for secondary defect) (▶ https://doi.org/10.1007/000-d4t)

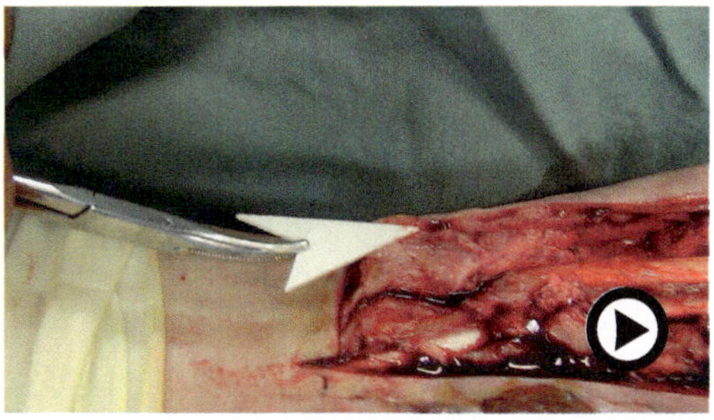

Fig. 3.33 Perforator ooze points from the suprafascial and infrafascial circulation on tourniquet release (Video 3.3 Perforator ooze points from the suprafascial and infrafascial circulation on torniquet release) (▶ https://doi.org/10.1007/000-d4v)

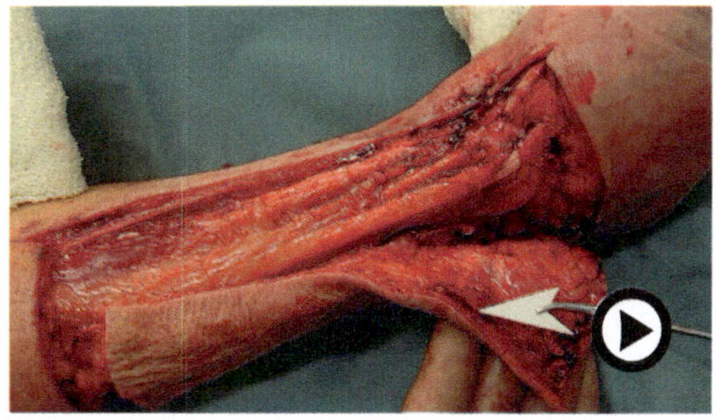

Fig. 3.34 The vascular flare on the release of tourniquet which starts in 15 min (Video 3.4 The vascular flare on the release of torniquet which starts in 15 min) (▶ https://doi.org/10.1007/000-d4w)

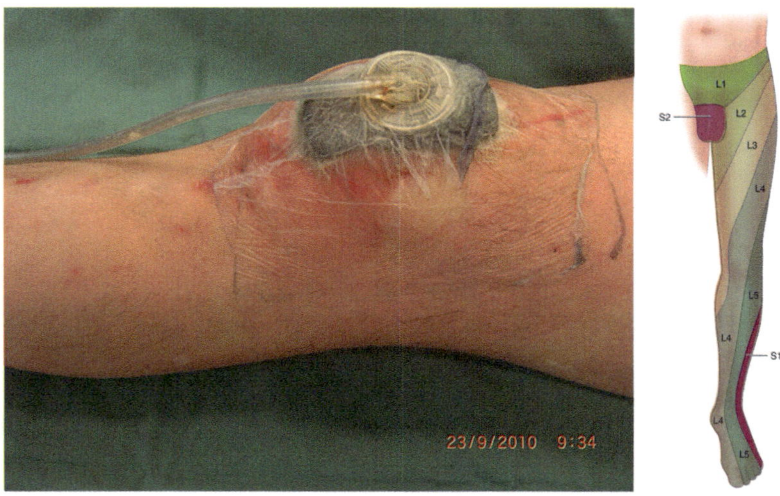

Fig. 3.35 Standard VAC dressing to create a granulation bed and offer the solution of a skin graft to reconstitute the integument—totally inappropriate. A limited option with a slow return of recovery and limited range of movement of the knee. The keystone provides an expeditious solution to such problems avoiding any techniques of skin grafting for wound closure over any ORIF reconstruction

3.1.3 Case 14: A Compound Patella After an ORIF Reduction with Exposed Wire and Bone—The Keystone Provides Integumentary Cover

This wound was closed directly under tension leading to tissue necrosis creating a subsequent defect with exposed metal 8 × 6 cm over the patella.

The clinical problem marred by complications of closure under tension (Figs. 3.35, 3.36, 3.37, 3.38, 3.39, 3.40, 3.41, 3.42, 3.43, 3.44, 3.45, 3.46, 3.47, 3.48, 3.49, 3.50, 3.51, 3.52, 3.53, 3.54, 3.55, 3.56, 3.57, 3.58, 3.59, 3.60, 3.61, and 3.62).

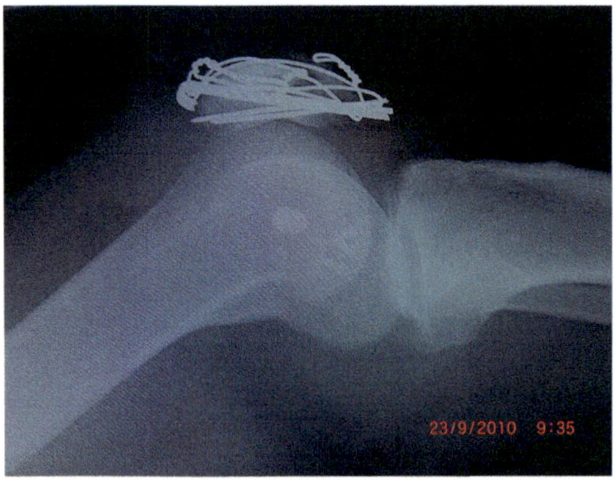

Fig. 3.36 An alternative free flap is a possible alternative reconstruction with one obvious drawback, because of the variability and concern of the microvascular anastomosis, the patient cannot bend their knee for a month or two. The keystone solution allows the patient home in a week without the restrictions of restricted movement and slow healing when a free flap reconstruction is used. With the keystone they are moving normally in a month exemplifying the P.A.C.E.S. characteristics—a suitable alternative to a microvascular repair and its limitations in limiting the range of movement initially which warrants no elaboration

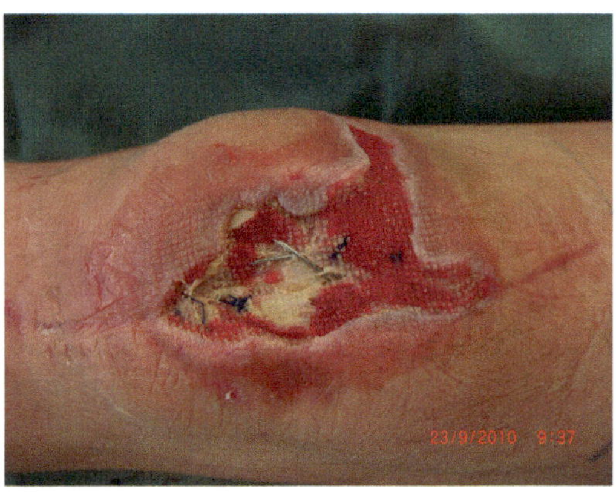

Fig. 3.37 Staged appearance of the success of the VAC dressing after 1 month to create granulation tissue and possibly a graft bed. The integrity of the ORIF has been maintained in preparation for the keystone reconstruction aligned along the L3/L4 dermatomes

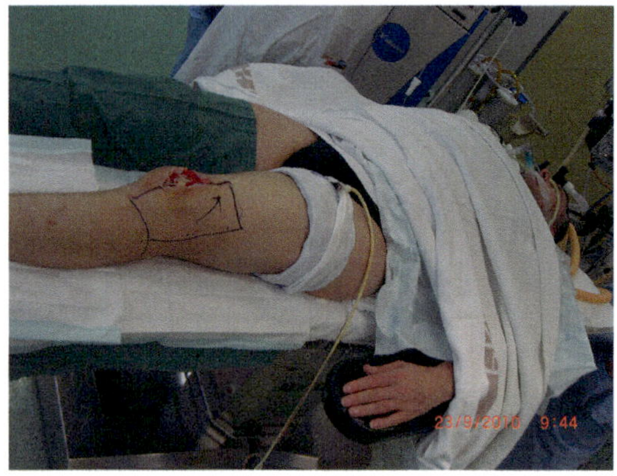

Fig. 3.38 Preoperative image with tourniquet applied before the preoperative scrub. The keystone in the L4/L5 dermatomes with the arrow indicating the level of undermining planned as long as it is fascial lined

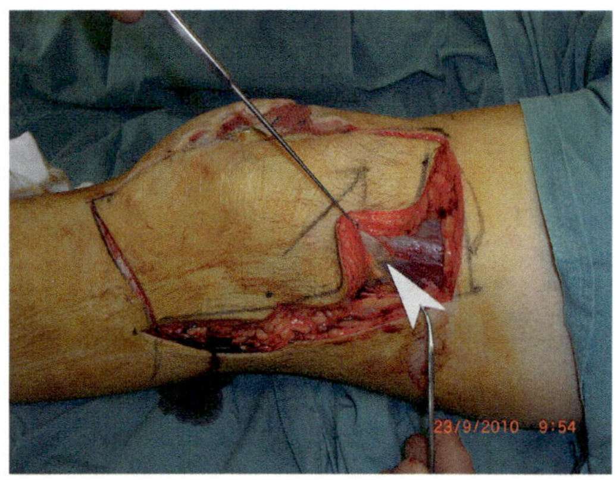

Fig. 3.39 Developing the plane for the fascial flap (arrowed)

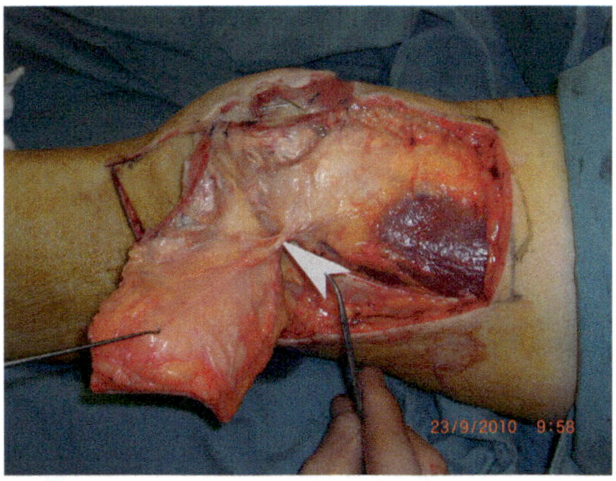

Fig. 3.40 Random perforators (arrowed) emerging during the blunt dissection of the fascial lined keystone which is not skeletonised to retain its perineural and perilymphatic support lines. The cost saving benefits of avoiding angiograms when the perforators can be visualised need no elaboration, i.e. when you see a perforator it is protected and discretely mobilised to facilitate advancement, rotation and transposition of the keystone island

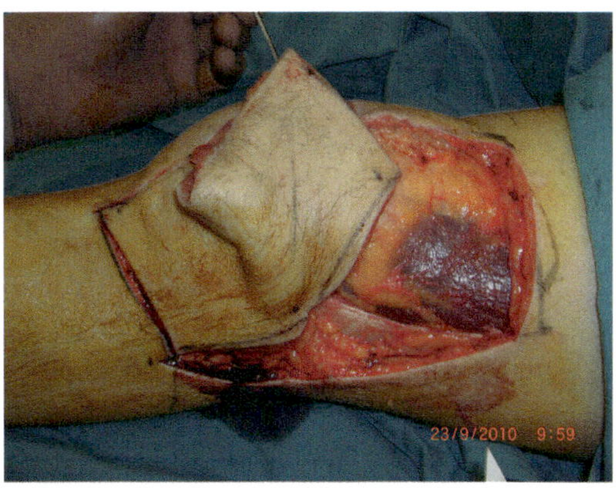

Fig. 3.41 Bony cover is achieved with raising of the keystone

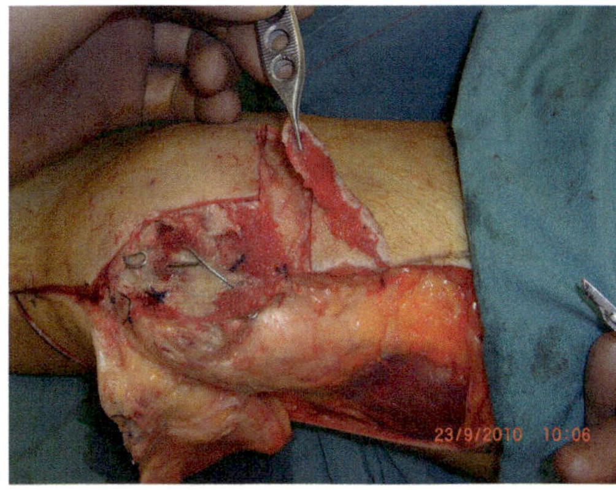

Fig. 3.42 Wound debridement to fit in alignment with the flap insertion site

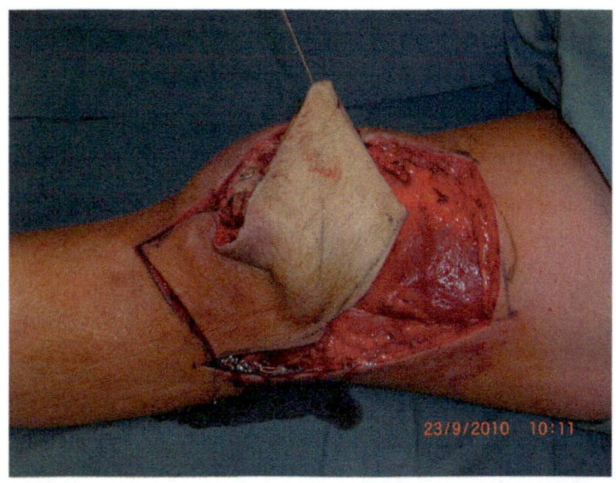

Fig. 3.43 Tourniquet release producing the dynamic vascular flare

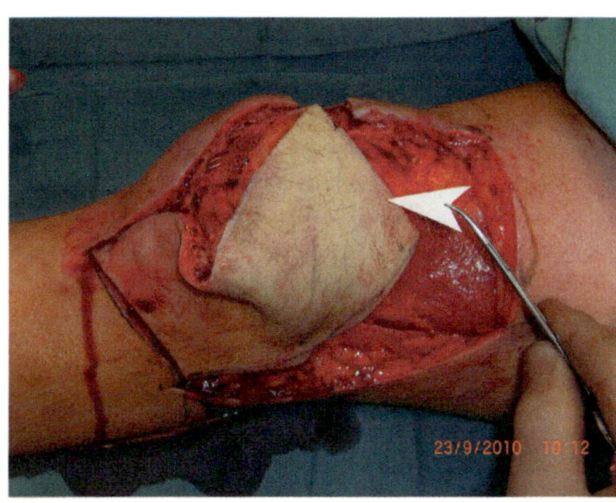

Fig. 3.44 The arrow indicates the perfusion is progressing to cover the apex of the keystone flap directly above the perforator site

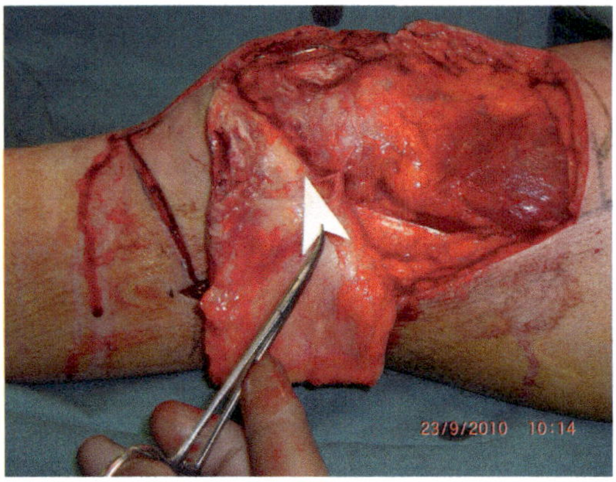

Fig. 3.45 Note the perforator presence on the arrow

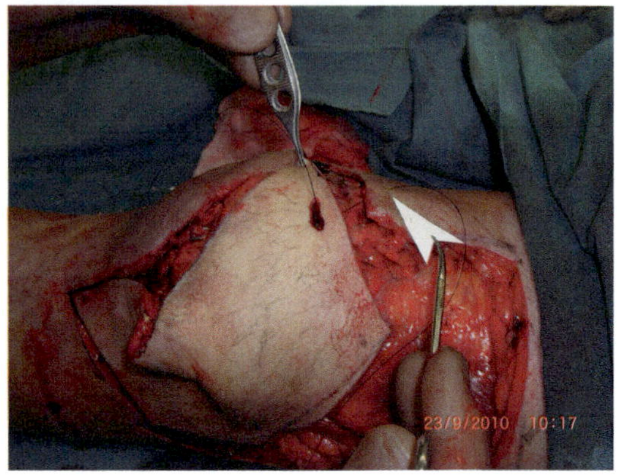

Fig. 3.47 Haemostasis: use microvascular clips. The keystone along the L3/L4 dermatomes is raised with sharp and blunt dissection to allow one to turn the flap across the patella defect. Preserve any obvious perforators that do not impede rotation. The flap is raised laterally along the patella ligament as far as the level of the tibial tuberosity. It is a fasciocutaneous island flap which supports the suprafascial and infrafascial circulation. Note the hypervascularity when the island design is completed and this hypothetical sympathectomy effect of an island flap is confirmed by the hypervascularity and the red dot sign with a vascular flare at the suture point where the island flap bleeds more than that of the receiving insertion margin. Slow perfusion in the epidermis is only temporary. The suprafascial and subfascial circulation intact. Note the arrow points to the perfusional sites of the deep fascia of the flap, the plane on which the flap is raised. Soft tissue cover of the exposed bone with reliable hypervascularised tissue and for skin grafting of any secondary defect in the lateral infrapatellar region (arrowed). The cyanotic colour of the blood reflects its slow vascular recovery

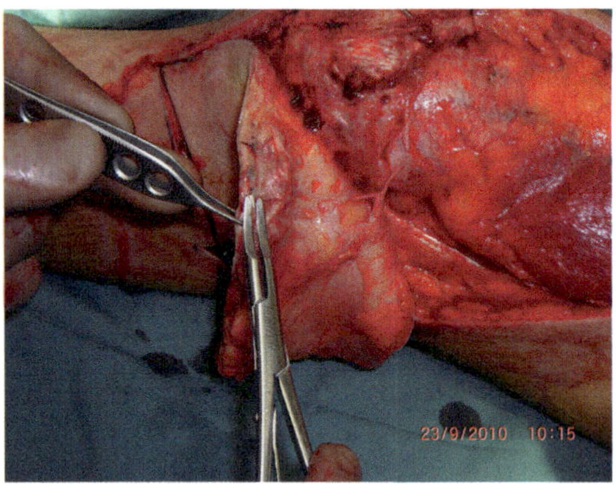

Fig. 3.46 Weck clips for haemostasis but no diathermy to avoid any necrosis

Fig. 3.48 The 3-phase locking mattress suture technique using 3/0 nylon closes the wound under some element of tension which is not a problem as the hypervascularity phase permits a fairly random pressure closure at the various suture points. The epidermal white lines of tension disappear because the circulation is based on suprafascial and infrafascial input

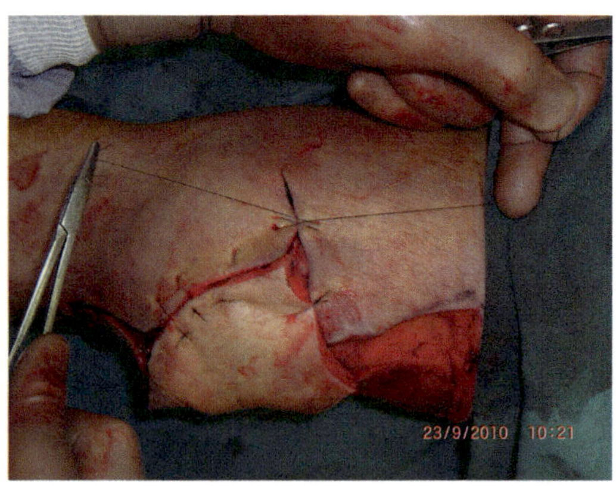

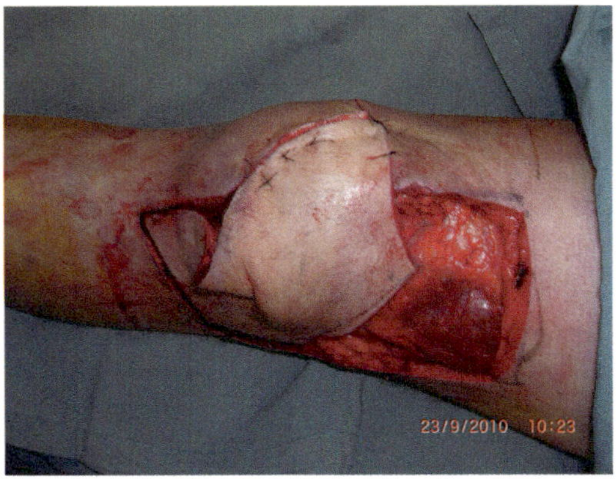

Fig. 3.49 After 10 min, the reactive hyperaemia phase is noted on the release of tourniquet. Closure under tension is not a contraindicaton. The secondary defect 6 × 8 cm is mesh grafted

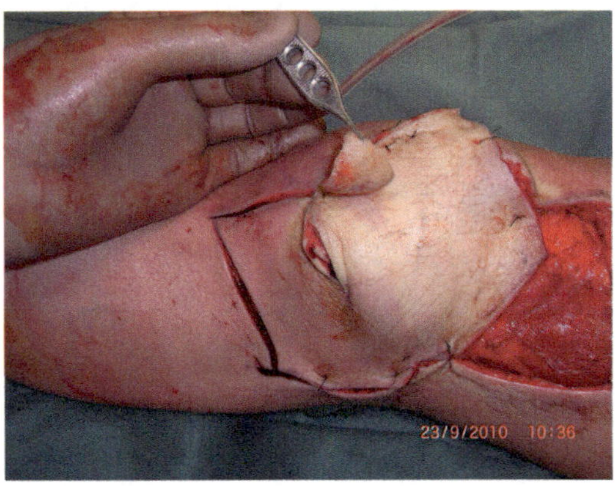

Fig. 3.50 The keystone allows dog ear revision in the acute phase because of the reliable fascial circulation

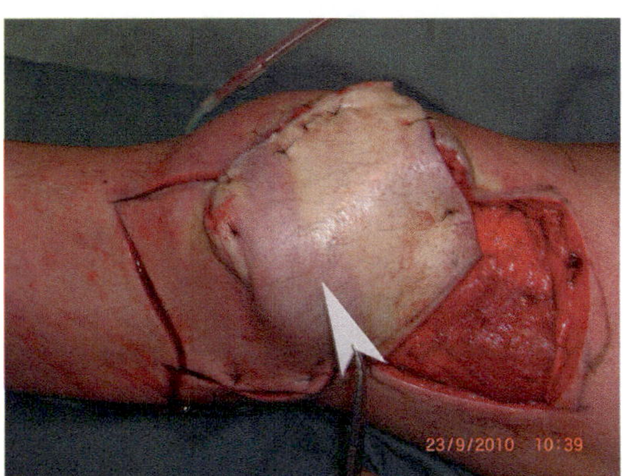

Fig. 3.51 The vascular perfusion in its recovery phase following the lines of various perforators in the suprafascial anastamoses before reaching the apex medially

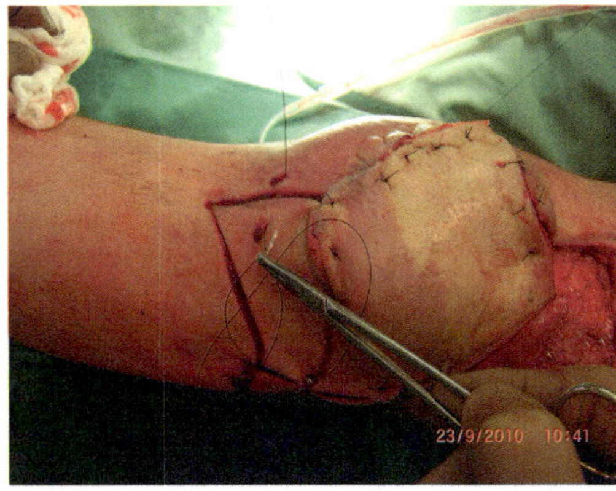

Fig. 3.52 A cyanotic phase of the red dot sign indicates a relative slugishness in the recovery phase of the circulation

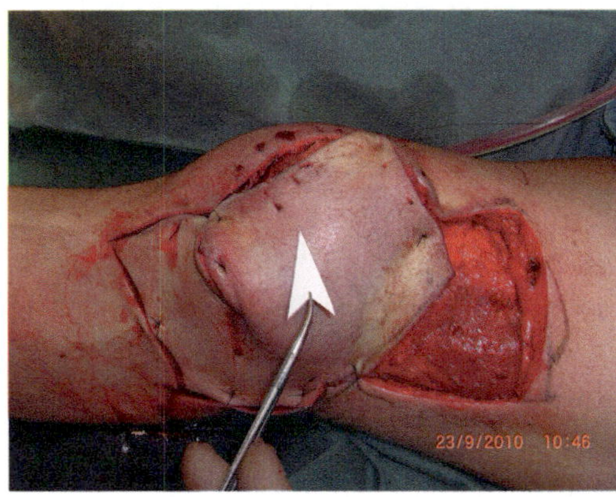

Fig. 3.53 Before the red dot sign subsequently becomes evident with full recovery

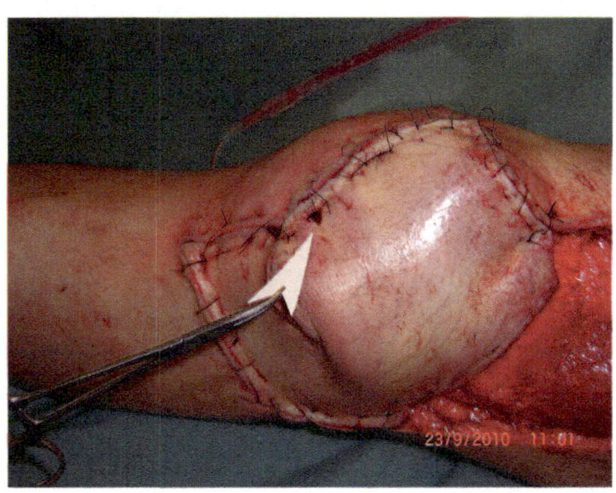

Fig. 3.54 The healing wound and the red dot sign and the somewhat irregular perfusional patterns on the patella flap prior to the mesh grafting of the secondary defect

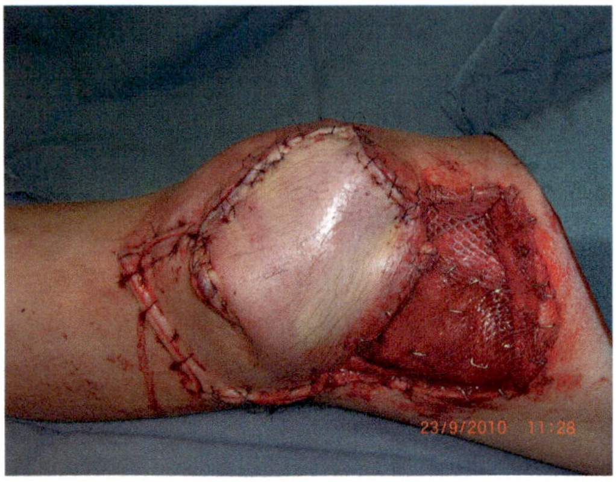

Fig. 3.55 The mesh grafting in situ with no evidence of any impending vascular necrosis demarkation

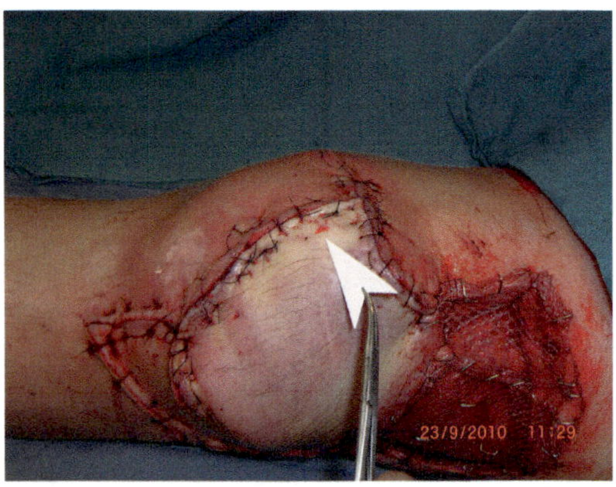

Fig. 3.56 The closure after 20 min. A free flap may take hours

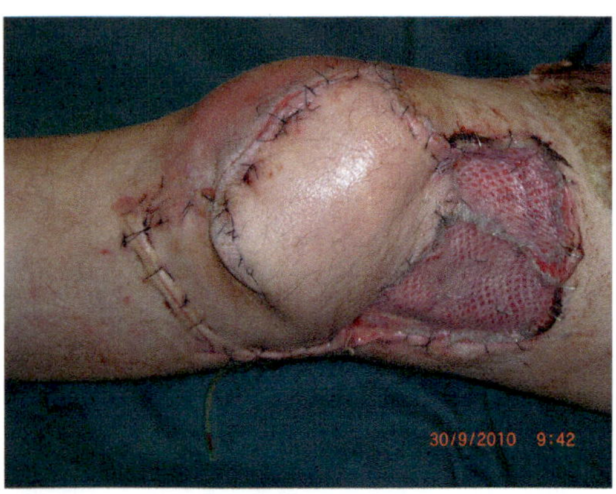

Fig. 3.57 Seven-day appearance

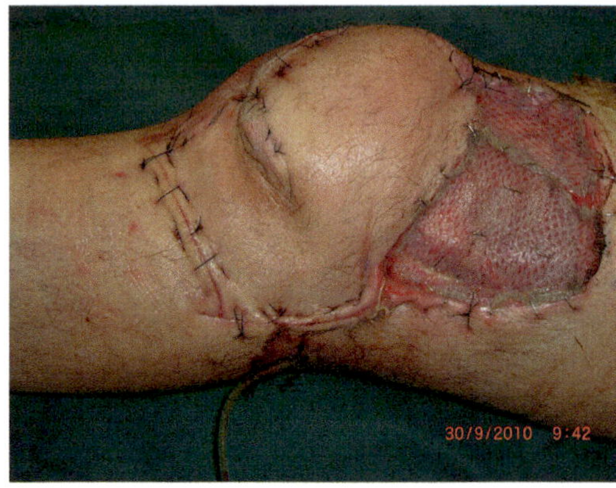

Fig. 3.58 Another view at 7 days of the healed wound. Note the dog ear has been trimmed intraoperatively

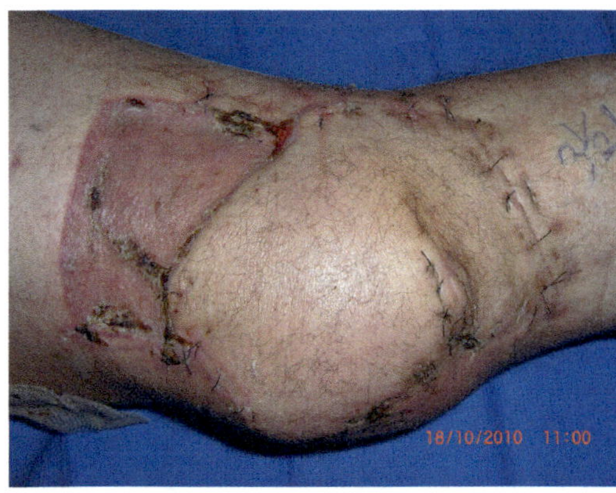

Fig. 3.59 3.5 week appearance. Patient satisfied, pain free, no complaints and the oedema is resolving

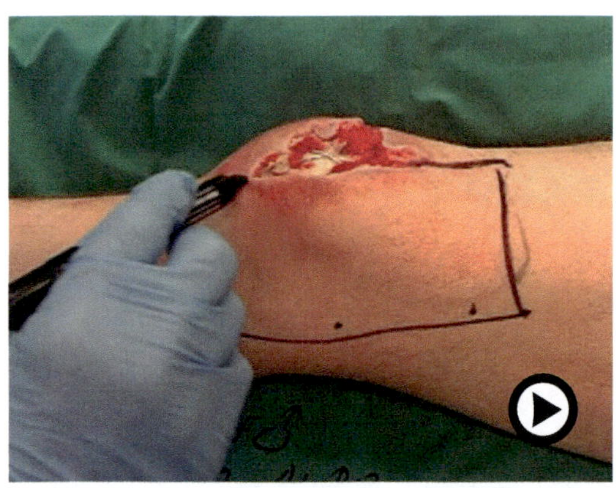

Fig. 3.60 The mark out of the fasciocutaneous island flap (keystone concept) parallel to the patella in the L3 dermatome (Video 3.5 The mark out of the fascio cutaneous island flap (keystone concept) parallel to the patella in the L3 dermatome) (▶ https://doi.org/10.1007/000-d4x)

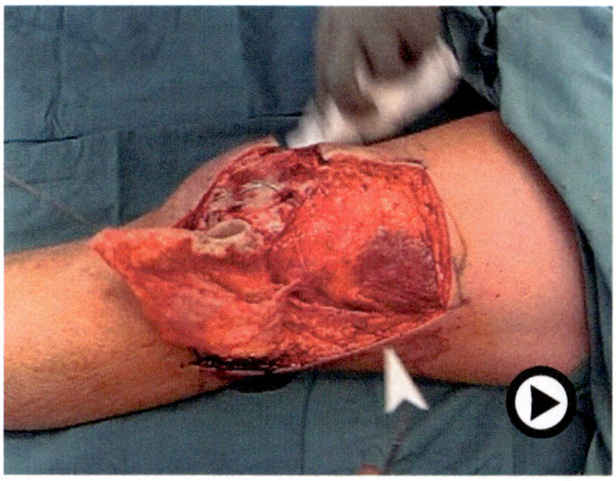

Fig. 3.61 Operative sequence in raising the parapatellar keystone in the L3 dermatome and finding incidentally the perforator support for the designated dermatome flap (without any angiograms and its implied cost saving) (Video 3.6 Operative sequence in raising the parapatellar keystone in the L3 dermatome and finding incidentally the perforator support for the designated dermatome flap (without any angiograms and its implied cost saving)) (▶ https://doi.org/10.1007/000-d4y)

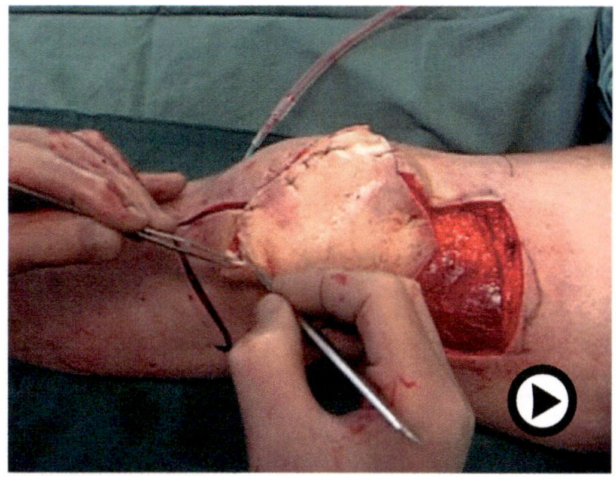

Fig. 3.62 Operative sequence and excision of dog ear at the epidermal level (Video 3.7 Operative sequence and excision of dog ear at the epidermal level) (▶ https://doi.org/10.1007/000-d4z)

3.1.4 Case 15: Traumatic Ulcer Over the Patella with Bone Exposed in an Obese Haemophiliac

This complicated case in a 65 year old with haemophiliac had a soft tissue defect following blunt trauma in an obese female of 120 kg. The issue of debridement in wound mangement and/or skin grafting provides a background of implicit complications in a person diagnosed with haemophilia. The chronic ooze reduces the success rate of any skin grafting, even when using a mesh technique. The keystone mark out, and its closure under tension characteristic provides a rapid solution for wound closure in this diabetic haemophiliac. The excess weight precludes expeditious recovery and the ongoing oozing with the development of wound haematomas is another impediment to rapid surgical healing (Figs. 3.63, 3.64, 3.65, 3.66, 3.67, 3.68, 3.69, 3.70, 3.71, and 3.72).

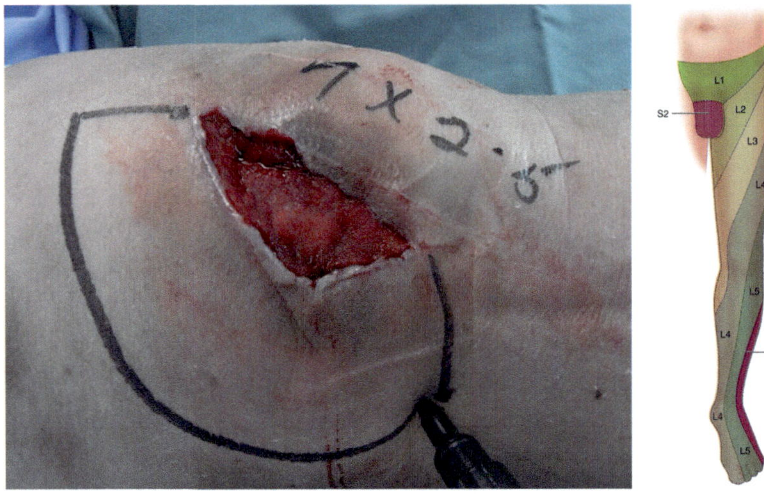

Fig. 3.63 This chronic ulcer of the lateral knee joint region in the lower third of the femoral complex at the level of the suprapatellar pouch. Patient was poorly compliant and resented VAC dressings, a fallback position to achieve healing. Any person who is non-compliant in relation to ongoing chronic dressings using a Redi-vac would be an indicator of long-term chornic healing phase with undue wound complications. Note the appearance of the poor quality surrounding tissue in this 7 × 2.5 cm defect. The haemophiliac bleeding tendency is reflected in the margins. The keystone design sits well in the superolateral quadrant of the peri-patella tissues

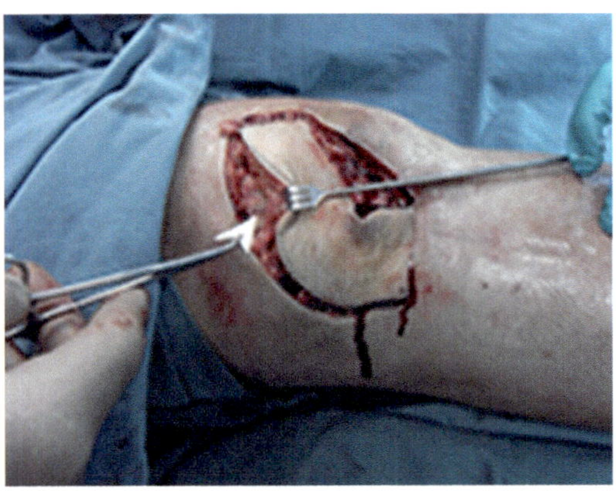

Fig. 3.64 Following debridement the arrow indicates the perforators for keystone support. The keystone attachment along the middle 1/3 of the design is the site of the random perforators

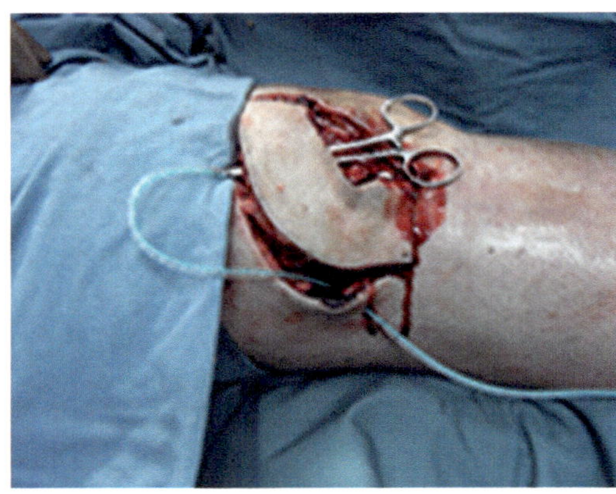

Fig. 3.65 Technique of Redi-vac tube insertion goes underneath the flap so both ulcers are drained by the Redi-vac tubing in a U-shaped manner. The tubing must be inserted below the flap randomly

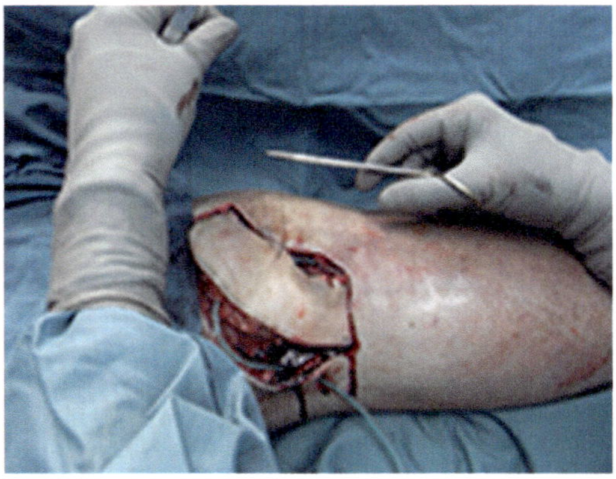

Fig. 3.66 The standard closure technique of locking mattress sutures at the convex and the concave sides of the keystone; further closure using ordinary mattress to achieve epidermal alignment in a single layer technique. The epidermal seal is achieved with a continuous nylon suture which stayed in 3 weeks because of the ooze along the suture line when the sutures were clipped, indicating a potential for wound breakdown—so another week of stabilisation did not hurt but achieved perfect healing

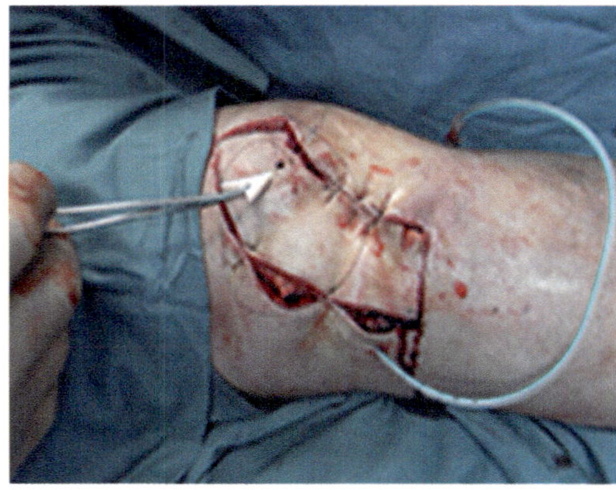

Fig. 3.68 The red dot sign is noted indicating hypervascularity in this sympathectomy outcome when an island flap is created. This red dot sign is a keystone characteristic. White lines of tension slowly subside following increase of perfusion of the subdermal plexus based on random perforators and the sympathectomy effect in routine reconstructive surgery, such white lines of tension raise an element of caution and are best avoided. The keystone seems to overcome these white lines of tension by the perfusional dynamics created by the islanding and hypothectically a sympathectomy effect by eliminating restrictions of the subdermal plexus perfusion—it just opens up channels. Hence, the observational findings of a red flap, the red dot sign and intact healing

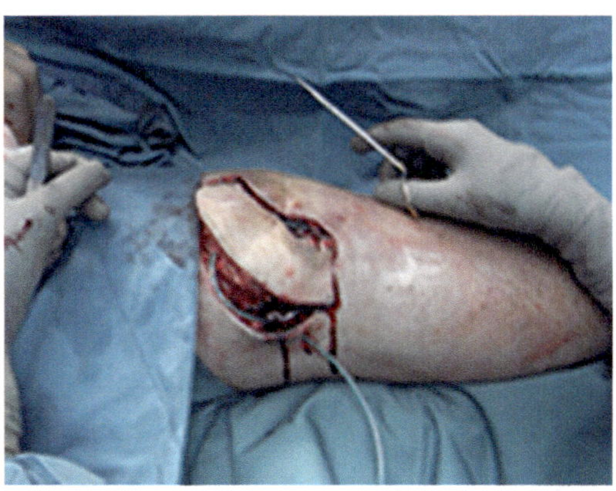

Fig. 3.67 The medial side closure is almost complete before focusing on the lateral side

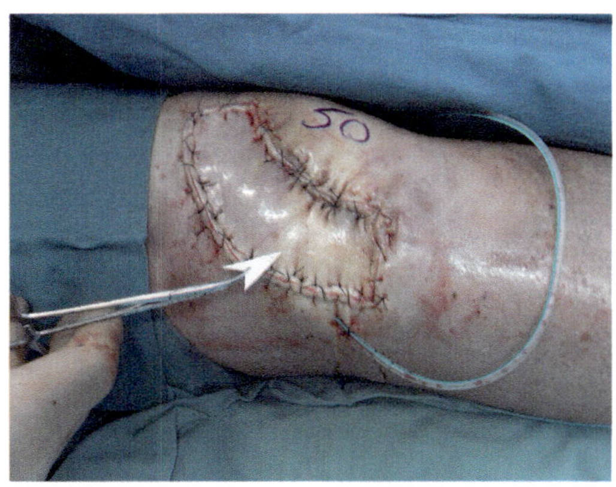

Fig. 3.69 Closure in 50 min. The cyanosis in the upper part of the wound is the predominant perforator blood supply in the proximal 1/3. Distal perfusion slowly recovering back to normal to give a intact, healed epidermal appearance which goes hand in hand with uncomplicated healing

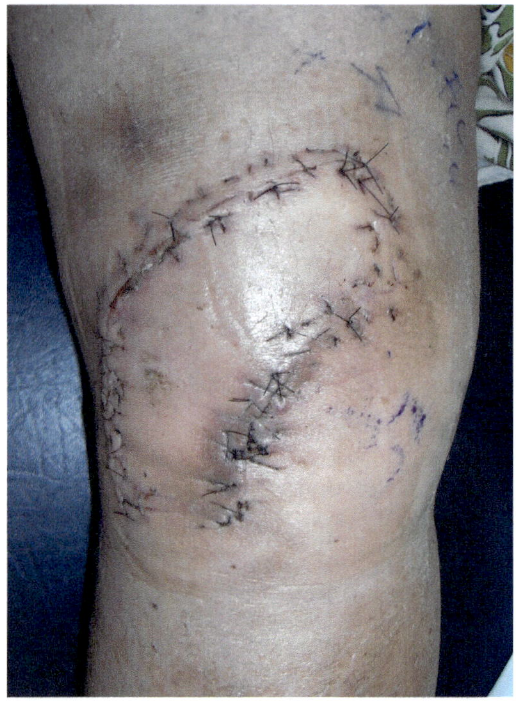

Fig. 3.70 Note the absence of any flap necrosis throughout the keystone consistent with the diagnosis and showing those characteristics of the keystone P.A.C.E.S. summarised below. Wound dressing technique at 3 weeks: cut the loops at 7–10 days. Some of the interrupted mattress at 14 days. Tension locking mattress sutures at least 21 days or longer if it bleeds. Any bleeding points in this haemophiliac indicate the need to leave intermittent sutures in longer

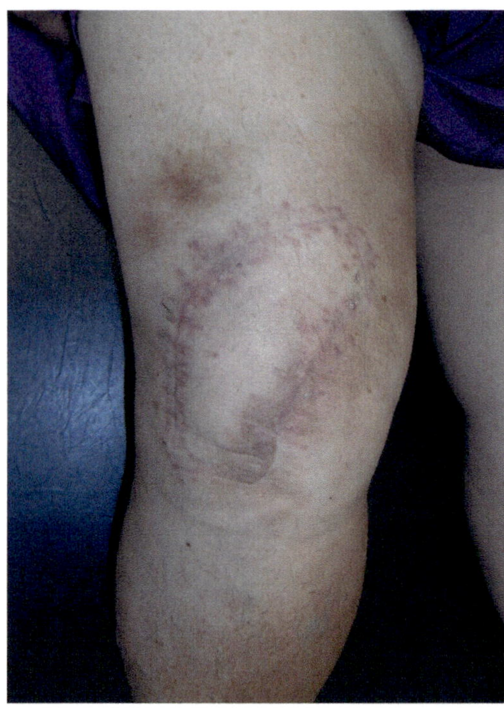

Fig. 3.71 Appearance at 6 weeks a satisfactory outcome. The patient is pain free, fully mobile and very satisfied with the operative outcome. The value of leaving the locking mattress sutures in for 6 weeks in this haemofiliac needs no elaboartion to avoid wound breakdown. Cross hatch marks are minimal in this obese leg, and a full functional knee joint range of movement was achieved reflecting the dramatic resolution of oedema, another keystone characteristic

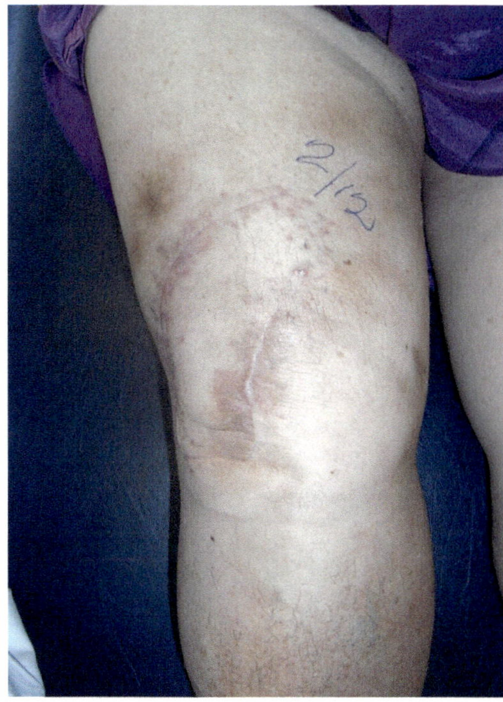

Fig. 3.72 Appearance at 2 months. The acronym P.A.C.E.S. is applied to describe the patient's clinical outcome: **P**ain: In this very anxious personality was almost totally absent. There was feeling of tightness which was of no concern which resolved spontaneously because of elastic release of tissue. **A**esthetics: An acceptable aesthetic outcome in this chronic wound when an alternative of skin grafting and healing by secondary intention were possible options when one considers her medical morbidities. **C**omplications: None recorded. **E**conomic: The timeframe for the surgical procedure and the short hospital stay all meeting with the patient's approval. **S**ensation: Returned with the resolution of swelling and oedema. It should be noted that this patient with long-term medical problems, the base is set for a complicated clinical story and the use of skin grafting and/or free flaps would have had an adverse effect on her psychological balance

3.1.5 Case 16: Infrapatellar Soft Tissue Loss Over the Tibial Tuberosity—The Resultant Defect After Debridement Solved with a Keystone

Closure over the patellar and knee region is a difficult reconstructive option and I quote now from the World Journal of Orthopaedic Surgery 2014 [3] 'A literature search focusing on flap knee reconstruction revealed much controversy regarding the optimal management of around the knee defects. Muscle flaps are the preferred option, mainly in infected wounds. Perforator flaps have recently been introduced in knee coverage with significant advantages due to low donor morbidity and long pedicles with wide arc of rotation. In the case of free flap, the choice of recipient vessels is the key point to the reconstruction. Taking the published experience into account, a reconstructive algorithm is proposed according to the size and location of the wound, the presence of infection and/or 3-dimensional defect'. Yet, the keystone perforator island flap simplifies the technique and seems to embrace multiple variations of random perforator island flap of the keystone concept (Figs. 3.73, 3.74, 3.75, 3.76, 3.77, 3.78, 3.79, 3.80, 3.81, 3.82, 3.83, 3.84, 3.85, 3.86, 3.87, 3.88, 3.89, 3.90, 3.91, 3.92, 3.93, and 3.94).

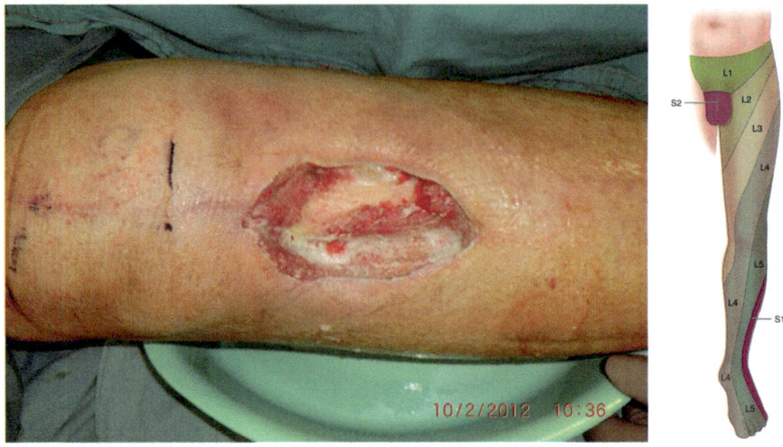

Fig. 3.73 This compound tibial fracture over the tibial tuberosity of the R knee following a motor vehicle accident. The red dots indicate the line of earlier scar which resulted in design modifications of the keystone design into a rectangle

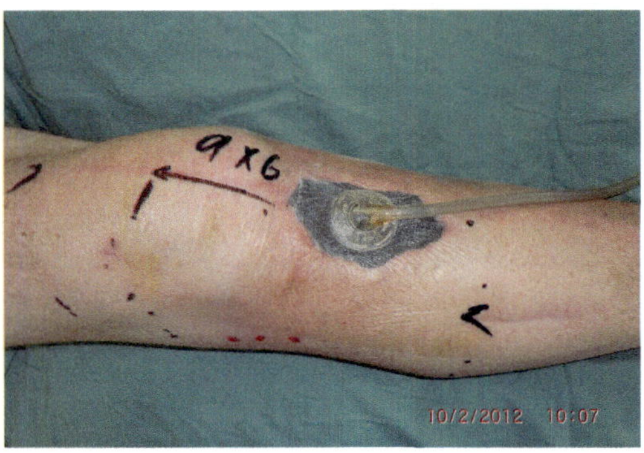

Fig. 3.74 The VAC dressing phase has been completed before the keystone reconstruction over the bony defect, the size of which is 9 × 6 cm. Rectangular mark out of keystone lateral to the patella is raised with blunt (digital) dissection to preserve the integrity of random perforators. This keystone procedure shows the limits to the fasciocutaneous island flap extending from the patella apex over the head of the fibula down the lateral compartment. Random perforators constitute the basis of vascular support. Angiographic investigations are not necessary. In the technique, it is imperative that 1/3 of the deep attachment is left intact. The fascial lined island design divides the skin down to the subcutaneous tissue proximally and distally. Surrounding scars have modified the keystone mark out

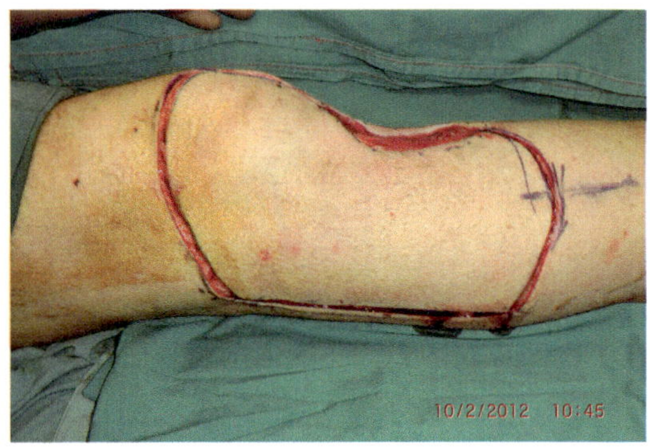

Fig. 3.75 The mark out of the keystone. The fascial plane is developed using the index finger so any perforators are protected from any sharp intrusion

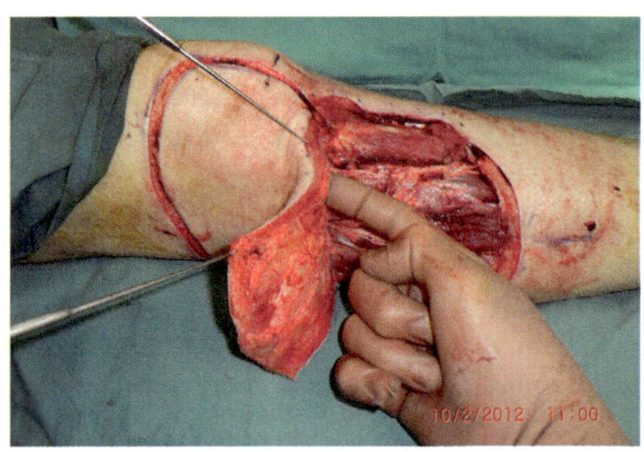

Fig. 3.76 The blunt dissection technique using the digit to preserve vascular integrity of any random perforators. Angiographic investigation is not required adding to the cost efficiency, sometimes necessary in microvascular repair

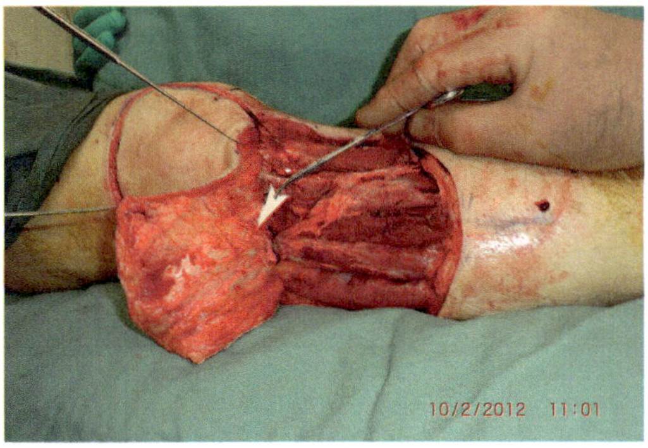

Fig. 3.77 The suprafascial and infrafascial circulation points are easily visualised (arrowed)

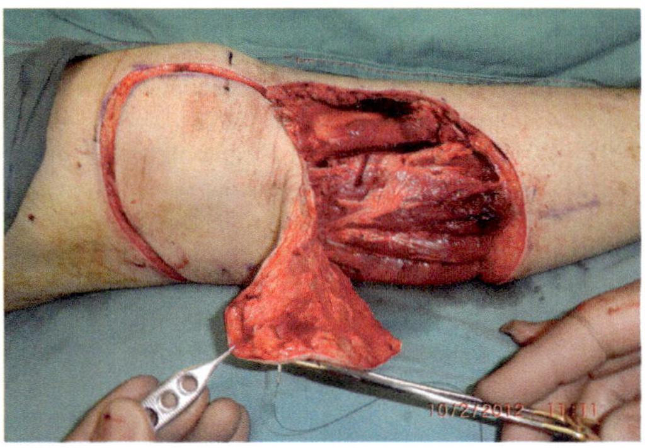

Fig. 3.78 Therefore on release of tourniquet there is full perfusion to the flap at the suprafascial and infrafascial levels prior to rotation and transposition over the exposed bony defect. Weck clip haemostasis is completed using micro clips as diathermy is avoided reducing the possibility of coagulative necrosis. The deep surface showing the vascular ooze prior to haemostasis using micro clips

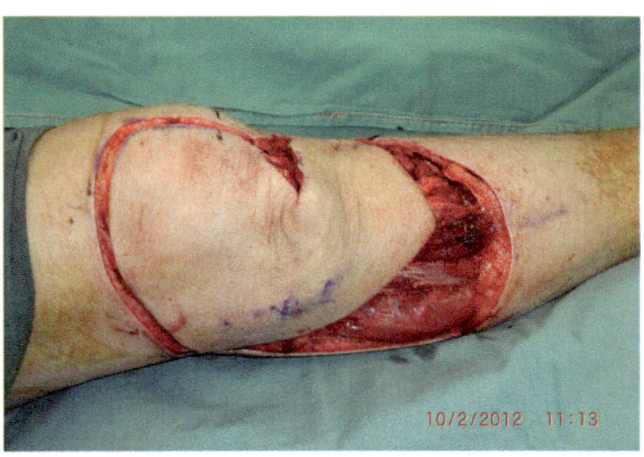

Fig. 3.79 The advancement rotation of the keystone over the bony defect. Staged reconstruction covering the exposed bony defect 9 × 6 cm over the tibial tuberosity. Note the keystone in the proximal aspect has skin and subcutaneous tissue divided only and the hyperaemic phase is evident in this upper section hypothesising as possibly a sympathectomy effect due to the island flap design. The distal 2/3 is the fascial lined component to close the bony defect. The tourniquet is released with recovery of perfusion

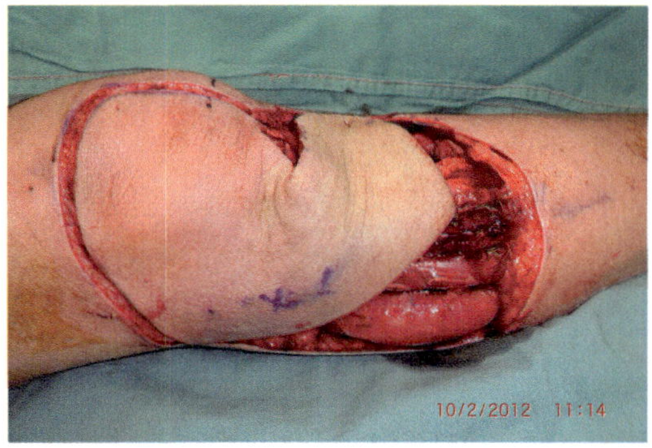

Fig. 3.80 The hyperaemic flare is noted and spreading distally. The island flap design eliminates any contribution from the subdermal plexus and focuses the vascularity on the random perforators. These clinical observations are noted regarding the reactive hyperaemia to produce the red dot sign over a short time frame which usually commences after 15 min—the basis of the red dot sign where the suture point bleeds more on the flap than along the inserted margin

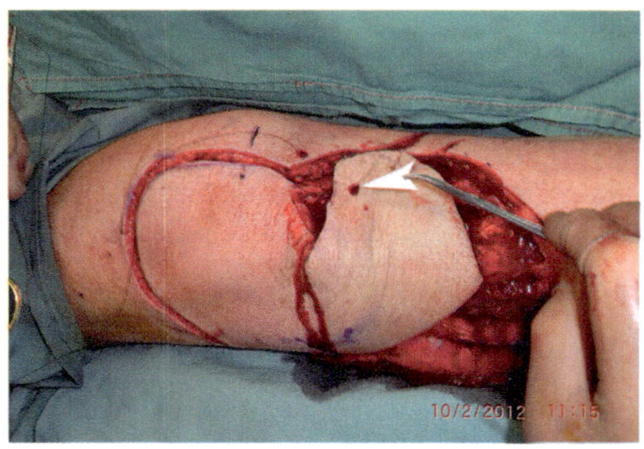

Fig. 3.81 Release of tourniquet and the hyperaemia in the flap helps to create the red dot sign a characteristic of the keystone based on these design techniques

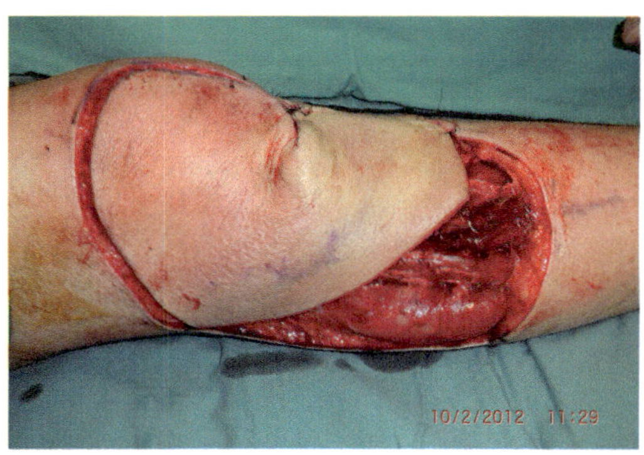

Fig. 3.82 Staged closure over the bone prior to the grafting of the secondary defect

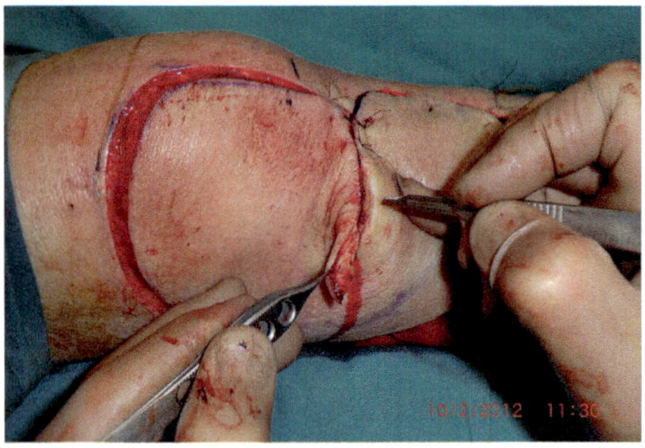

Fig. 3.83 Trimming the dog ear intraoperatively, a reflection of the keystone's reliable vascular perfusion

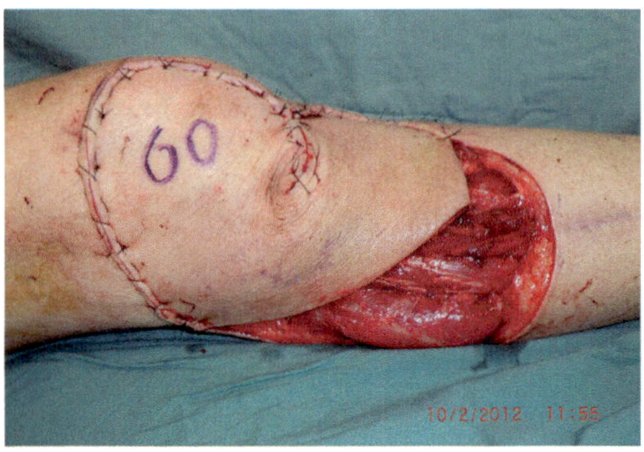

Fig. 3.84 Timeframe of 60 min as indicated and the microvascular reconstruction would be measured in hours

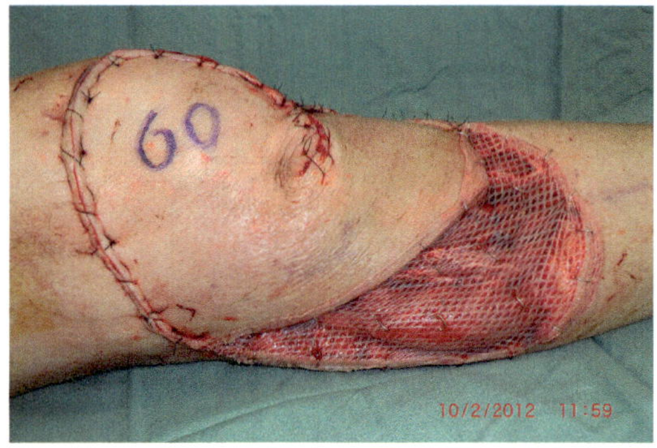

Fig. 3.85 Mesh grafting from the opposite limb completes the procedure. The secondary defect is mesh grafted. The random use of perforators with blunt dissection is quite a timesaver and without delineation of individual named perforators, these non-specific perforator sources can retain the somatic and autonomic supply from the dermatome which becomes an application of the embryological basis to account for the observed clinical findings. And microvascular procedures, sometimes an acceptable alternative, have a different timeframe depending on the experience of the operator but these embryological factors contribute to the observed characteristics of the keystone P.A.C.E.S. Pain free postoperatively (apart from the donor site for the split skin graft). Aesthetically a like-for-like match has been achieved. Complications from a vascular point of view were not evident as the flap healed perfectly. Economics from investigation and speed of surgical repair are self-evident. Sensory recovery returns in 2–3 weeks as the same timeframe as the resolution of oedema. It is the somatic nerves up the neurovascular axes which facilitate this recovery as the perforators are not skeletonised to facilitate cover

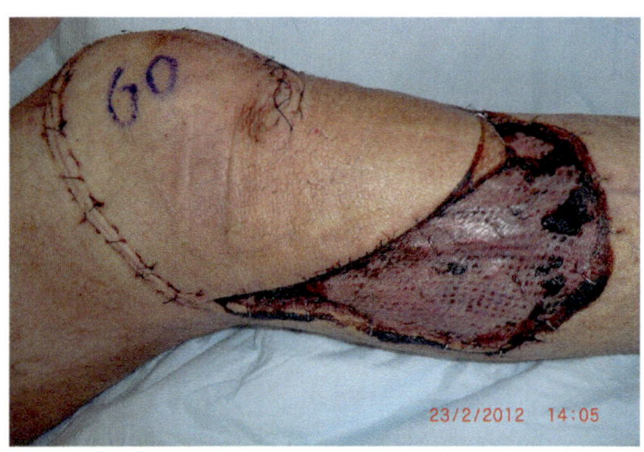

Fig. 3.86 Healed appearance at 2 weeks. The postoperative video supplement reveals the patient's satisfaction, once more illustrating the keystone characteristics from a patient's point of view as well as the documented images

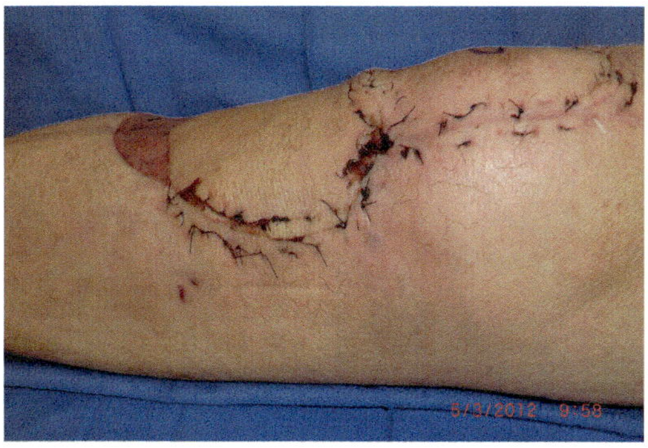

Fig. 3.87 Postoperative appearance at 10 days with the locking mattress sutures in situ for at least 3 weeks

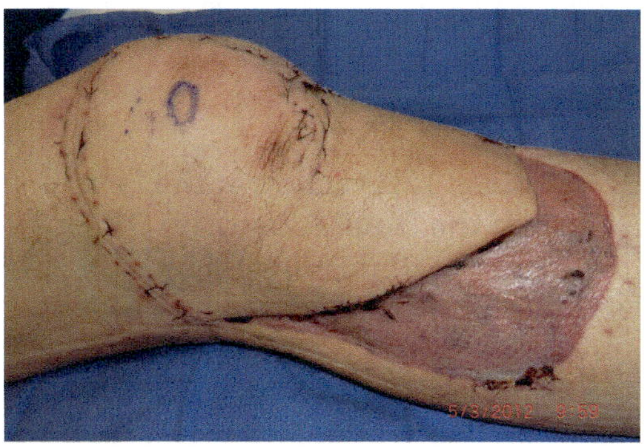

Fig. 3.88 Another view of postoperative appearance at 10 days, patient very grateful and the only pain he has is in the skin graft donor site

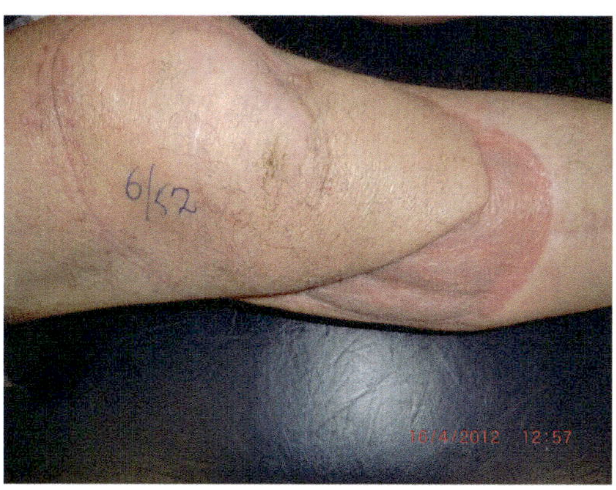

Fig. 3.89 Postoperative appearance at 6 weeks and the videos summarise the patient's satisfaction

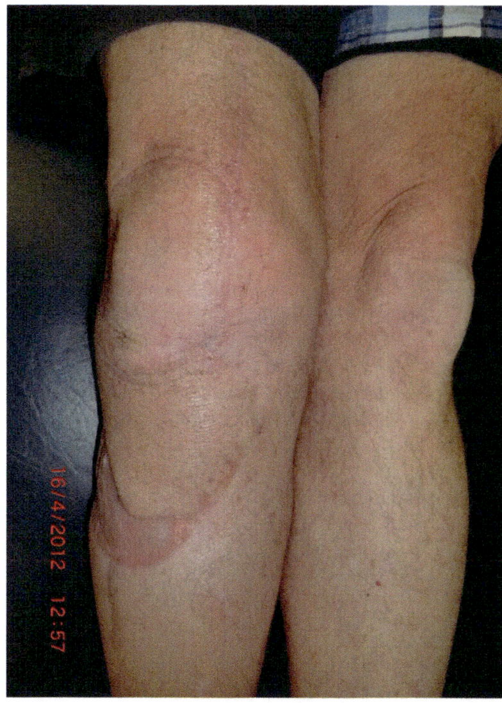

Fig. 3.90 Postoperative appearance at 6 weeks with the P.A.C.E.S. characteristics exemplified and the patient's satisfaction in the videos needs no elaboration

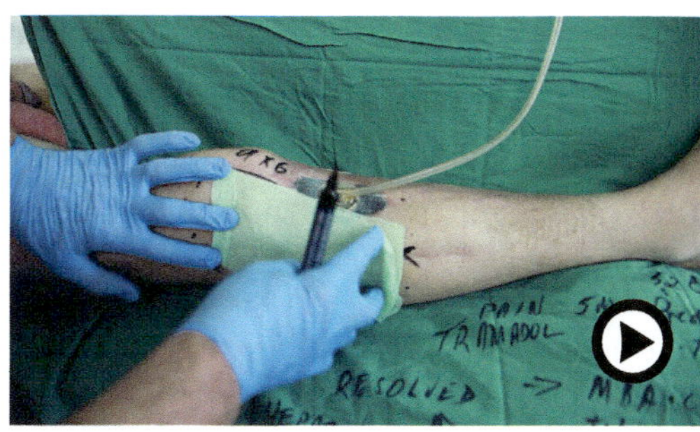

Fig. 3.91 Planned operative sequence of an FCIF in a keystone manner (Video 3.8 Planned operative sequence of an FCIF in a keystone manner) (▶ https://doi.org/10.1007/000-d50)

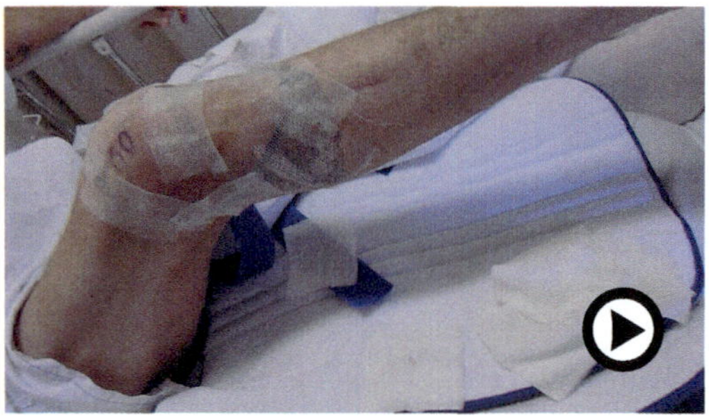

Fig. 3.92 Early postoperative patient response revealing the patient's satisfaction and contentment with the surgery which was pain free (apart from the graft site) (Video 3.9 Early postoperative patient response revealing the patient's satisfaction and contentment with the surgery which was pain free (apart from the graft site)) (▶ https://doi.org/10.1007/000-d51)

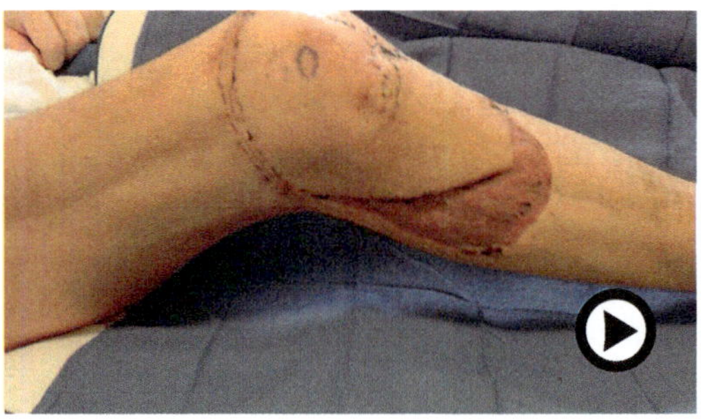

Fig. 3.93 Postoperative patient response with a healed graft site and exercising under supervision (Video 3.10 Postoperative patient response with a healed graft site and exercising under supervision) (▶ https://doi.org/10.1007/000-d52)

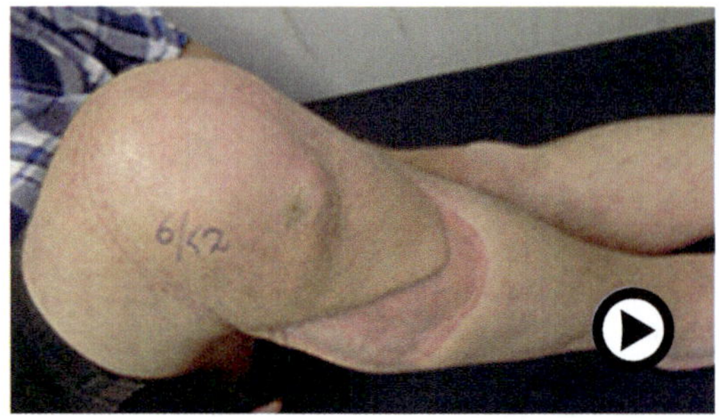

Fig. 3.94 Patient assessment at 6 weeks on completion of healing indicating his satisfaction and of course further illustrations of the keystone characteristics of P.A.C.E.S. and the rapid healing (Video 3.11 Patient assessment at 6 weeks on completion of healing indicating his satisfaction and of course further illustrations of the keystone characteristics of P.A.C.E.S. and the rapid healing) (▶ https://doi.org/10.1007/000-d53)

3.1.6 Case 17: Fracture at the Level of the Tibial Tuberosity ORIF in the USA Followed by Wound Breakdown on Return

This skiing injury of a fractured upper 1/3 tibia and fibular had a meticulous soft tissue cover resulting in subsequent necrosis / osteomyelitis and the need for Redi-vac suction following transfer back to Australia from the USA. The overuse of very fine nylon as was the habit in the USA could have been contributory to tissue necrosis and flap breakdown (Figs. 3.95, 3.96, 3.97, 3.98, 3.99, 3.100, 3.101, 3.102, 3.103, and 3.104).

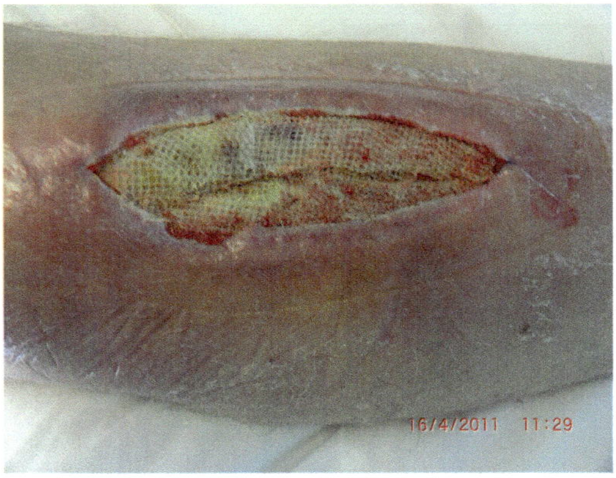

Fig. 3.95 This 10 × 4 cm defect over the tibial tuberosity extending down along the proximal 1/3 of the anterior tibial line. Necrosis following an ORIF in the USA. The images of the necrosis were unavailable as this was conducted by the orthopaedic team. Following Redi-VAC suction dressings completed the debridement over a 3-week period. The ORIF plate is not on view hence not removed. The keystone procedure salvaged this orthopaedic breakdown, avoiding an amputation

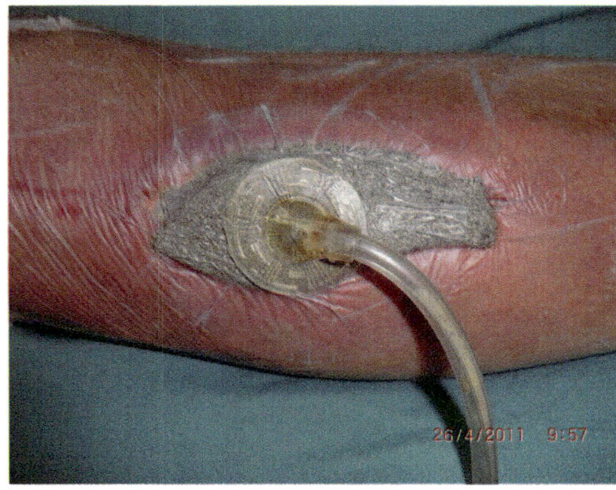

Fig. 3.96 VAC dressings by the local orthopaedic unit

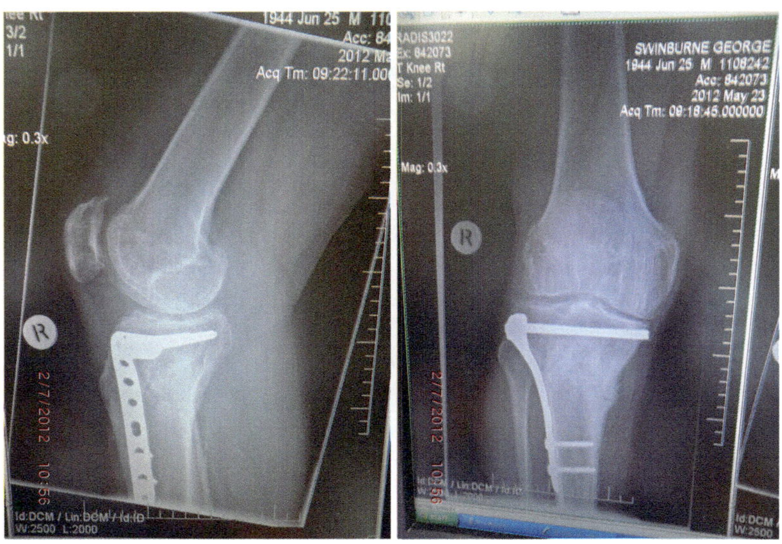

Fig. 3.97 The ORIF procedure performed in the USA. Lateral and AP views on X-ray of April 2012

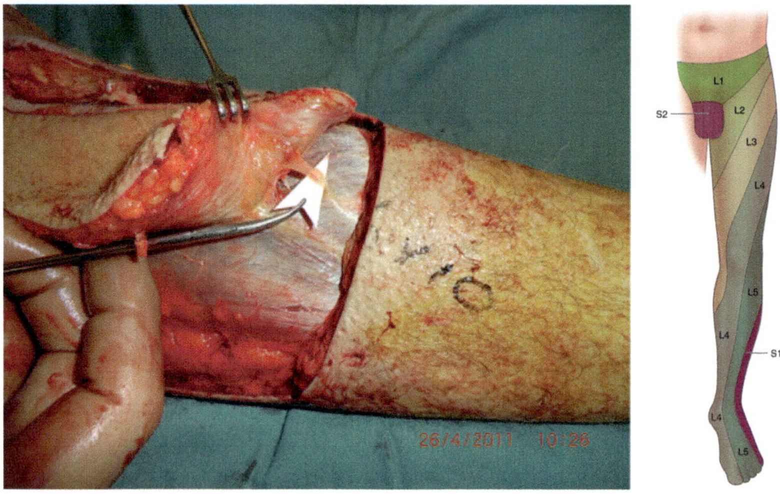

Fig. 3.98 The keystone design in the L5 dermatome to cover a 10 × 4 cm anterior tibial defect and removal of the ORIF procedure needed an external fixateur to stablise the fracture. The keystone soft tissue mark out when turned almost on itself at 180° constitute what we have termed the Omega variant Ω for this horseshoe shaped flap repair to achieve bony cover with vascularised fascial lining. The standard blunt dissection technique creates the plane of dissection with a fascial lined keystone preserving filamentous perforators and avoiding any damage of these vital lifelines that perforate the fascia from the underlying muscular compartment of the lateral peroneal complex of L5 dermatome

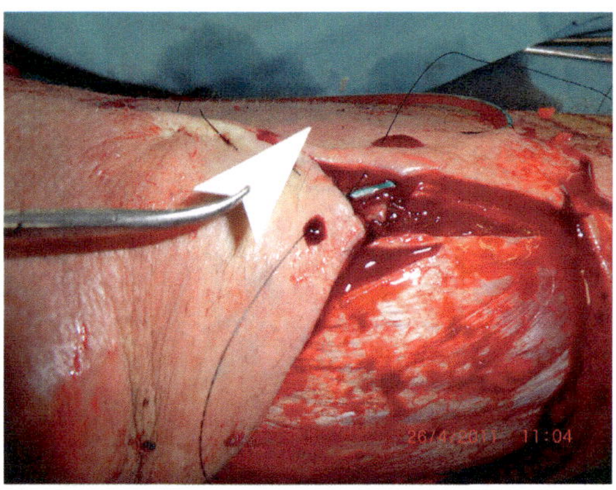

Fig. 3.99 The tourniquet release red dot sign is evident in this random perforator keystone in its hyperaemic phase. Hypothetically, this is attributed to a sympathectomy manifestation, a consequence of the island flap design on a fascial base. It ensures vascular integrity to optimise healing. Experimental evidence to confirm the red dot sign in oxygenated blood is overcome by simply observing the intensity of the red dot, and the oxygen tension in the blood is evidence enough of its hyperaemic reliabilty. Hence, if any incredulous minds offer criticism just look at the photograph. Angiography is not necessary with this keystone technique, another economic cost saving

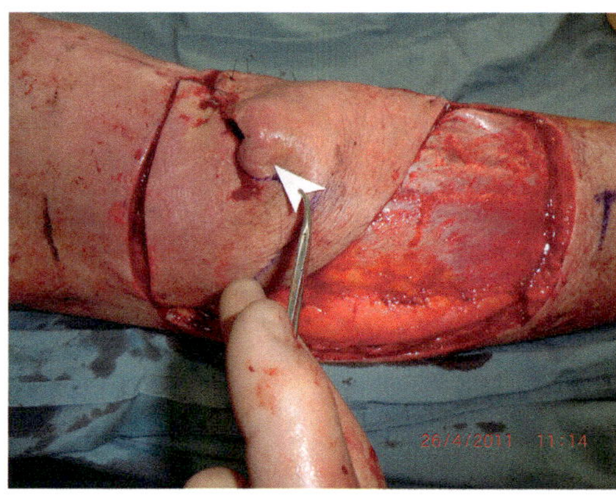

Fig. 3.100 Another phase of the hyperaemic reliability, who would ever dream of trimming a dog ear in a flap reconstruction where circulation could only be regarded as precarious. The fact that this is clinically successful at the dermal epidermal level and the tissues are buried for epidermal closure is a significant indicator of its clinical reliability. Another observation finding repeated on umpteen occaisions over the years which is again contraray to plastic surgical reconstructive flap thinking. The arrow indicates the subdermal perfusion to achieve wound closure. This is achieved by excising skin at the dermal epidermal level and the suprafascial circulation maintains the flap integrity

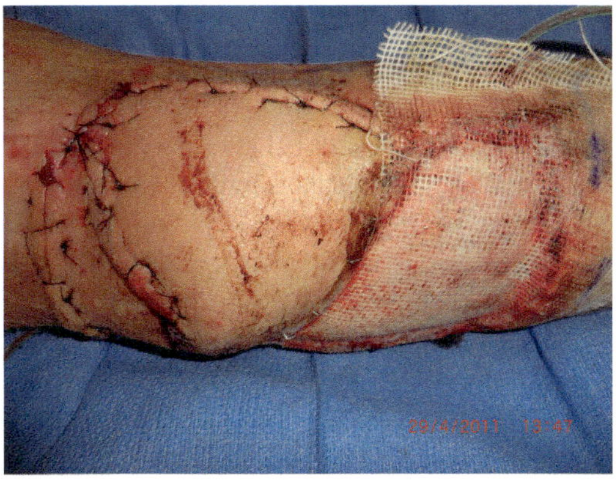

Fig. 3.101 P.A.C.E.S. illustrated again at 3rd day appearance with no pain, aesthetically acceptable, no flap necrosis, economically sound and too early to comment on the resolution of oedema and the return of sensation for this exposed bony defect at the tibial tuberosity which may take 4–5 weeks to become clinically evident as all my findings are based on clinical observations and documented with accompanying dated images

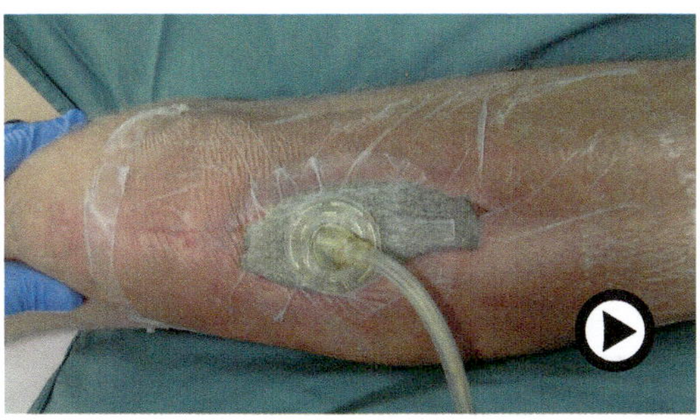

Fig. 3.102 Clinical referral under Redi-vac dressing the orthopaedic unit referral and their debridement (Video 3.12 Clinical referral under Redi-vac dressing the orthopaedic unit referral and their debridement) (▶ https://doi.org/10.1007/000-d54)

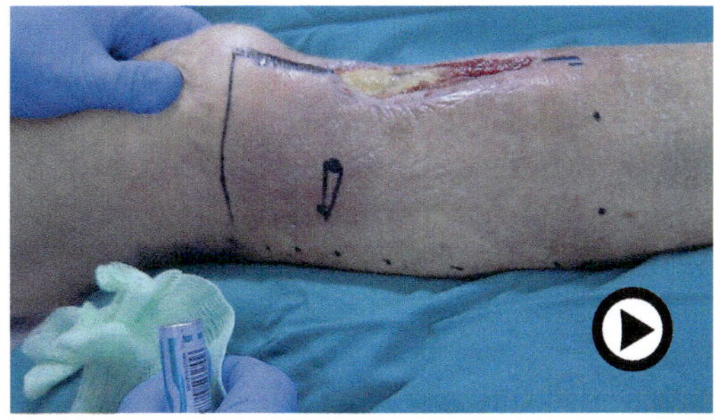

Fig. 3.103 The flap mark out in the L5 dermatome and the surface marking of the lateral popliteal nerve as a precaution (Video 3.13 The flap mark out in the L5 dermatome and the surface marking of the lateral popliteal nerve as a precaution) (▶ https://doi.org/10.1007/000-d55)

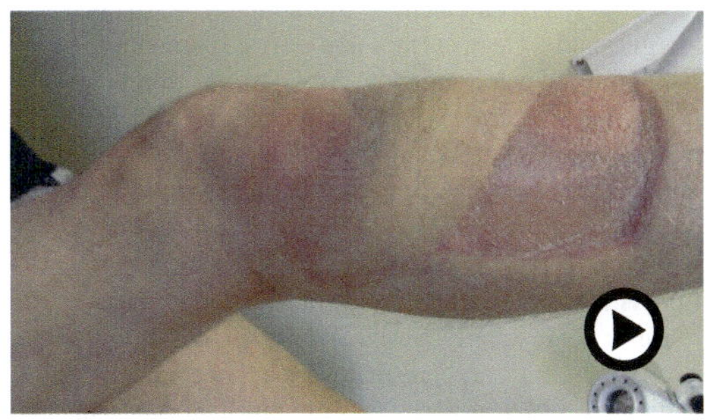

Fig. 3.104 Patient response revealing his satisfaction with the surgical outcome and recovery of full range of movement and pain free (Video 3.14 Patient response revealing his satisfaction with the surgical outcome and recovery of full range of movement and pain free) (▶ https://doi.org/10.1007/000-d56)

3.1.7 Case 18: Chronic Osteomyelitis in the Upper 1/3 Tibia Following a Failed Myocutaneous Gastrocnemius Flap for a Wound Closure over a Tibial Fracture

This case illustrates one basic principle in reconstructive surgery of a muscle flap reconstruction being the bed for a successful skin graft over bone. If a muscle flap is used and its neurovascular integrity is at risk, the muscle supply nerve will end up with a fibrous tissue replacement and the contractile nature of the muscle flap has been forfeited. This may have been the explanation of this particular case. The summary from the Indian Journal of Orthopaedics [4] gives an overview of the problems and possible solutions to such complicated cases. However, the keystone soft tissue flap ended up as a salvation technique for this wound, developing chronic osteomyelitis, an element of non-union and a sinus to the open marrow cavity (Figs. 3.105, 3.106, 3.107, 3.108, 3.109, 3.110, 3.111, 3.112, 3.113, 3.114, 3.115, 3.116, 3.117, 3.118, 3.119, and 3.120).

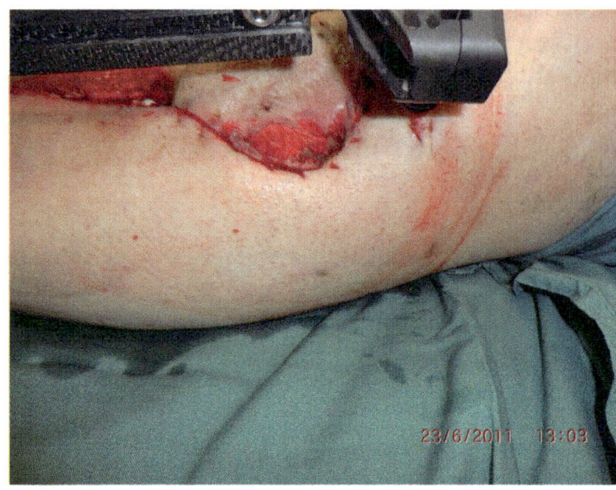

Fig. 3.105 Debridement of wound to create fresh margins and a clean surface and a freshly lined cavity with minimal contamination. An ORIF for tibial fracture was covered with a gastrocnemius [5] myocutaneous flap. Wound breakdown and non-union with chronic osteomyelitis were the resultant complications. External fixateur stabilisation was needed. The gastrocnemius muscle flap reverted to a fibrous mass because of damage or deficiency of the intrinsic nerve supply. Surgical debridement at this site was like cutting carpet as there was no normal tissue and the fibrous scar tissue was the resultant outcome

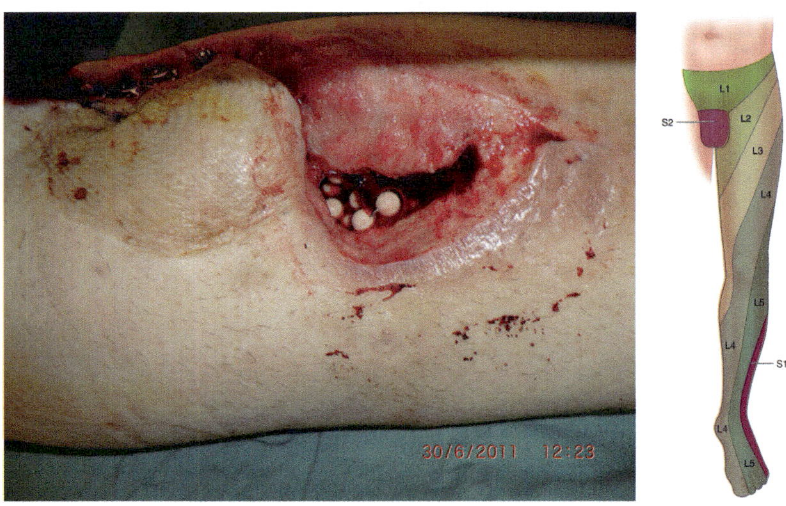

Fig. 3.106 Subsequently the orthopaedic team debrided the bone and installed gentamycin beads into the marrow cavity filled with granulation tissue for the management of the chronic osteomyelitis defect. The keystone reconstruction which is illustrated in the next video designed along the L5 dermatome was used to cover the defect

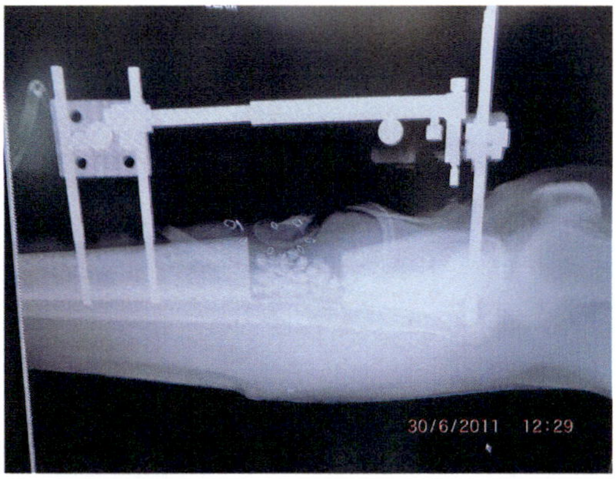

Fig. 3.107 The gentamycin beads are evident in the marrow cavity on this X-ray film. An external fixateur stabilises the wound

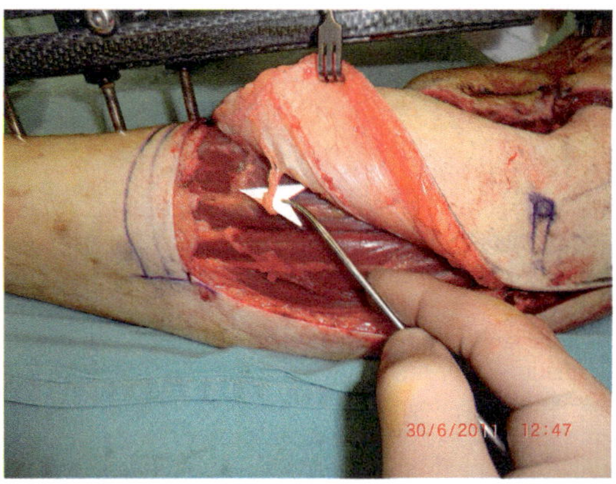

Fig. 3.108 Random muscular perforators are preserved when exposed with blunt dissection—the best method of raising the fascial lined flap (arrow)

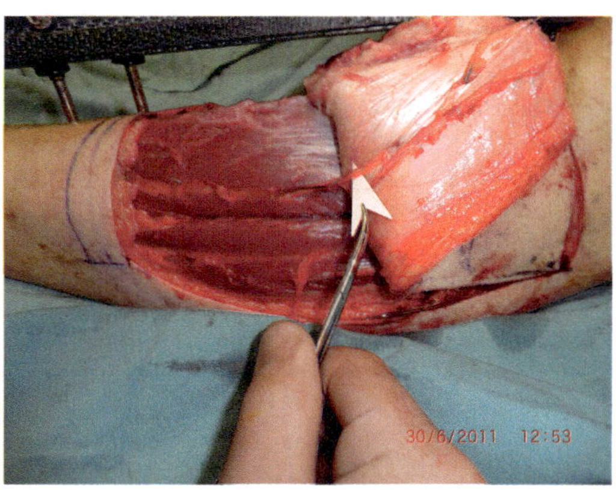

Fig. 3.109 A perforator site (arrow) from the peroneal compartment raised with blunt dissection to preserve its integrity before advancement, roation and transposition to cover the osteomylitic defect in bone

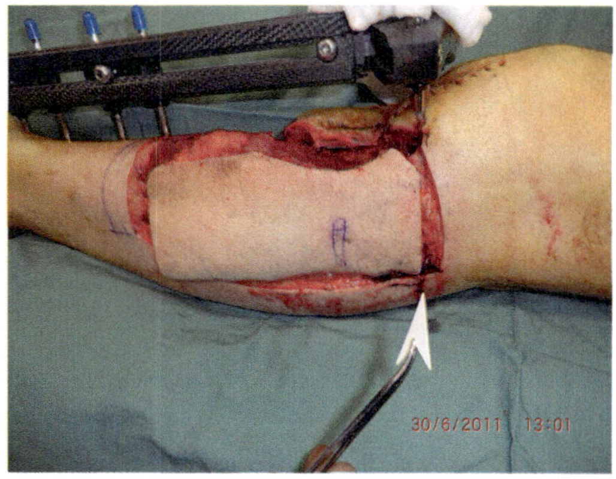

Fig. 3.110 The hyperaemic phase on release of tourniquet

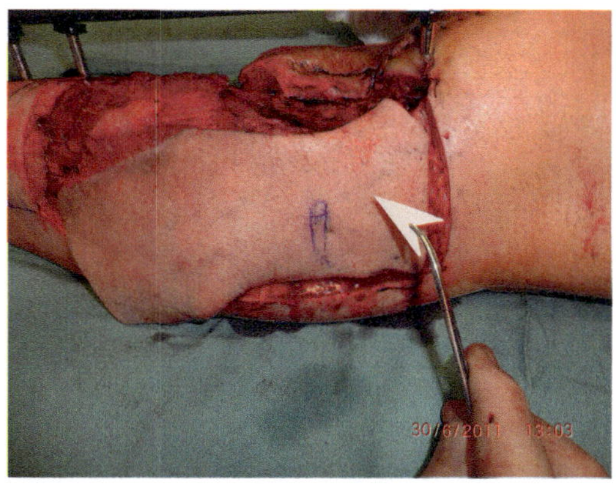

Fig. 3.111 This keystone along the L5 dermatome measures ~10 × 20 cm. The distal part of the flap is undermined with fascial lining to advance, rotate and transpose (ART) to cover the tibial defect. The video confirms the surgical techniques employed in this reparitive procedure. Angiographic evidence was not required as long as one stays within the L5 dermatome. The hyperaemic phase of the keystone is evident confirming vascular integrity. The keystone characteristics became evident as the procedure developed. The distal part is undermined and rotated to cover the vital/bony structures. The arrow points to the reactive hyperaemia in this island keystone once the tourniquet is released. One presumes this reflects the possible sympathectomy effect when these dermatomally aligned fascially based and only partically detached adjacent to the perforator sites coming through within the L4 dermatome

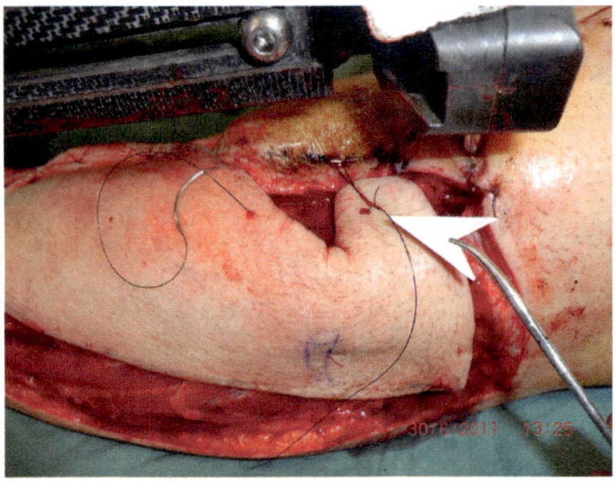

Fig. 3.112 This omega variant Ω is really a keystone bent on itself in the shape of a horseshoe. The red dot signs confirm its vascular integrity

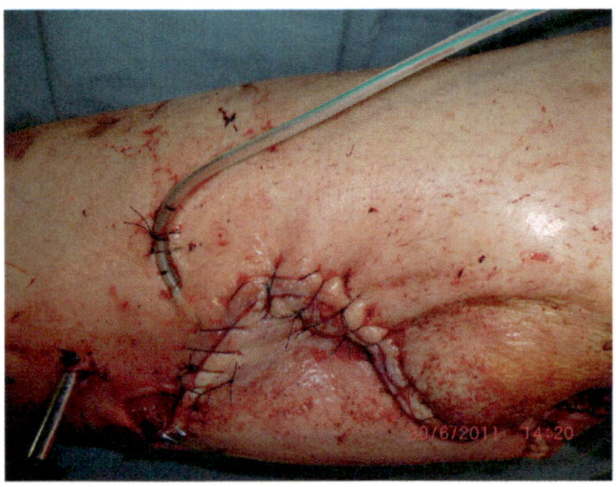

Fig. 3.113 On completion with Redi-vac drainage. No vascular impedance with the use of suction drainage which contrasts with free flap use

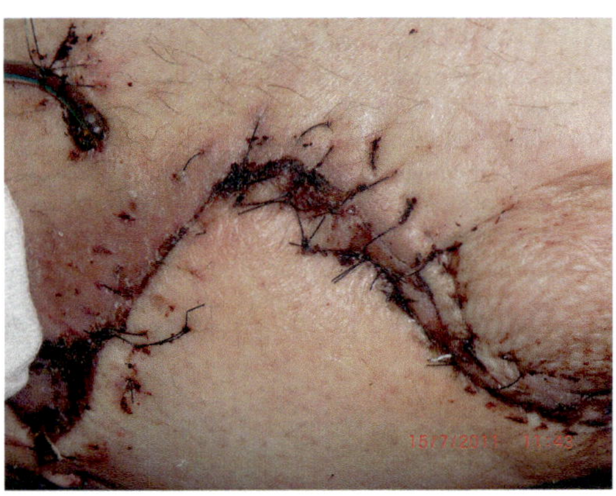

Fig. 3.114 Early postopersative image beneath the fixateur without any vascular impediment and signs of inflamation in the keystone

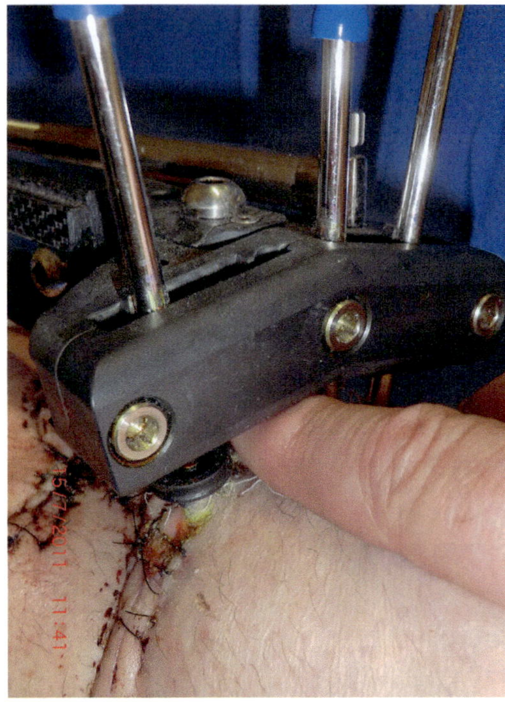

Fig. 3.115 This case is the definitive example of the resolution of oedema characterising the keystone with the P.A.C.E.S. acronym. Even by creating more scar tissue with the keystone, the oedema resolution in 24 h was quite dramatic. As illustrated my index finger could fit beneath the external fixateur frame which was not possible preoperatively because of tight alignment. As we hypothesise about the hyperaemic effect to cause the Red Dot Sign, could a similar effect be focussed at the lymphatic level with dilatation facilitating increased drainage of oedema fluid? Total volume of the index finger (Length × Width × Height) could give an estimate of the volume reduction with the resolution of oedema under the fixateur the patient just simply said 'it feels better'. Others may argue it was the resolution of infection—but such a speedy reduction of oedema overnight and the control of infection would be certainly longer than a 24 h timeframe

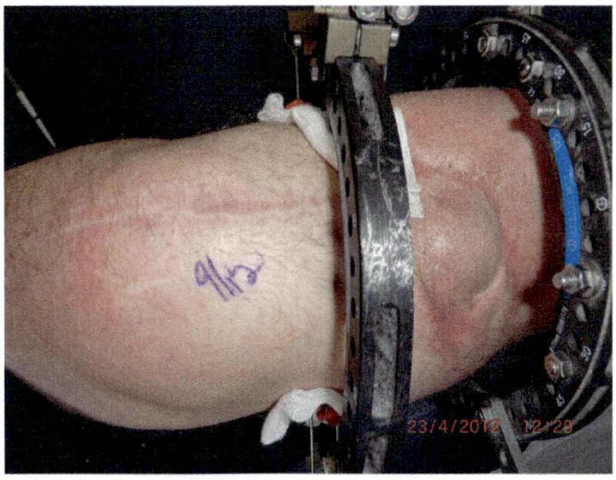

Fig. 3.116 Appearance at 9 months fully healed. The acronym P.A.C.E.S. is again verfied in this case with a strong focus on pain relief and resolution of oedema

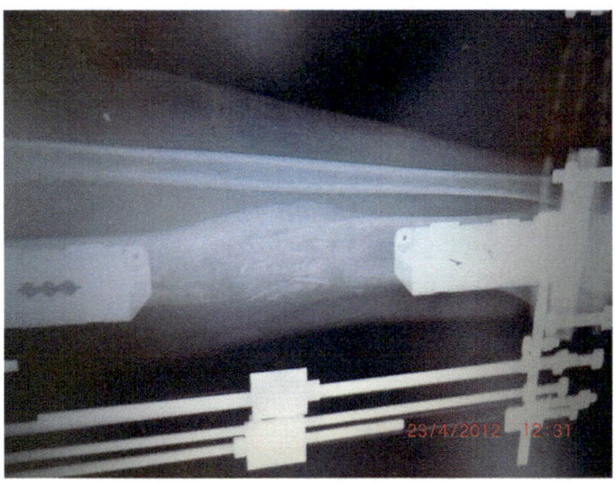

Fig. 3.117 The X-ray showing the Ilizarov [6] bone healing technique of callous formation of the divided ends of the tibial fracture an essential ingredient to bone healing with the resolution of the osteomylitis and the use of gentamycin beads

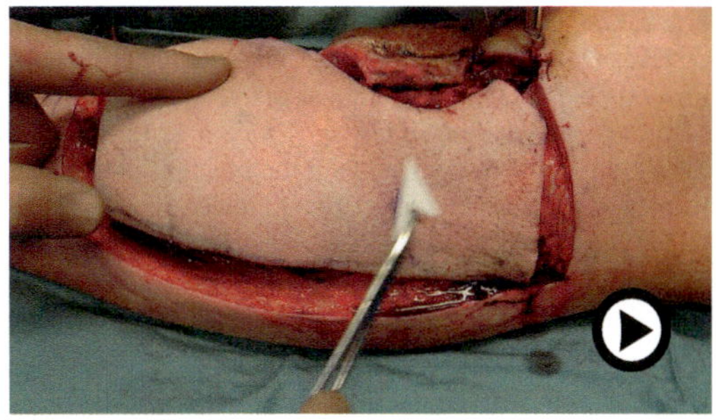

Fig. 3.118 The hyperaemic phase on release of tourniquet of the fasciocutaneous keystone flap showing full vascular integrity (Video 3.15 The hyperaemic phase on release of torniquet of the fascio cutaneous keystone flap showing full vascular integrity) (▶ https://doi.org/10.1007/000-d57)

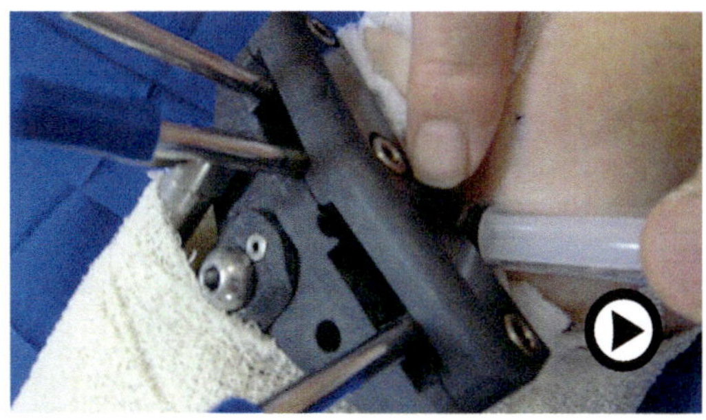

Fig. 3.119 The patient's reaction to the success of the operation is summarised. Healing has been achieved with increased mobility and resolution of oedema almost overnight. My index finger could not fit under the external fixateur preoperatively but postoperatively a 1.5 cm space was created allowing my index finger to fit underneath the fixateur. The patient's satisfaction is recorded (Video 3.16 The patient's reaction to the success of the operation is summarised. Healing has been achieved with increased mobility and resolution of oedema almost overnight. My index finger could not fit under the external fixateur preoperatively but postoperatively a 1.5 cm space was created allowing my index finger to fit underneath the fixateur. The patient's satisfaction is recorded) (▶ https://doi.org/10.1007/000-d58)

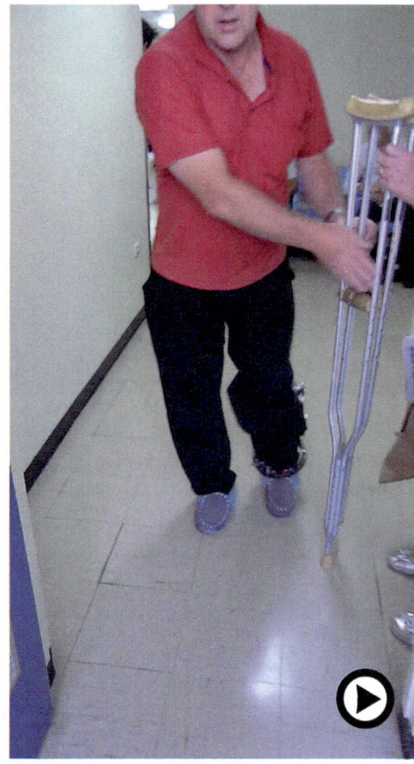

Fig. 3.120 Postoperative mobilisation and dispensing with the crutches on full weight bearing. An acceptable alternative to lower limb amputation which was offered to him initially. The keystone technique saved his leg (Video 3.17 Post-operative mobilisation and dispensing with the crutches on full weight bearing. An acceptable alternative to lower limb amputation which was offered to him initially. The keystone technique saved his leg) (▶ https://doi.org/10.1007/000-d59)

3.1.8 Case 19: R Tibia with 20 Years of Chronic Osteomyelitis from a War Injury in Sudan (Figs. 3.121, 3.122, 3.123, 3.124, 3.125, 3.126, 3.127, 3.128, 3.129, 3.130, 3.131, 3.132, 3.133, 3.134, 3.135, 3.136, 3.137, and 3.138)

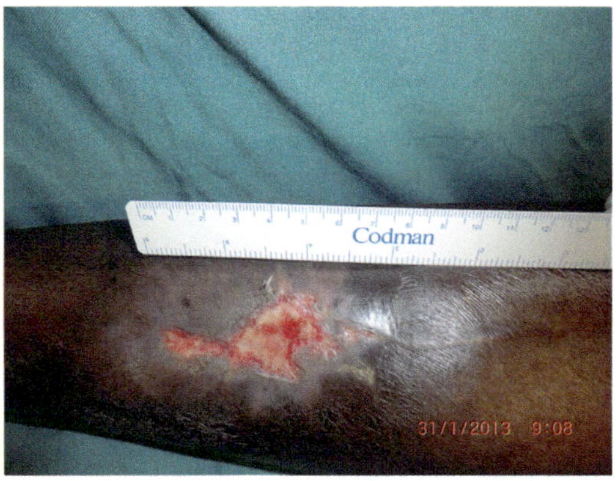

Fig. 3.121 In this 55-year-old male with chronic osteomyelitis of the R tibia following an accident in Sudan 20 years ago and likewise followed by 20 years of dressings. Anatomical site middle 1/3 tibia. A duet orthopaedic procedure in association with Mr Ian Harris at the Western Hospital, Melbourne

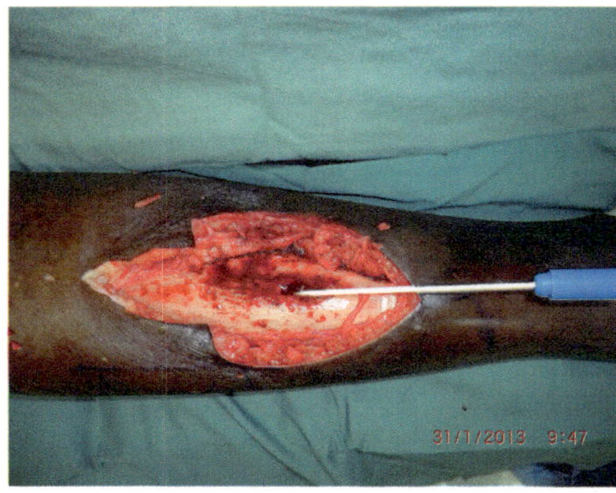

Fig. 3.123 Broaching the marrow cavity in preparation for cortical bone matrix cement

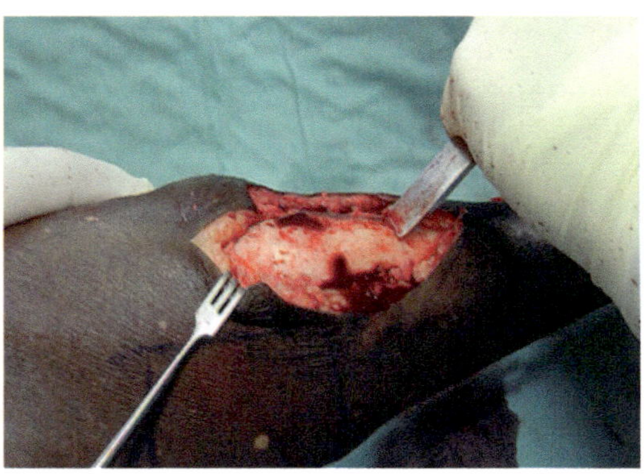

Fig. 3.122 Debridement at the cortical bone level in association with the orthopaedic department

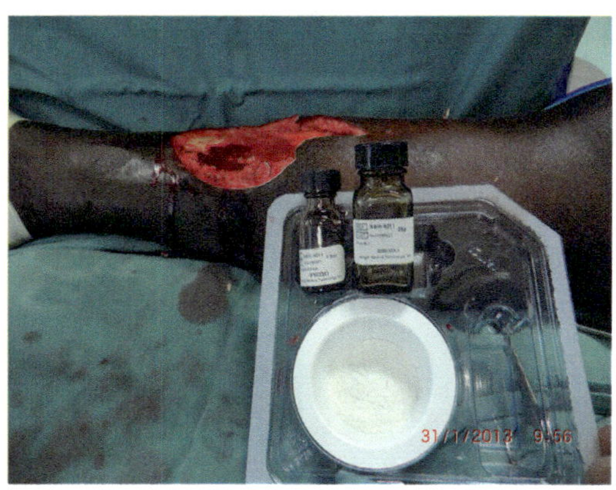

Fig. 3.124 Bone matrix cement to be used in preparation for reconstituting the cortical defect in the tibia

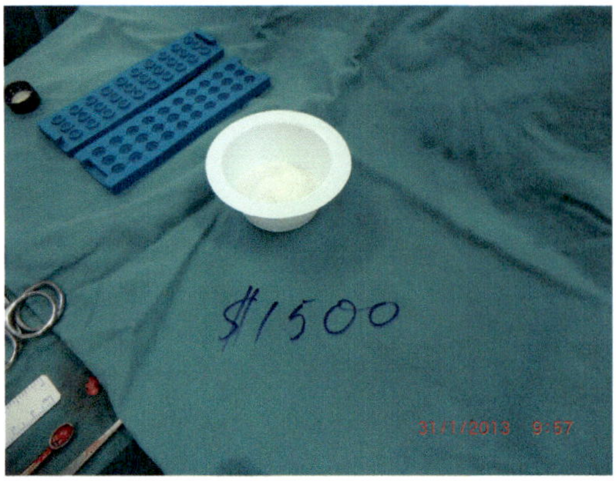

Fig. 3.125 This two-part mixture is blended to become a solid cortical replacement for the osteomyelitic deficiencies that have gone on for 20 years

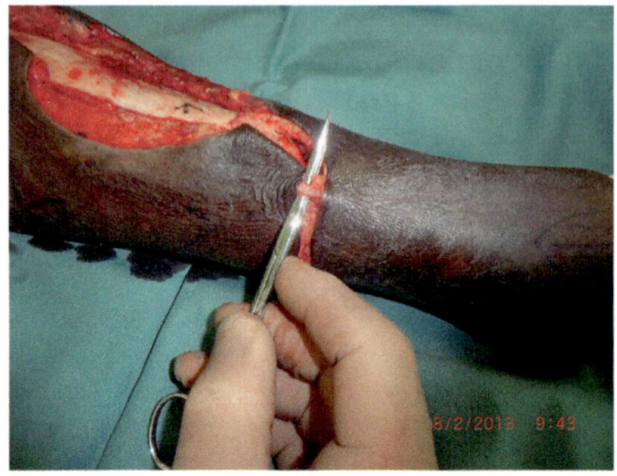

Fig. 3.127 The nerve is anatomically dissected off the base of the keystone in the L5 dermatome to preserve its integrity, not restrict rotation and avoiding sequelae of somatic dysfunction of sensory changes to the distal foot

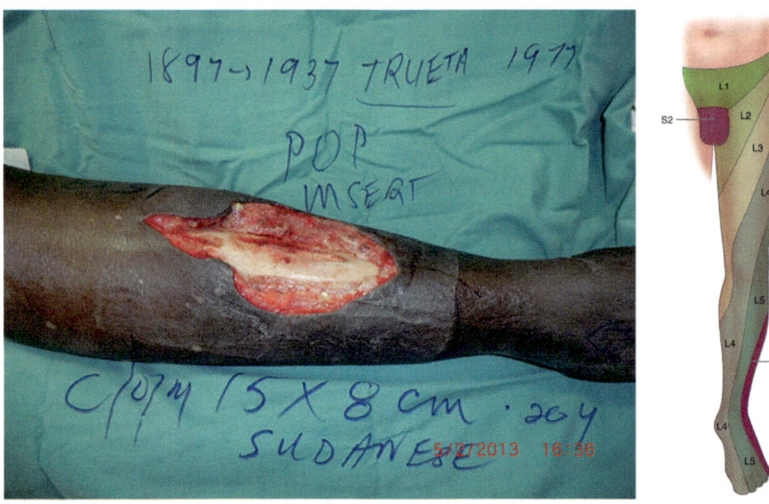

Fig. 3.126 Defect is 15 × 8 cm along the anterior tibial line. Keystone flap repair is designed within the L5 dermatome with random perforators along the line of the superficial peroneal nerve which is preserved. These perforators are not skeletonised but left as random support units for the flap

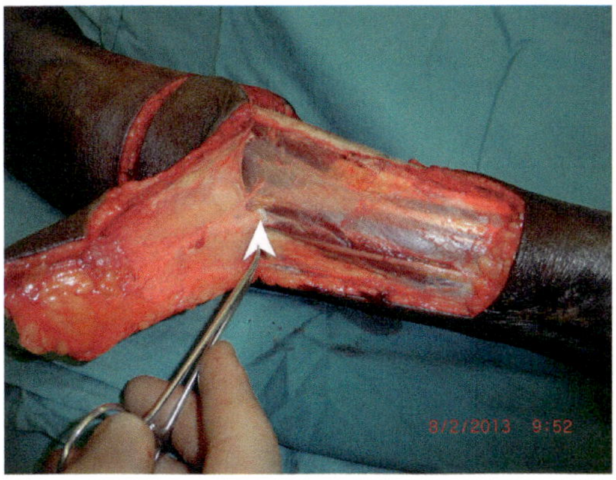

Fig. 3.128 The white arrow indicates the perforator vascular support and exit point of the superficial peroneal neurovascular system. The island flap design divides the dermis and epidermis only without breaking or harming any of the longitudenal structures which have an important contribution to neural sensation and lymphatic drainage. Proximally located is the incision that creates the island fascial principle when the dermis epidermis only is divided. This preserves in continuity any longitudenal neurovascular structure which helps the postoperative oedema, autonomic neural supply, venous drainage with lymphatic backup. The preservation of the superficial peroneal nerve is an essential requirement for retaining somatic and autonomic sensation to the foot and presumably assisting in lymphatic drainage as the oedema resolves after a few weeks following such chronic injuries. It is hypothesised that the sympathectomy effect of using an island flap increases the vascular flow which becomes evident by 15 min on release of tourniquet. This incisional peripheral wound has no part in the flap viability and is closed directly. Closure under tension is one of the surgical characteristics of the keystone reflecting its hyperaemic vascularity

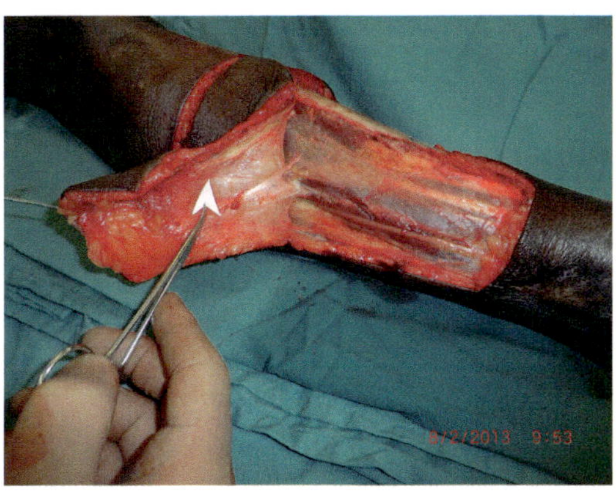

Fig. 3.129 The white arrow sits on the sites where the subfascial circulation oozes from the fascial bed. Diathermy is avoided, and haemostasis is achieved using micro clips

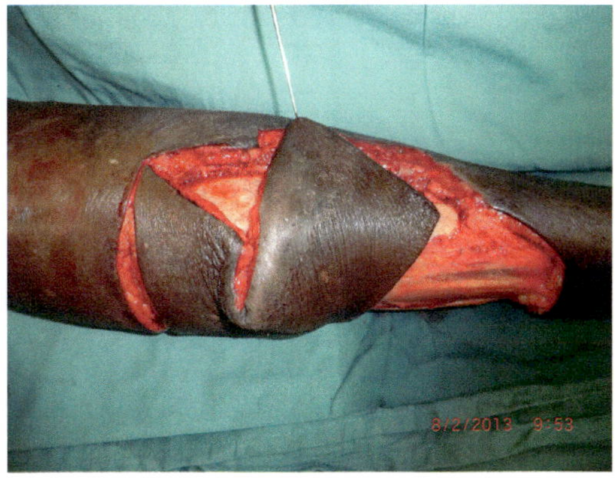

Fig. 3.130 The Omega variant allows the flap to be turned on itself in a u-shaped manner as the fascial base ensures vascular integrity over and above any issues with the subdermal complex. An essential design requirement is that 1/3 of the keystone design is left attached to deeper structures without any undermining. Again, the dog ear trim can be done in continuity because of this reliable circulartory dynamic which is really a bit heretical in flap reconstruction unless there is an intact suprafascial and infrafascial vascular intergrity. The 3-phase locking mattress suture technique closes the integument with Redivac drainage installed

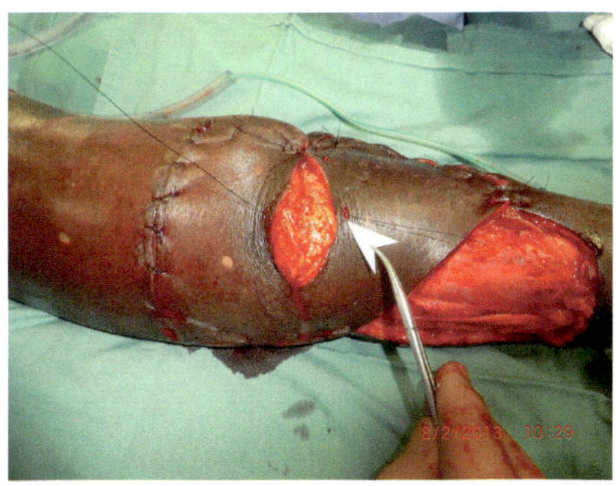

Fig. 3.131 The arrow indicating the red dot sign and the hypervascularity indicates the safety of the repair when the keystone is folded on itself in what we have published as its omega variant

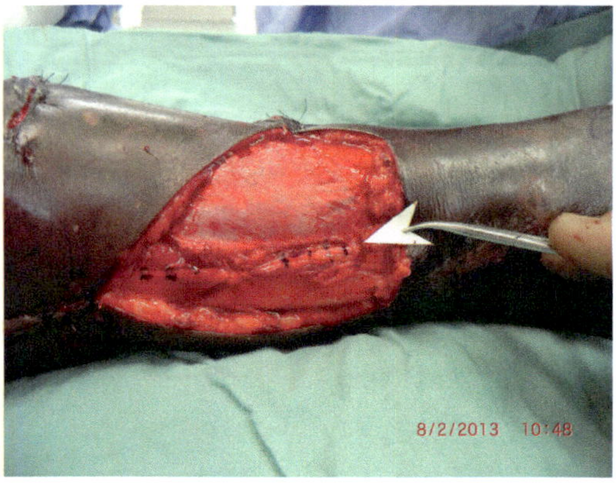

Fig. 3.132 The wound closure is completed, and the secondary defect is mesh grafted

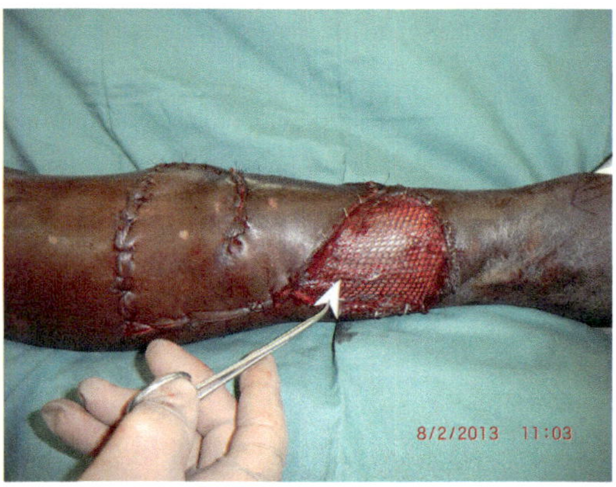

Fig. 3.133 Mesh grafting of the secondary defect in theatre and providing healing for the first time in 20 years

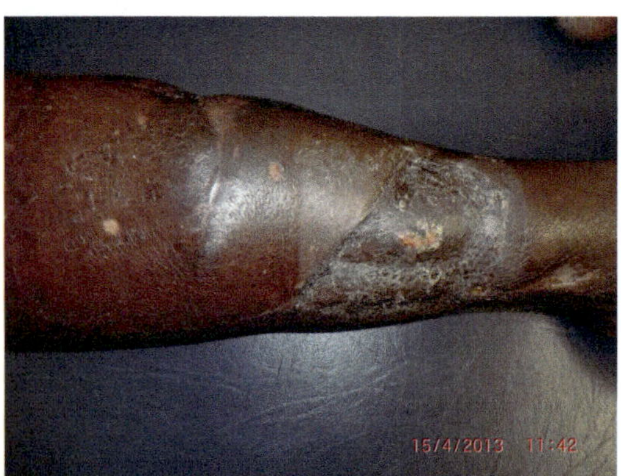

Fig. 3.136 Nine-week postoperative view. The patient is pain free with an aesthetic match, no wound complications, in an economic timeframe, with intact somatic sensation all contributing to the resolution of oedema

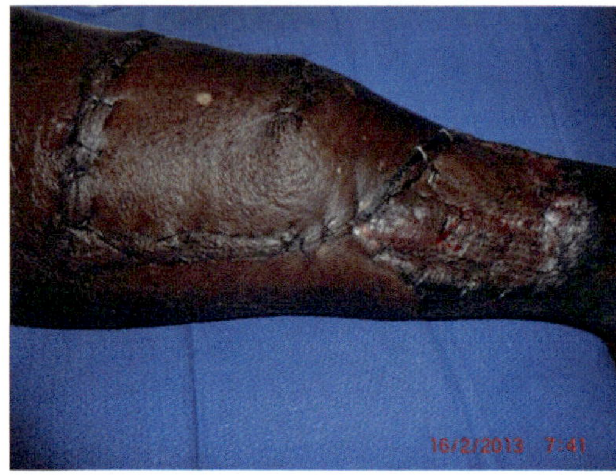

Fig. 3.134 This appearance at 8 days of the fully healed wound with a 20 year history of a chronic ulcer

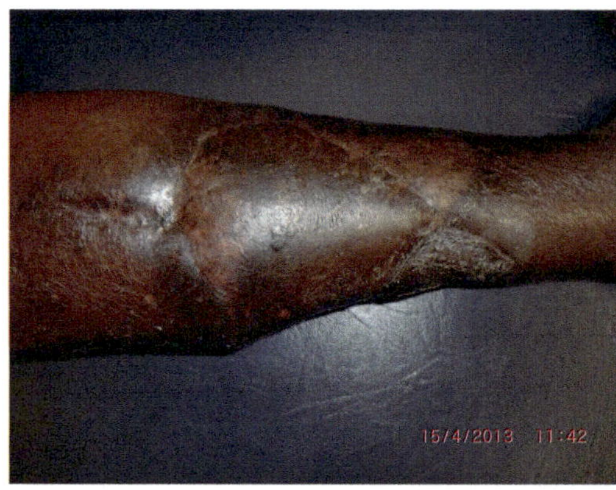

Fig. 3.135 Postoperative appearance at 9 weeks and the P.A.C.E.S. characteristics of the keystone are once more exemplified

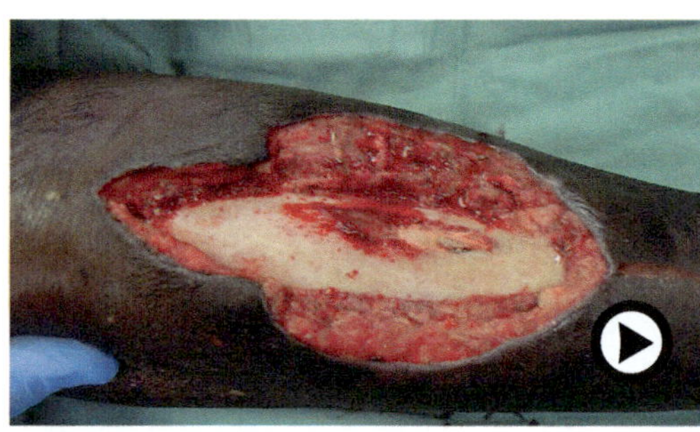

Fig. 3.137 The clinical history on video of this case spanning 20 years from war torn Africa where lack of medical attention results in chronic ulceration with osteomyelitis (Video 3.18 The clinical history on video of this case spanning 20 years from war torn Africa where lack of medical attention results in chronic ulceration with osteomyelitis) (▶ https://doi.org/10.1007/000-d5a)

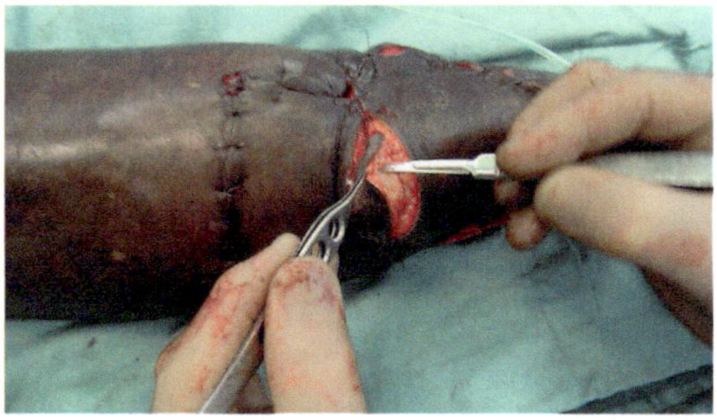

Fig. 3.138 Dog ear removal and the hypervascularity in the subdermis which guarantees flap integrity—all random perforator based

3.1.9 Case 20: Closure of ORIF Defect of Lower Limb Middle 1/3 Tibia (Figs. 3.139, 3.140, 3.141, 3.142, 3.143, 3.144, 3.145, 3.146, 3.147, 3.148, 3.149, 3.150, and 3.151)

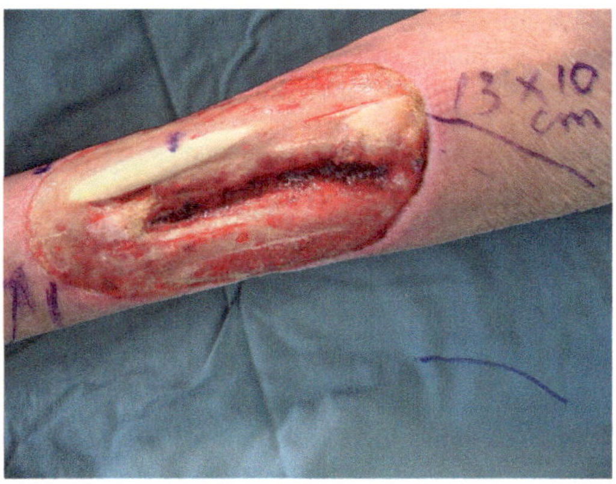

Fig. 3.139 The clinical defect 13 × 10 cm and the ORIF metal is in the depths of the wound as in Fig. 3.140

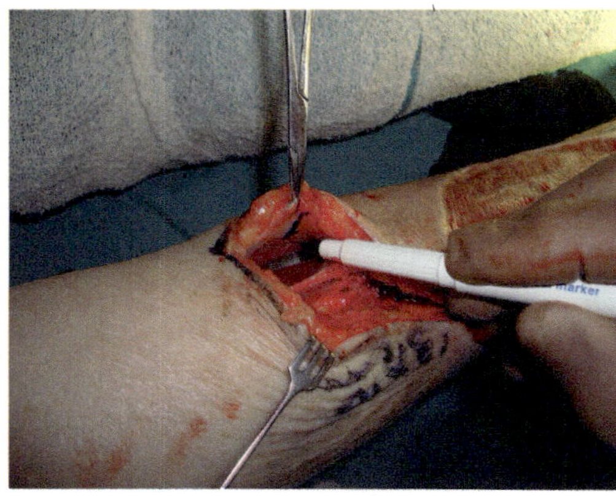

Fig. 3.140 Flap preparation of the tissue marker viewing the deep fascial line on the deep surface of the keystone to ensure its vascular viability with a suprafascial and infrafascial circulation [7] to cover the metal exposed

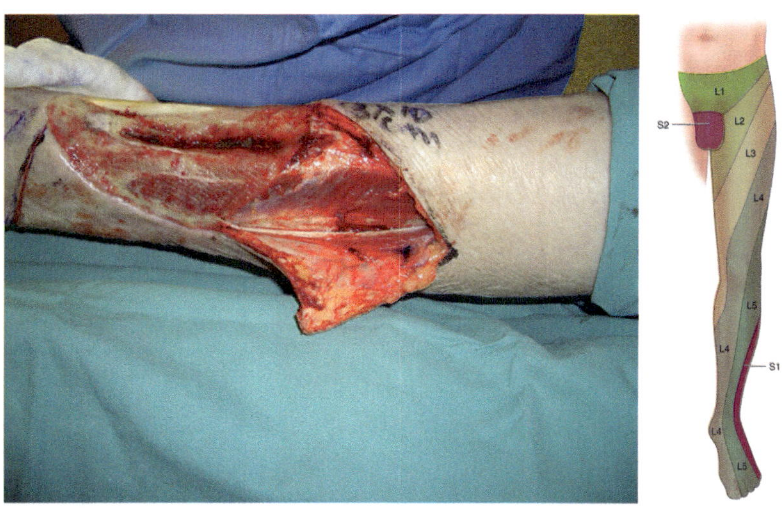

Fig. 3.141 The sural nerve is visualised in the raising of the flap to preserve its integrity to ensure neural continuity to the innervation of the foot in the L4 dermatome. The fascial attachments are detached along the nerve to allow advancement, rotation and transposition

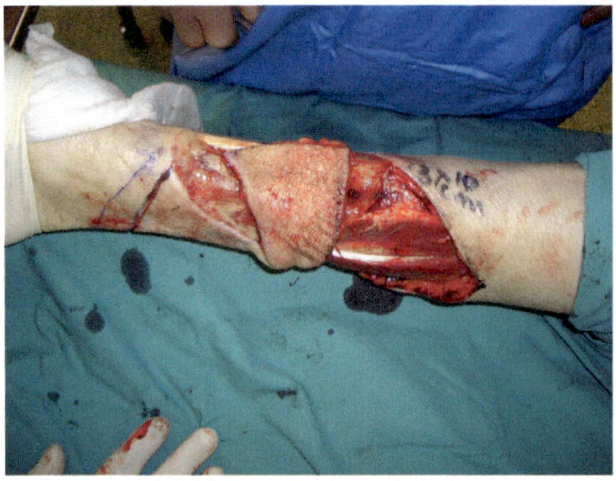

Fig. 3.142 Partially closed procedure prior to mesh grafting

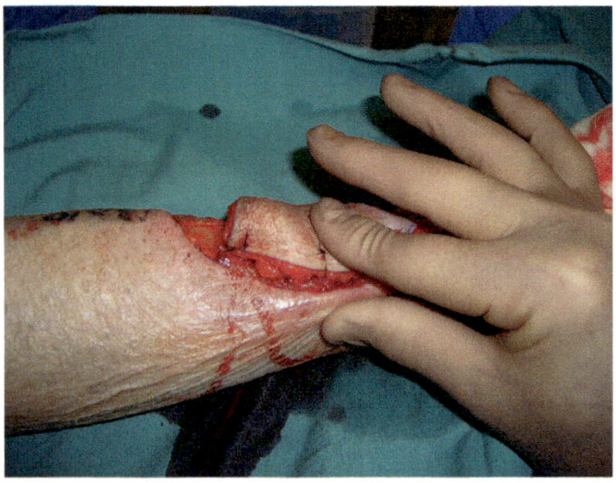

Fig. 3.143 V-Y closures of the loose tissue tails of the keystone flap and reducing the size of any secondary defect prior to mesh grafting. Such closure under tension does exist but this does this does not preclude its use because of the reliability of the hypervascularity, a sympathectomy effect creating the red dot sign facilitating closure under tension

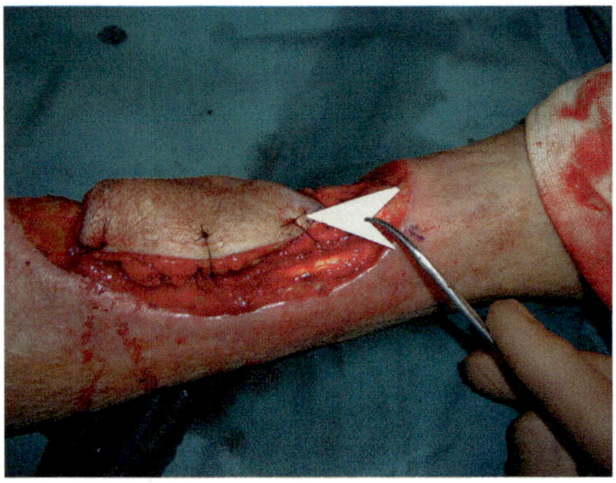

Fig. 3.144 Tensional closure with locking mattress sutures and the red dot sign at the arrow point ensures vascular perfusion and integrity

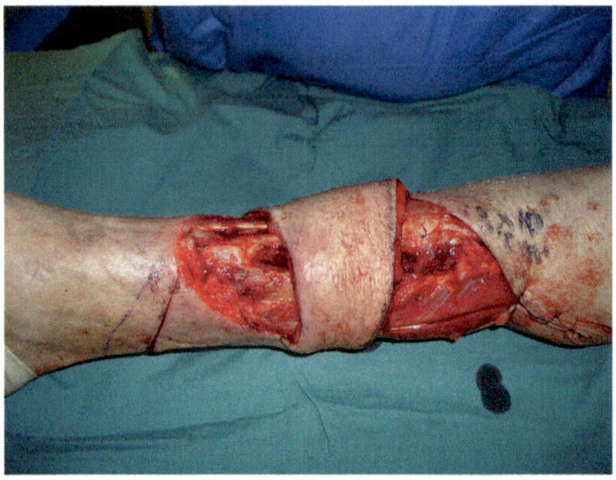

Fig. 3.145 The flap is pink (the sympathectomy effect), and the red dot sign indicates this increased vascular perfusion facilitating healing in association with closure under tension and mesh grafting

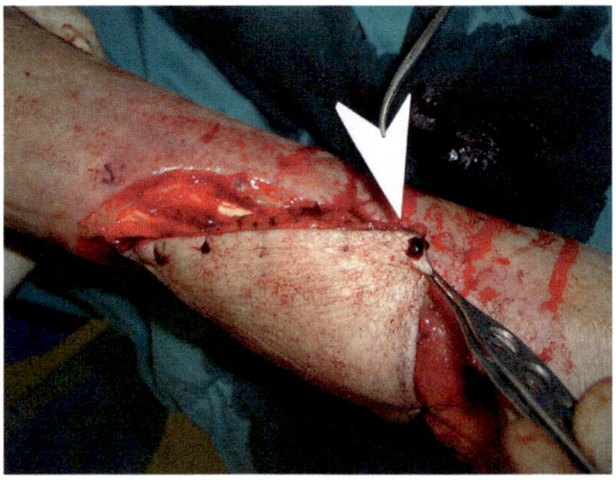

Fig. 3.146 A red dot sign, a little cyanotic in this case but this does not detract from the clinical observation that there is increased vascular flow and this cyanotic phase subsides as time progresses. It is not a contraindication to flap reconstruction and caution

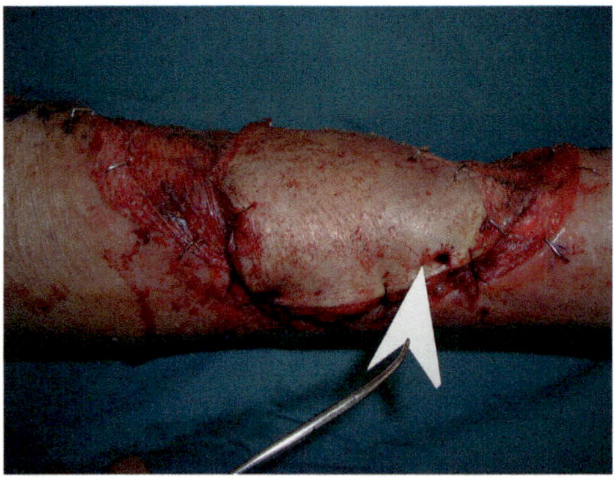

Fig. 3.147 Another view of the same prior to dressings and the completion of mesh grafting ensures wound healing. The red dot sign on the arrow head is a complementary indicator of its vascular integrity

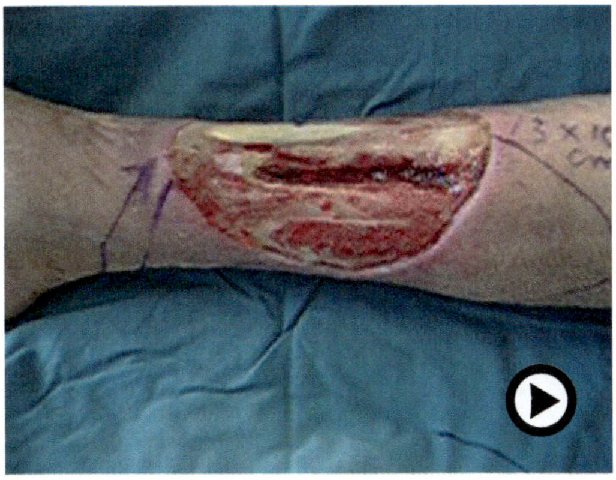

Fig. 3.148 Preoperative appearance with the keystone mark out indicated and based on the L5 dermatome (Video 3.19 Preoperative appearance with the keystone mark out indicated and based on the L5 dermatome) (▶ https://doi.org/10.1007/000-d5b)

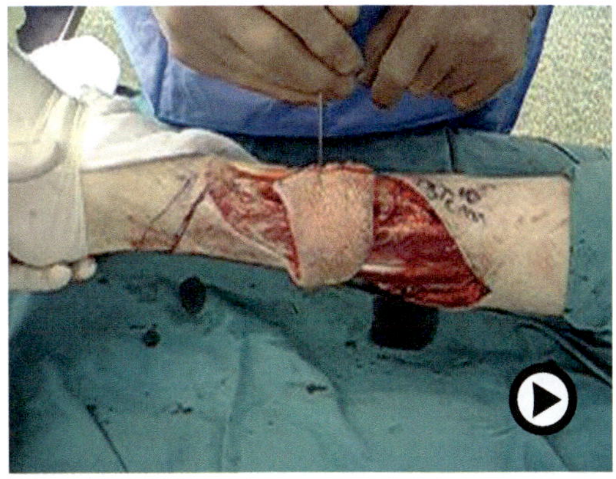

Fig. 3.150 The reliability of the flap being turned at right angles to cover the metal in the depths of the wound (Video 3.21 The reliability of the flap being turned at right angles to cover the metal in the depths of the wound) (▶ https://doi.org/10.1007/000-d5d)

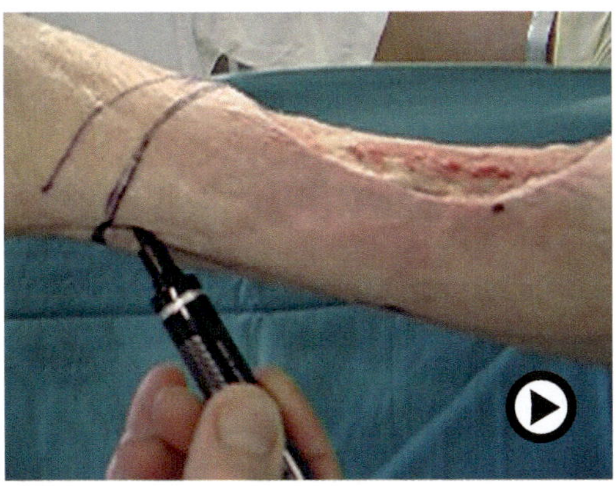

Fig. 3.149 The mark out of the keystone design (Video 3.20 The mark out of the keystone design) (▶ https://doi.org/10.1007/000-d5c)

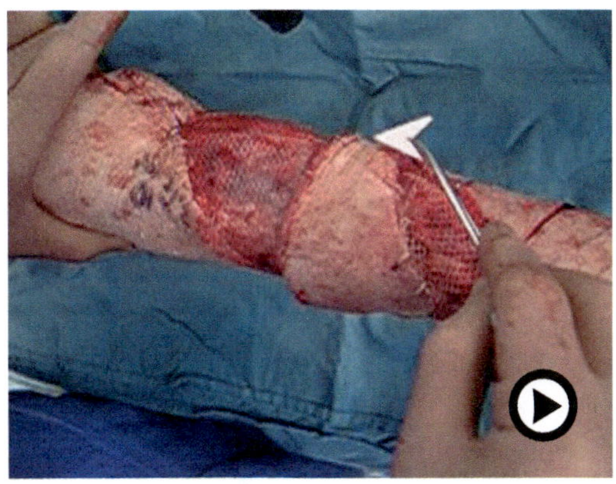

Fig. 3.151 The red dot sign (arterialised blood) on the arrow confirms reliable vascularity and perfusion to ensure healing of the wound to cover the exposed metal (Video 3.22 The red dot sign (arterialised blood) on the arrow confirms reliable vascularity and perfusion to ensure healing of the wound to cover the exposed metal) (▶ https://doi.org/10.1007/000-d5e)

3.1.10 Case 21: Closure of a Post-Traumatic Chronic Osteomylitic Ulcer After 32 Years and 14 Operations Sited Along the Anterior Tibial Line

A Keystone solution to a 32 year old compound tibial fracture in a 45-year-old industrial worker who had undergone 14 procedures over that timeframe to the patient's absolute frustration. He even initially refused my suggestion that I could solve the problem when his previous orthopaedic surgeon said there was no other solution from a reconstructive point of view to salvage his leg apart from an amputation. Hence, one can appreciate this lack of acceptance of another reconstructive option to help salvage the leg, including grafting which had failed repetitively (Figs. 3.152, 3.153, 3.154, 3.155, 3.156, 3.157, 3.158, 3.159, 3.160, 3.161, 3.162, 3.163, 3.164, 3.165, and 3.166).

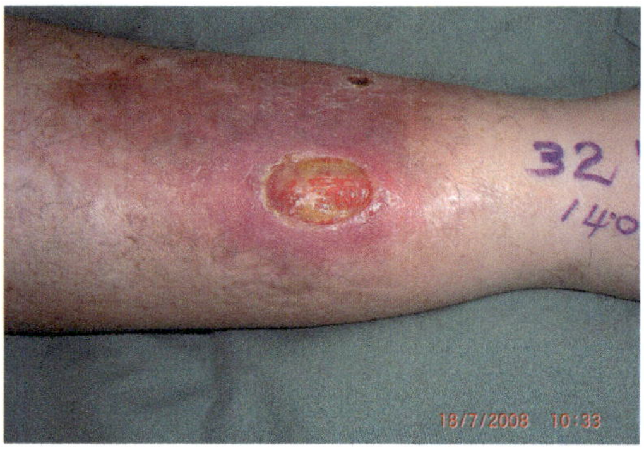

Fig. 3.152 Fourteen operations over 32 years following a compound tibial injury and was told nothing further could be done and the keystone became the solution to this chronic problem to the patient's absolute disbelief initially

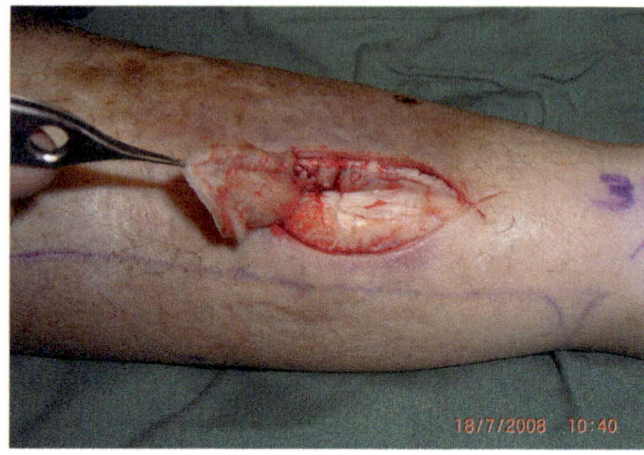

Fig. 3.153 A standard debridement and the thickness of the surrounding cavity help give an indication of the amount of peripheral oedema and swelling which became the bain of the patient's life. He could not stand up at a workbench at work and the restrictions of the oedema meant he always had to buy two pairs of shoes to accommodate the foot on the oedematous lower limb. As part of the debridment procedure, the superficial cortical layers of the tibial bone completed the debridement of the R tibia

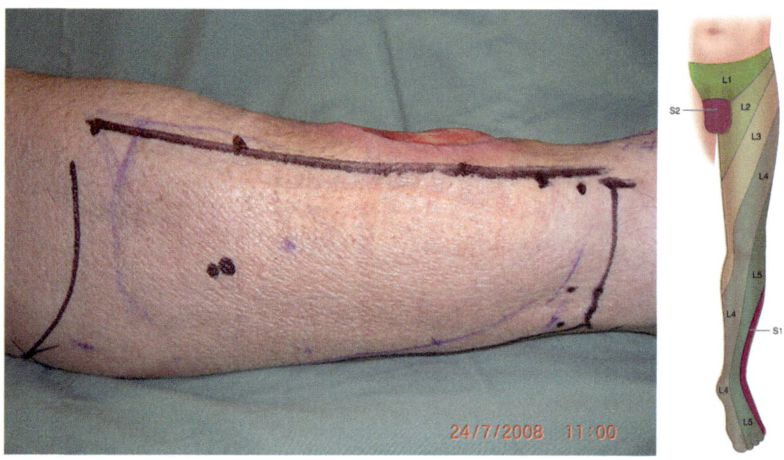

Fig. 3.154 A fasciocutaneous island flap, a design variant of the keystone. Instead of being in an arc, it is longitudinally aligned in the L4 dermatome along the line of the superficial peroneal nerve

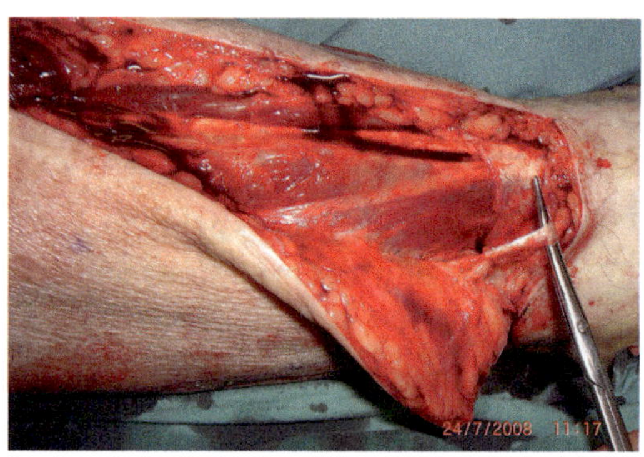

Fig. 3.155 A branch of the superficial peroneal nerve is defined, cleared from the flap to facilitate transposition from the flap base

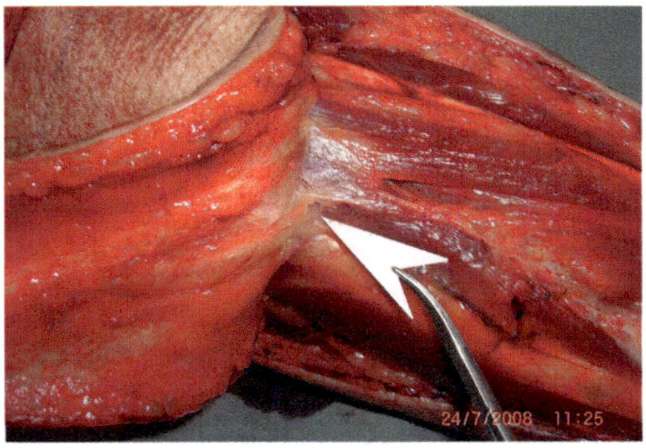

Fig. 3.156 Raising the flap with a fascial base using mainly blunt dissection allows one to define specific perforators from the peroneal compartment which are not individually skeletonised to protect their neural, autonomic, somatic and lymphatic embryological input. In other words, one does not have to skeletonise the perforators to achieve keystone closures. The fasciocutaneous island flap lined with fascia is raised up to the level of the superficial peroneal nerve exit point through the deep fascia in the lateral compartment in the L5 dermatome which becomes the axis of rotation and transposition

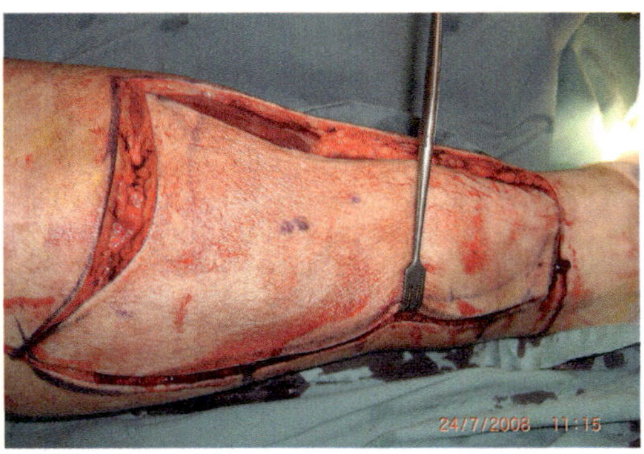

Fig. 3.157 The outline of the island flap and in its proximal extent the incision of the island flap is at the dermal epidermal level, nothing deeper to preserve any longitudinal running structures of a venous or lymphatic nature

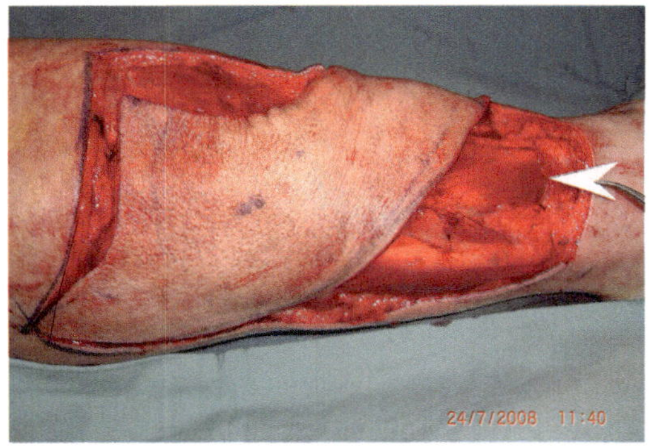

Fig. 3.158 The art of closure—advancement, rotation and transposition of the flap to cover the tibial defect of 32 years duration. Repetitive skin grafts were the inadequate solution to achieve wound cover which was not clinically satisfactory to the patient because of repetitive failures

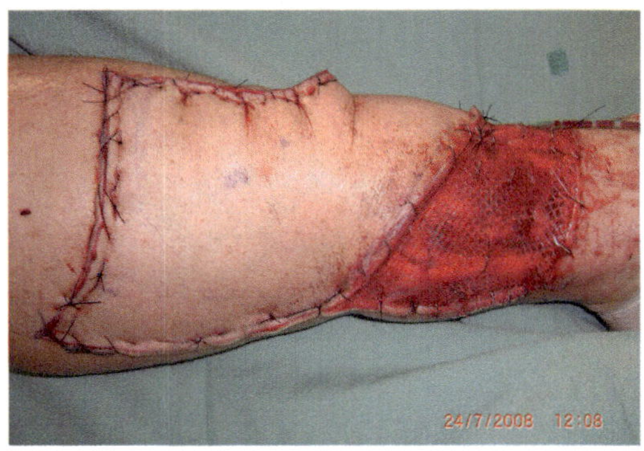

Fig. 3.159 Staged repair with the standard 3-phase locking mattress sutures in their definitive position closing the superior part of the wound and the posterior margin in the wound. The defect above the lateral malleolous has been mesh grafted contributing to the final healing phase

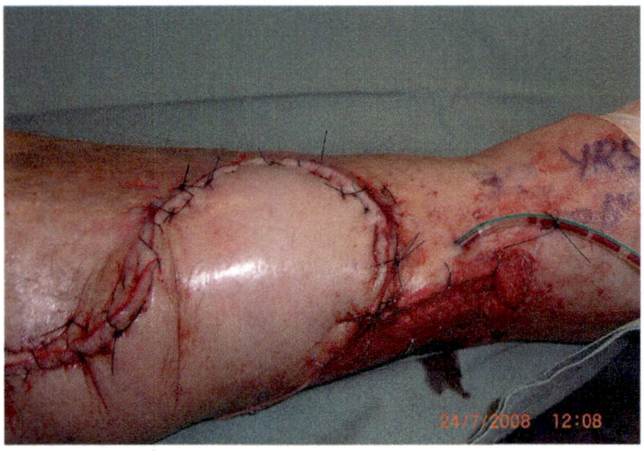

Fig. 3.160 Finished product with Redi-vac drainage under the flap

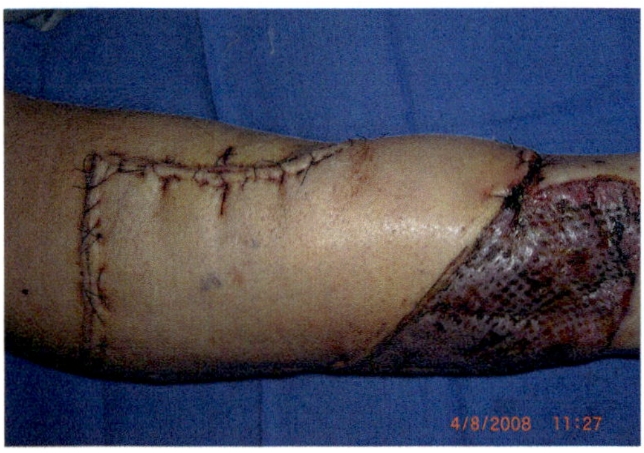

Fig. 3.161 Eleven days postoperative appearance and the healed graft appearance

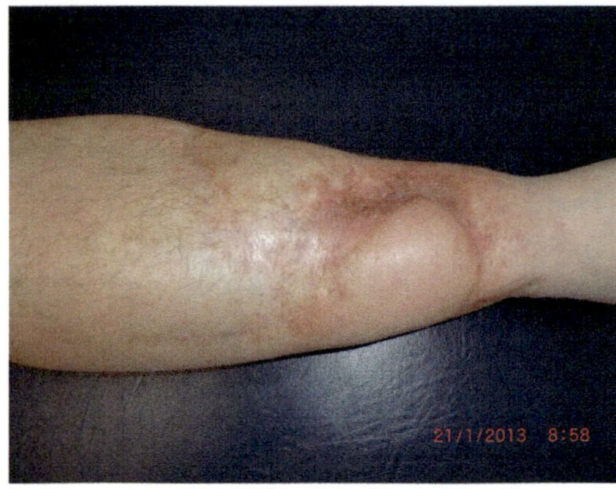

Fig. 3.162 The postoperative appearance years later. A secondary scar revision was completed again using keystone principles to reduce the scar medially. More importantly, an important contribution to oedema management and resolution of the swollen limb were only appreciated lately when the patient admitted his former habit of having to buy 2 sizes of shoes to allow him to walk normally. This has now ceased. Even after a day back at work standing all day swelling was no longer a problem and he reverted back to almost a normal lifestyle for which he was eternally grateful. He smiled gratefully at outpatients during these postoperative reviews knowing he indicated to me he was reluctant to have further surgery previously. He had 14 procedures prior to 2008 before the keystone and was told nothing could be done for his leg barring amputation. Timeframe of keystones from July 2008 to the eventual outcome of January 2013. Other may think doing microvascular lymphovenular anastamosis over an extended period of time is bypassed by the use of the keystone principle where random anastamotic links help to resolve peripheral oedema

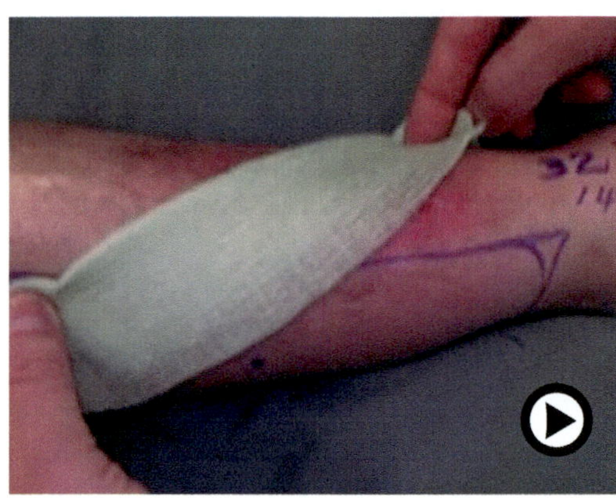

Fig. 3.163 Planned operative procedure (Video 3.23 Planned operative procedure) (▶ https://doi.org/10.1007/000-d5f)

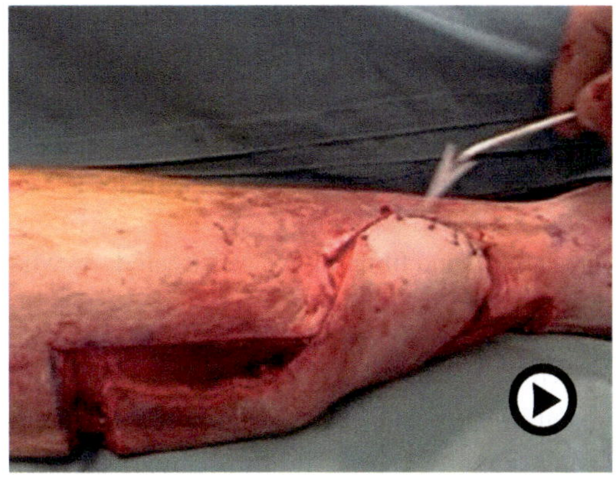

Fig. 3.164 Nearing completion and the perfusion reading to the limits of the flap (white arrow) confirming its potential healing state—not bad after 32 years and 14 procedures (Video 3.24 Nearing completion and the perfusion reading to the limits of the flap (white arrow) confirming its potential healing state—not bad after 32 years and 14 procedures) (▶ https://doi.org/10.1007/000-d5g)

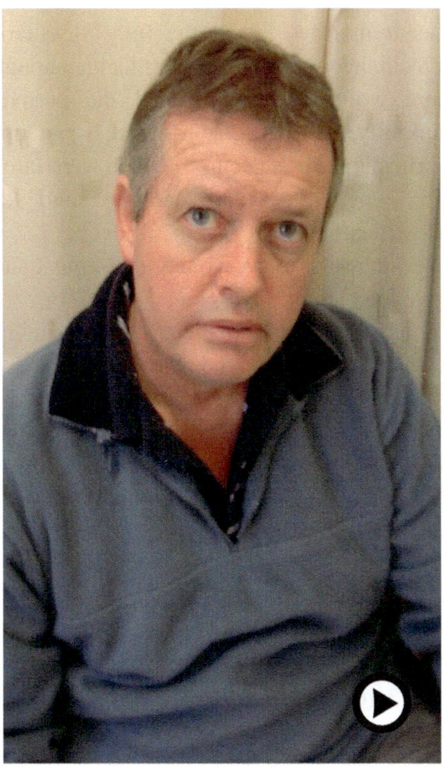

Fig. 3.165 The patient's video response to the keystone solution to the chronic problem. All the swelling of the limb has disappeared, he can stand up at a workbench all day with no problem and he is pleased to be back at work with a single sized pair of shoes and avoiding the use of support stockings (Video 3.25 The patient's video response to the keystone solution to the chronic problem. All the swelling of the limb has disappeared, he can stand up at a workbench all day with no problem and he is pleased to be back at work with a single sized pair of shoes and avoiding the use of support stockings) (▶ https://doi.org/10.1007/000-d5h)

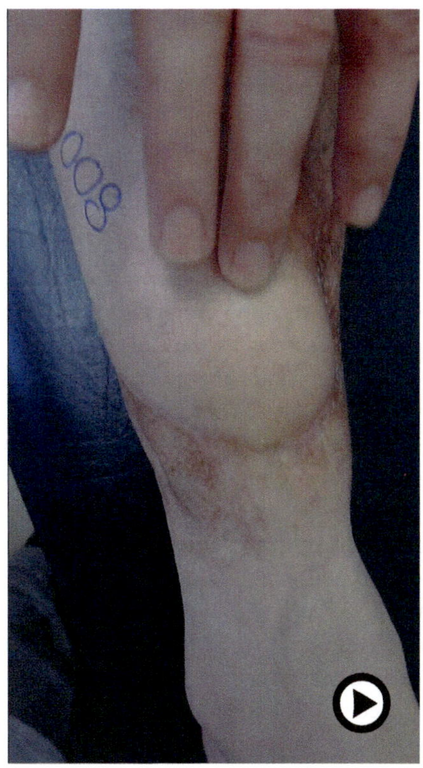

Fig. 3.166 The patient's personal recollections at a subsequent outpatient review of his satisfaction of the outcome, being initially hesitant of further surgery with recovery of sensate tissue and improvement in lymphatic drainage reducing peripheral oedema (Video 3.26 The patient's personal recollections at a subsequent outpatient review of his satisfaction of the outcome, being initially hesitant of further surgery with recovery of sensate tissue and improvement in lymphatic drainage reducing peripheral oedema) (▶ https://doi.org/10.1007/000-d5j)

3.1.11 Case 22: Chronic Osteomyelitis of the Tibia—The Keystone Salvage Avoiding Amputation After Three Microsurgical Failures

This compound tibial injury was treated, by what was then the current trend in surgical reconstruction for orthopaedic problems of the lower limb.

All three microvascular free flaps—lat dorsi, radial forearm and gracilis—all failed in spite of being done by experts in the field in what was regarded at the time that Melbourne was the microsurgical 'mecca' of the world. With Ian Taylor's contribution doing the first published free flap and the Bernie O'Brien Institute establishing a microsurgical research centre at St Vincent's Hospital.

One of the contacts knew of my success in the use of fasciocutaneous island flaps in lower limb reconstructions which was the metamorphosis for stage 1 before the development of the keystone design.

This chronic granulating wound became a problem for the patient emotionally, and the option of a lower limb amputation for a former jogger was regarded as the only option. It was one of the registrars in the unit at the Alfred Hospital where he was ensconced and it was suggested by Mr. David Hunter-Smith that he can be transferred to my unit at The Western General Hospital for a fasciocutaneous island flap because of my expertise. It was done in association with the orthopaedic unit, including Mr. Ray Crowe. Standard orthopaedic debridement was done enlarging the dead space but removing infective elements as a precaution. Dead space must be eliminated in all surgical procedures to bypass that focus of fluid accumulation becoming the focus of an infected development. The skin alignment of the incision mark out is determined by the non-tensional onlay of the flap so any element of tension can be avoided so as not to create additional vascular problems. To eliminate the dead space, an iliac crest bone graft was used in spite of superficial osteomyelitis. The fibular malunion stabilised the lower limb. This bone grafting into an infected wound caused criticism but there is one surgical factor that became evident, dead space creates problems and must be eliminated. Hence the radical decision to do a bone graft in infected tissue.

As time developed and with Redi-vac drains installed when the debridement extended to the adjacent marrow cavity, the fully vascularised fasciocutaneous island flap was viable enough to ensure wound healing around the periphery. Thankfully, the Redi-vac worked, some minor superficial necrosis occurred which went into the drain tube for future culture and drug sensitivities.

Yes, it healed to everyone's amazement and to relieve the patient's symptoms.

A subsequent debridement of the wound margin was completed and the videos show the extent of successful rehabilitation back to a normal full walking gait, stable enough to dispense with the crutches.

The patient was discharged and successfully returned to his exercise jogging habits doing long distance running with no adverse sequelae developing. He returned to work at Australia Post delivering mail and was forever grateful he had 2 legs to use on his delivery bicycle (Figs. 3.167, 3.168, 3.169, 3.170, 3.171, 3.172, 3.173, 3.174, 3.175, 3.176, 3.177, 3.178, 3.179, 3.180, 3.181, 3.182, 3.183, 3.184, 3.185, and 3.186).

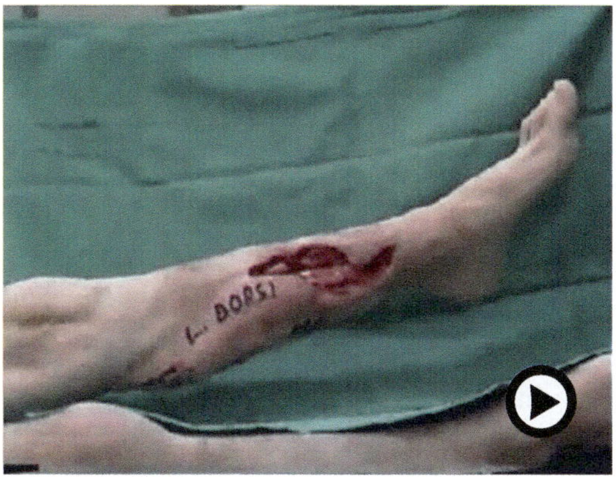

Fig. 3.167 The dead space defect osteomyelitis cavity of the tibia following 3 failed microvascular free flaps because the basic surgical principle of filling dead space was not respected and I used an iliac bone crest, some would say questionably to fill the space and with VAC drainage healing was achieved contravening the principles of bone graft in the presence of infection but the suction drain tube saved the day. In other words, dead space is a killer (Video 3.27 The dead space defect osteomylitic cavity of the tibia following 3 failed microvascular free flaps because the basic surgical principle of filling dead space was not respected and I used an iliac bone crest, some would say questionably to fill the space and with VAC drainage healing was achieved contravening the principles of bone graft in the presence of infection but the suction drain tube saved the day. In other words, dead space is a killer) (▶ https://doi.org/10.1007/000-d5k)

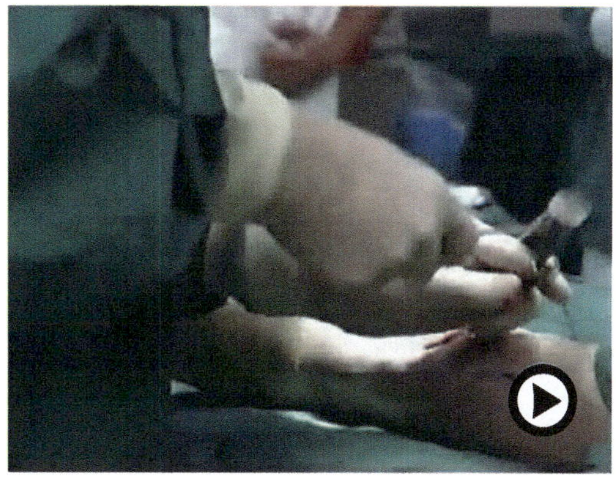

Fig. 3.169 After an initial skin debridement, further bony debridement occurred before the FCIF staged reconstruction (Video 3.29 After an initial skin debridement further bony debridement occurred before the FCIF staged reconstruction) (▶ https://doi.org/10.1007/000-d5n)

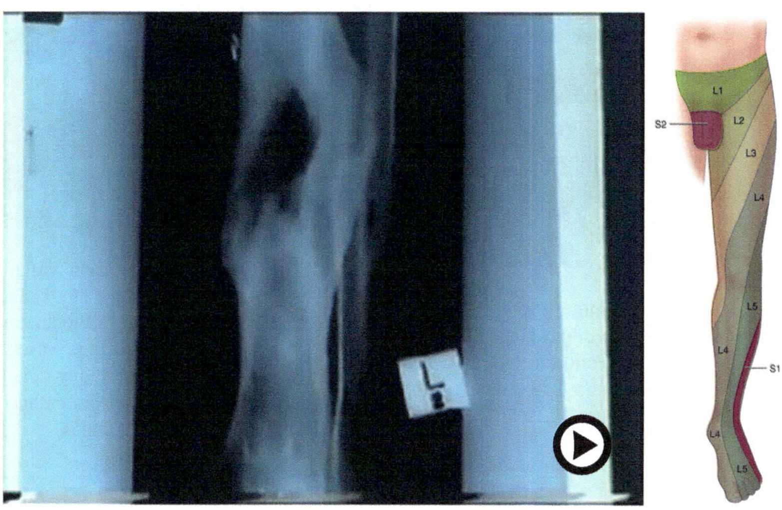

Fig. 3.168 A 55-year-old male with a compound tibial fracture. Three microvascular free flaps all failed—lat dorsi free flap, radial forearm free flap and gracilis. The 8 × 6 cm osteomyelitic cavity is revealed with its malunion and crateriform defect on X-ray (Video 3.28 A 55 year old male with a compound tibial fracture. Three microvascular free flaps all failed—Lat dorsi free flap, radial forearm free flap and Gracilis. The 8 × 6 cm osteomyelitic cavity is revealed with its malunion and cratiform defect on X-ray) (▶ https://doi.org/10.1007/000-d5m)

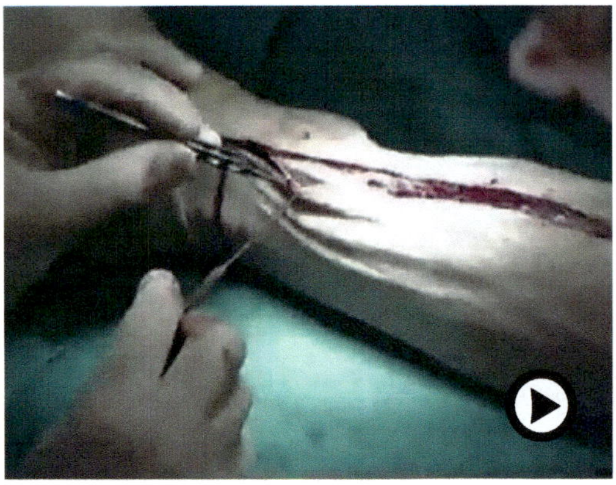

Fig. 3.170 The mark out of the fasciocutaneous island flap based on the superficial peroneal nerve dermatome of lateral calf of L5 and the debridement of the defect margin throughout. Please note that any scars in situ in the FCIF is not a vascular impedance factor initiating flap necrosis—part of regular plastic surgical teaching (Video 3.30 The mark out of the fascio cutaneous island flap based on the superficial peroneal nerve dermatome of lateral calf of L5 and the debridement of the defect margin throughout. Please note that any scars insitu in the FCIF is not a vascular impedance factor initiating flap necrosis—part of regular plastic surgical teaching) (▶ https://doi.org/10.1007/000-d5p)

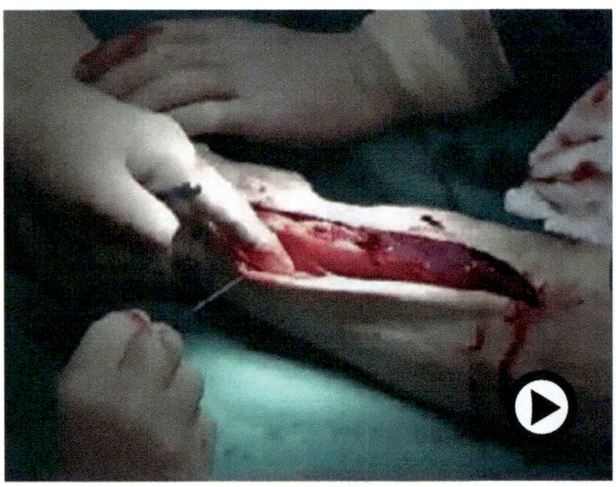

Fig. 3.171 Blunt dissection technique using the index finger to minimise any sharp dissection damage to any perforators (Video 3.31 Blunt dissection technique using the index finger to minimise any sharp dissection damage to any perforators) (▶ https://doi.org/10.1007/000-d5q)

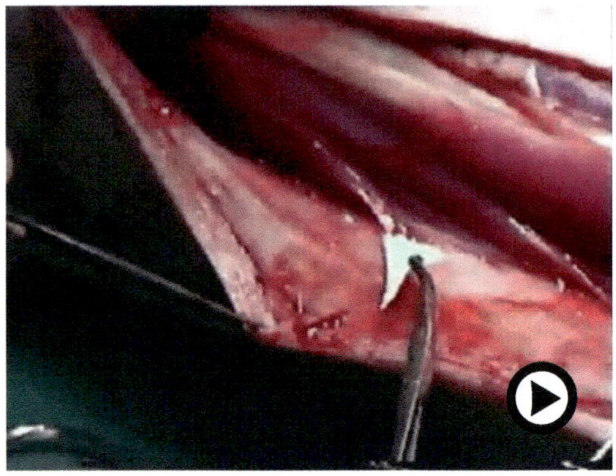

Fig. 3.172 Indicating the superficial peroneal nerve (white arrow marker) which initially was divided to facilitate the flap transfer with subsequent cases. This was removed from the deep fascial attachment to retain distal foot innervation (Video 3.32 Indicating the superficial peroneal nerve (white arrow marker) which initially was divided to facilitate the flap transfer with subsequent cases. This was removed from the deep fascial attachment to retain distal foot innervation) (▶ https://doi.org/10.1007/000-d5r)

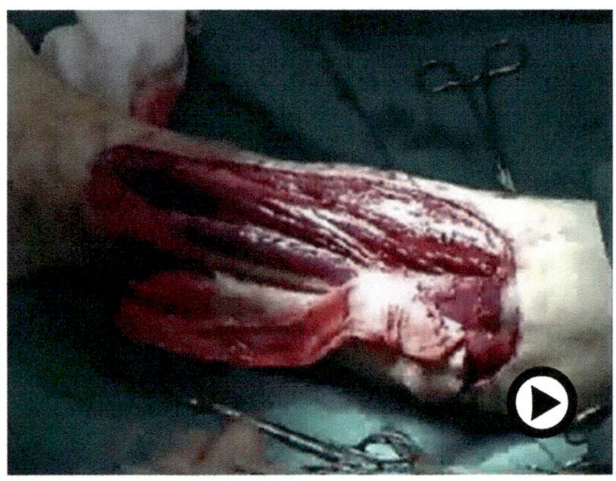

Fig. 3.173 The subfascial fascia vascular points were sealed with micro clips to save any coagulative necrosis on the deep surface of this fasciocutaneous island flap (Video 3.33 The subfascial fascia vascular points were sealed with micro clips to save any coagulative necrosis on the deep surface of this fascio cutaneous island flap) (▶ https://doi.org/10.1007/000-d5s)

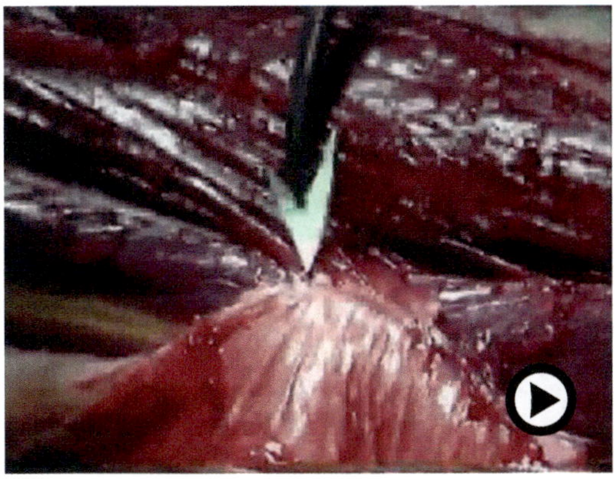

Fig. 3.174 Microcirculation focal points before haemostasis (Video 3.34 Microcirculation focal points before haemostasis) (▶ https://doi.org/10.1007/000-d5t)

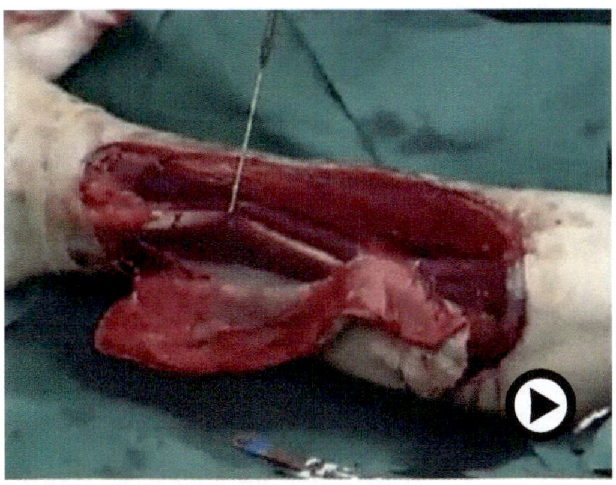

Fig. 3.175 The fasciocutaneous flap raised and the superficial peroneal nerve is seen emerging from the distal limit (Video 3.35 The fascio cutaneous flap raised and the superficial peroneal nerve is seen emerging from the distal limit) (▶ https://doi.org/10.1007/000-d5v)

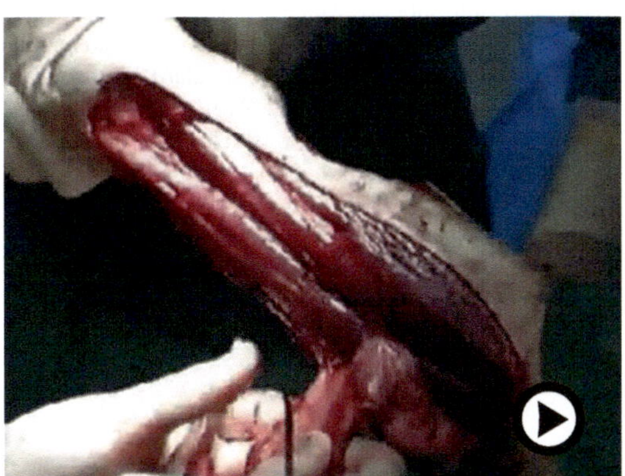

Fig. 3.176 Operative sequence (Video 3.36 Operative sequence) (▶ https://doi.org/10.1007/000-d5w)

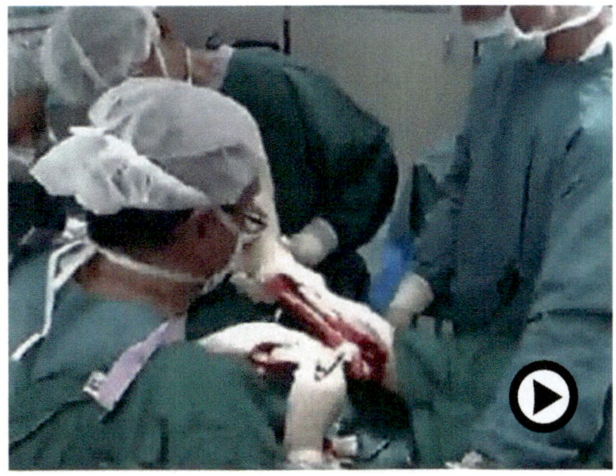

Fig. 3.177 Operative sequence (Video 3.37 Operative sequence) (▶ https://doi.org/10.1007/000-d5x)

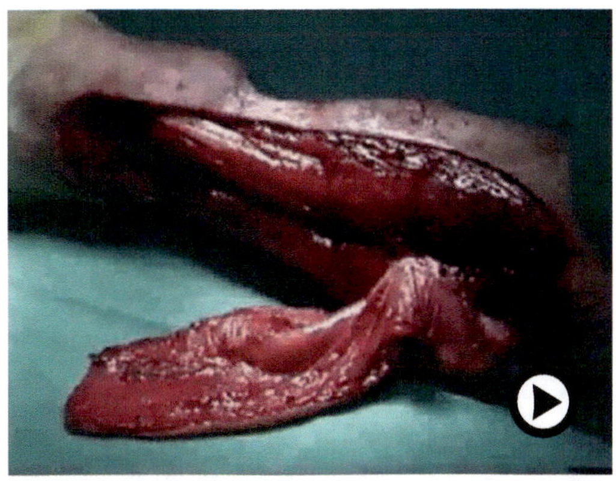

Fig. 3.178 The flap elevated to cover the compound tibial fracture site (Video 3.38 The flap elevated to cover the compound tibial fracture site) (▶ https://doi.org/10.1007/000-d5y)

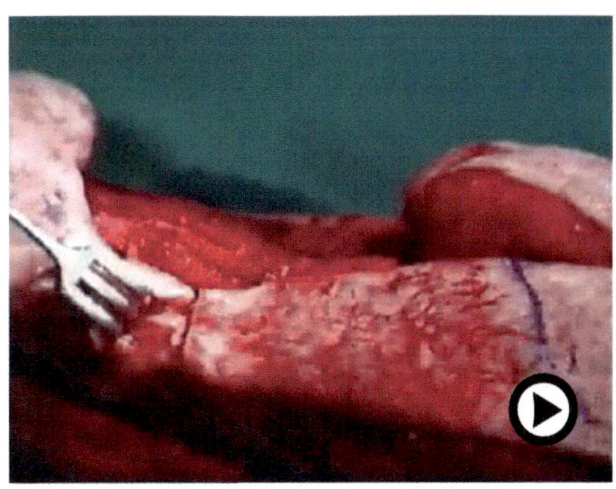

Fig. 3.179 Debriding the tissue and de-epithelialising a section to fit underneath the bridge of surrounding tissue over the bony defect (Video 3.39 Debriding the tissue and de-epithelialising a section to fit underneath the bridge of surrounding tissue over the bony defect) (▶ https://doi.org/10.1007/000-d5z)

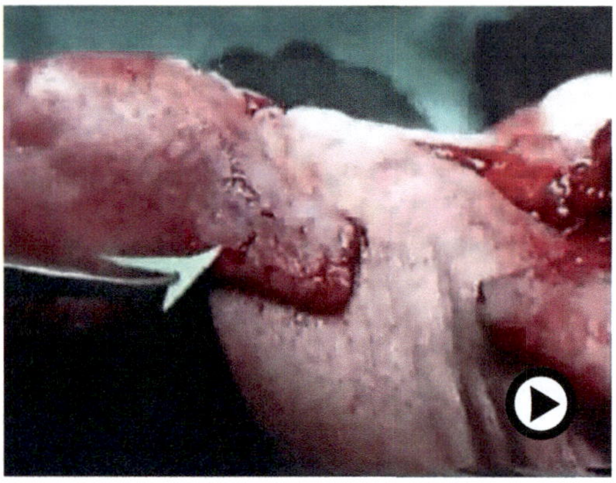

Fig. 3.180 The flap underneath the bridge of tissue which has been aligned to fit in with the flap margin to subsequently cover the defect and the bone graft (Video 3.40 The flap underneath the bridge of tissue which has been aligned to fit in with the flap margin to subsequently cover the defect and the bone graft) (▶ https://doi.org/10.1007/000-d60)

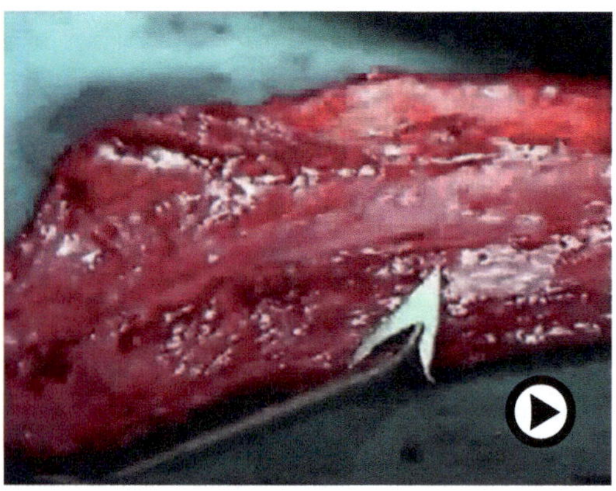

Fig. 3.181 The deep surface of the flap with the arrow showing areas of micro perfusion and oozing which are sealed with Weck clips to save any necrosis from diathermy (Video 3.41 The deep surface of the flap with the arrow showing areas of micro perfusion and oozing which are sealed with weck clips to save any necrosis from diathermy) (▶ https://doi.org/10.1007/000-d61)

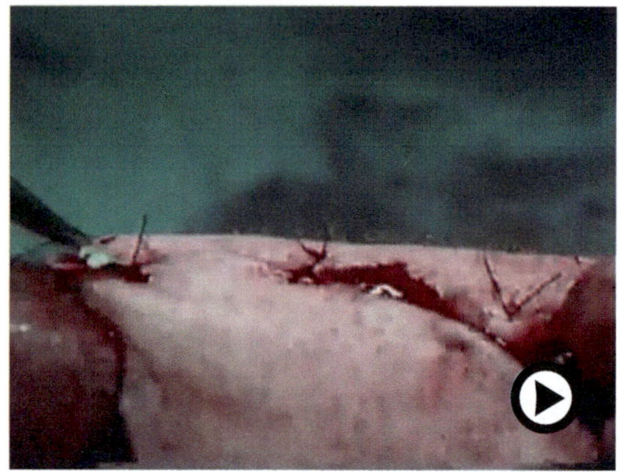

Fig. 3.182 The red dot sign at the suture points of the locking mattress sutures confirming intact vascular perfusion (Video 3.42 The red dot sign at the suture points of the locking mattress sutures confirming intact vascular perfusion) (▶ https://doi.org/10.1007/000-d62)

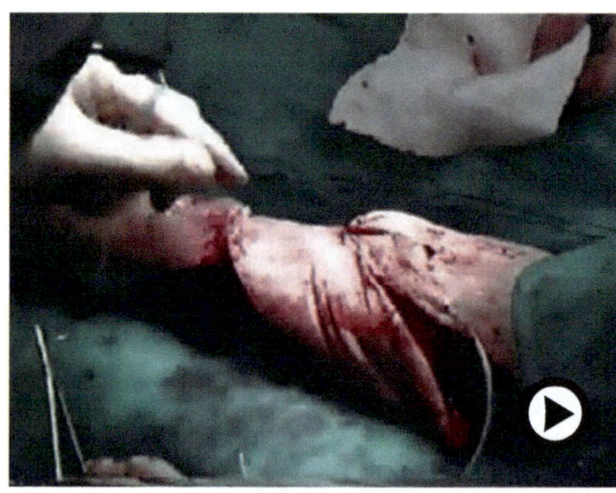

Fig. 3.183 Closing the wound after debridement using the standard 3-phase locking nylon mattress sutures with Redi-vac drain support which produced no more than 10–15 ml of serosanguinous ooze (Video 3.43 Closing the wound after debridement using the standard 3-phase locking nylon mattress sutures with Redi-vac drain support which produced no more than 10–15 ml of serosanguinous ooze) (▶ https://doi.org/10.1007/000-d63)

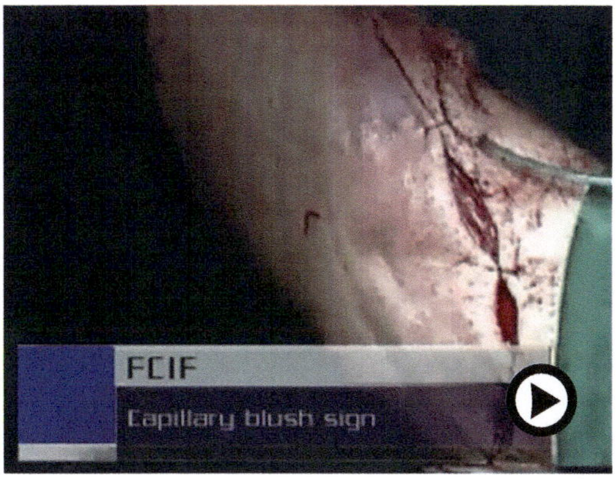

Fig. 3.184 Staged completion of wound closure using the standard 3-phase locking nylon mattress sutures, full viability in the flap with the vascular flare (Video 3.44 Staged completion of wound closure using the standard 3-phase locking nylon mattress sutures, full viability in the flap with the vascular flare) (▶ https://doi.org/10.1007/000-d64)

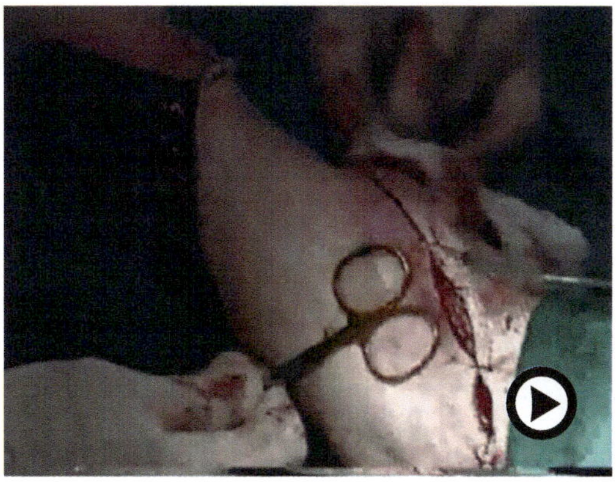

Fig. 3.185 Prior to completion, the scissors are used as a compression test to assess the vascular integrity when pressure is applied to the suprafascial and infrafascial vascular support. This is before the wound is completely repaired (Video 3.45 Prior to completion the scissors are used as a compression test to assess the vascular integrity when pressure is applied to the suprafascial and infrafascial vascular support. This is before the wound is completely repaired) (▶ https://doi.org/10.1007/000-d65)

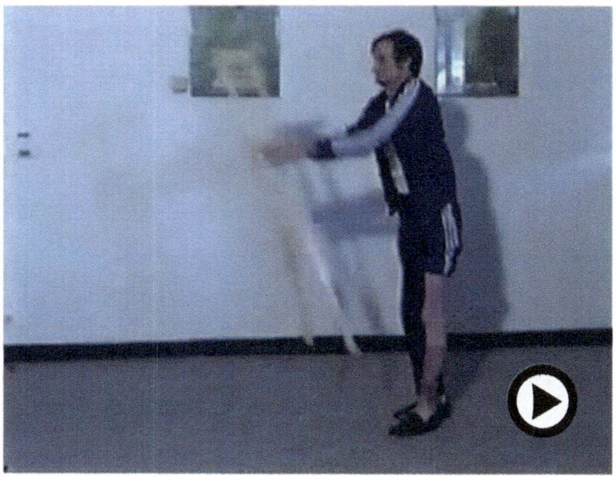

Fig. 3.186 His return to normal walking and dispensing with the crutches, something he had not done for months. Full weight bearing at 14 days. No infection evident. The proposed below knee amputation was avoided, and the patient was back to jogging in 3 months. The fasciocutaneous island flap, the basis of the keystone concept was the salvage procedure in allowing the patient to return to normal lifestyle (Video 3.46 His return to normal walking and dispensing with the crutches, something he had not done for months. Full weight bearing at 14 days. No infection evident. The proposed below knee amputation was avoided and the patient was back to jogging in 3 months. The fascio cutaneous island flap, the basis of the keystone concept was the salvage procedure in allowing the patient to return to normal lifestyle) (▶ https://doi.org/10.1007/000-d66)

3.1.12 Case 23: Compound Tibia and the ORIF Closure

Again the same principles apply that the fasciocutaneous island flap based on random perforators from the vicinity of the superficial peroneal nerve without defining and stripping the perforators so they are somatic, autonomic, neural and lymphatic support based on embryology as they are all outlined withint the dermatomal precincts (Figs. 3.187, 3.188, 3.189, 3.190, and 3.191).

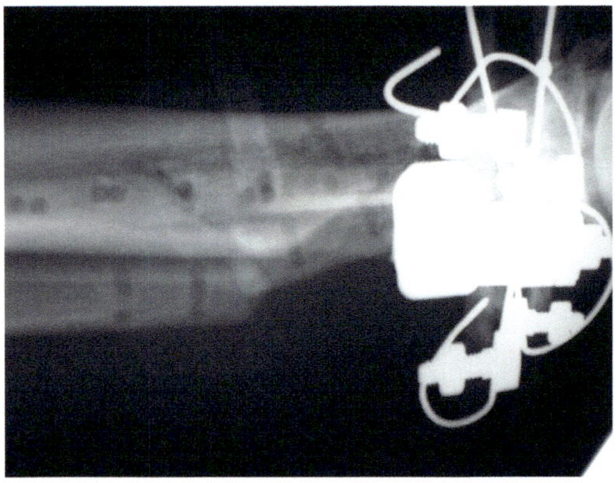

Fig. 3.187 With the evident ORIF stabilising metalware on X-ray

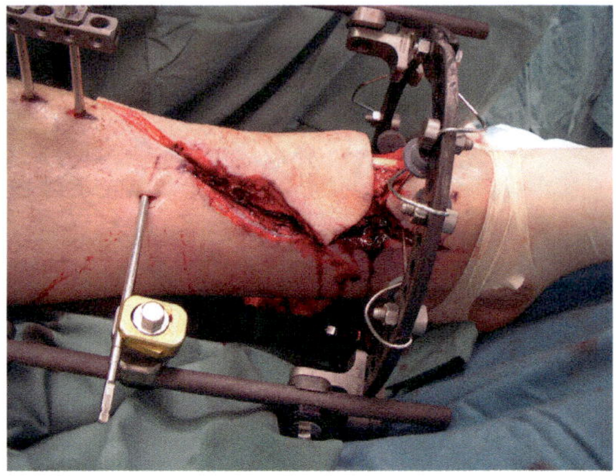

Fig. 3.189 Staging the reconstruction prior to definitive insertion to cover the defect

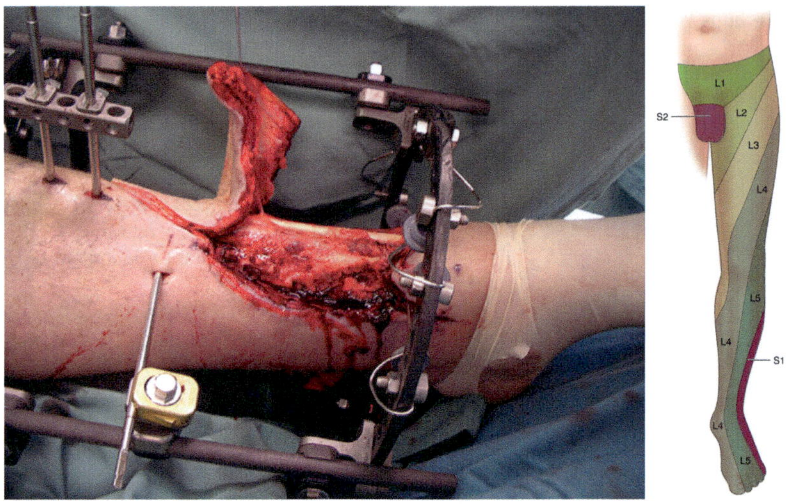

Fig. 3.188 Raising the fasciocutaneous keystone island flap along the L4 dermatome with the external fixateur in situ to cover the chronic open wound and the osteomyelitic cavity

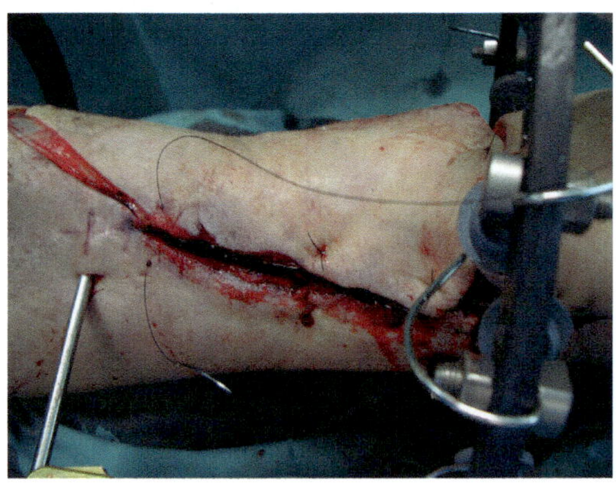

Fig. 3.190 The red dot sign is confirmatory evidence of the hypervascular perfusion

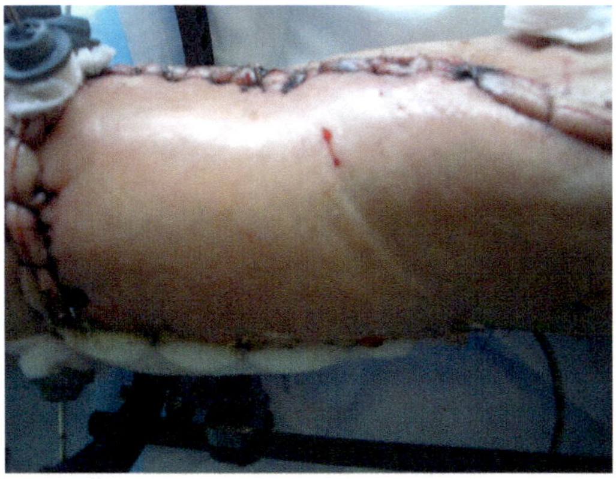

Fig. 3.191 The reliable vascularity does not preclude the use of Redi-vac suction drainage which is usually precluded in microsurgical procedures

3.1.13 Case 24: Compound Tibia (Figs. 3.192, 3.193, 3.194, 3.195, 3.196, 3.197, 3.198, 3.199, 3.200, 3.201, and 3.202)

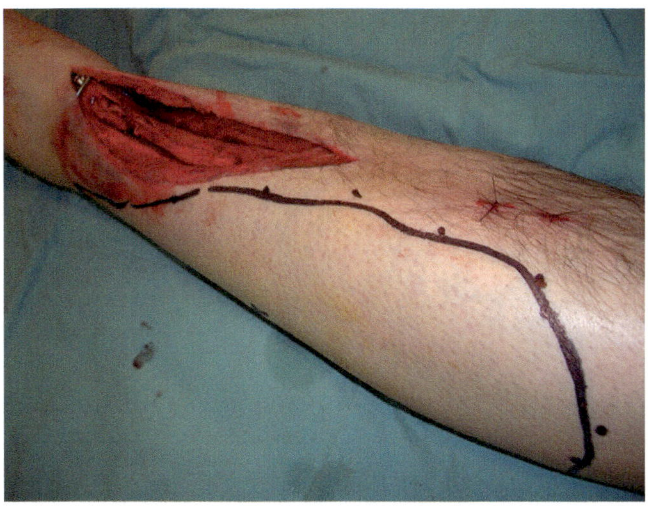

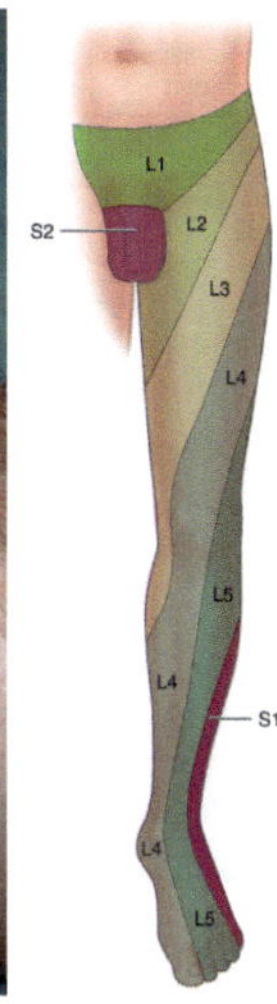

Fig. 3.192 The fascial lined fasciocutaneous island flap along the L5 dermatome is marked out and proximally the skin and subcutaneous tissue is divided to ensure the island flap design has been maintained

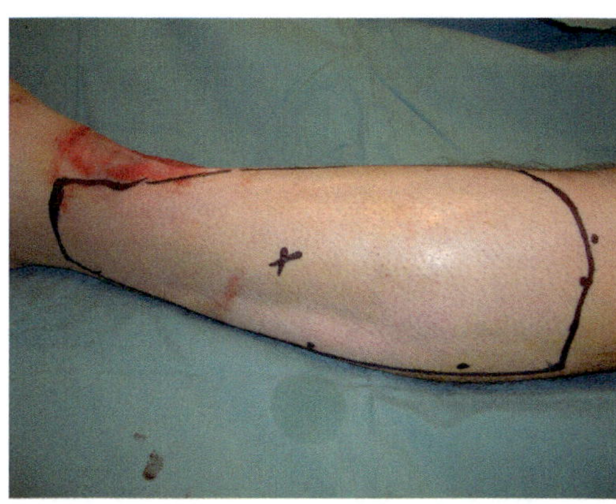

Fig. 3.193 Advancement, rotation and transposition of the fascial lined island flap covers the compound fracture—why create an island by dividing the proximal epidermis where it is hypothesised this contributes to the sympathectomy effect, increasing vascular flow to produce the red dot sign clinically and the vascular flare, an indicator of potential success

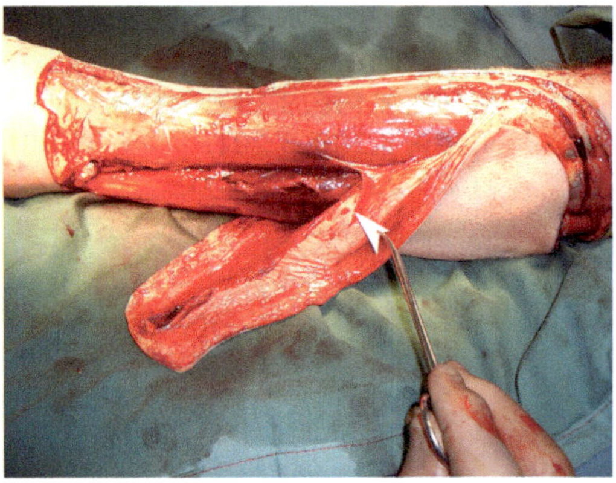

Fig. 3.194 The deep surface of the fascial lined flap is indicated by the arrow and the microperforators which may be divided need haemostatic closure with clips and not diathermy. The deeper perforator above the white arrow is the lifeline for flap viability

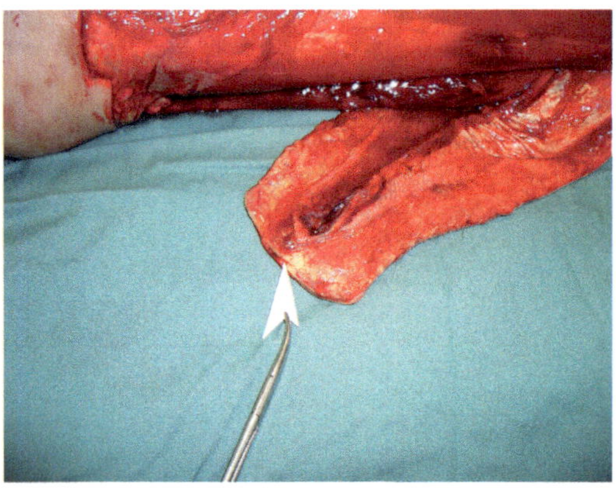

Fig. 3.195 The fully raised island flap with distal subdermal perfusion indicated at the arrowhead

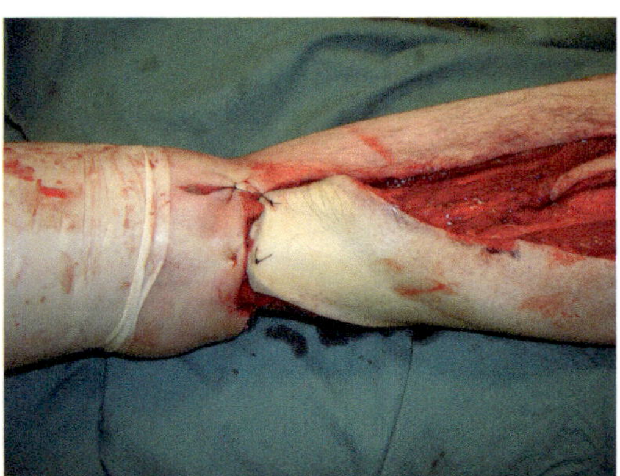

Fig. 3.196 Closure of the compound tibia

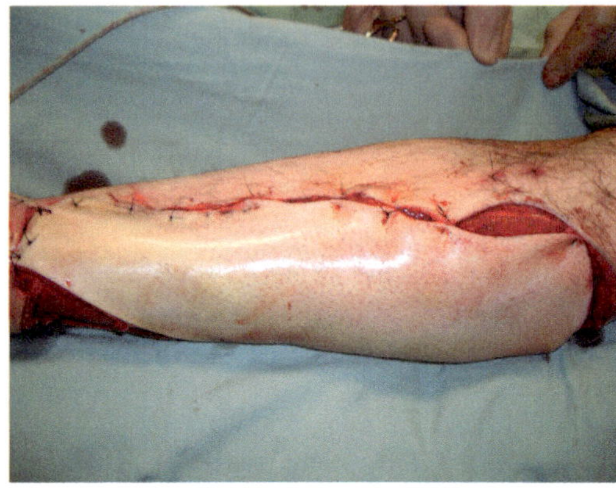

Fig. 3.197 Full vascular perfusion under the following conditions aligned along the L5 dermatome, fascial lined island flap which is rotated and advanced over the exposed bone. On the release of tourniquet, these delayed sympathectomy observations become evident and the hyperperfusion phase usually starts at the 15 min interval

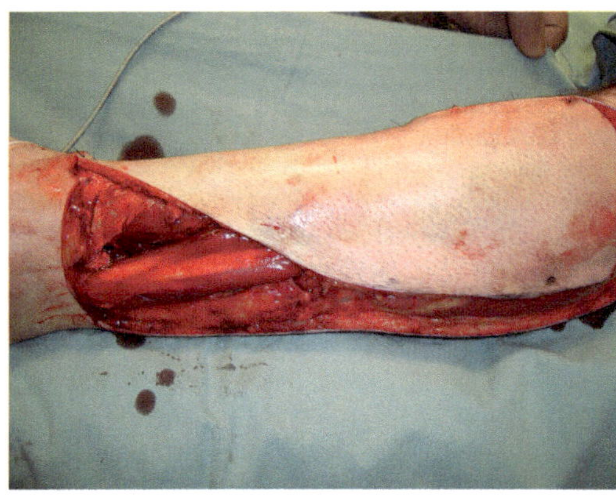

Fig. 3.198 Prior to mesh grafting of the secondary defects

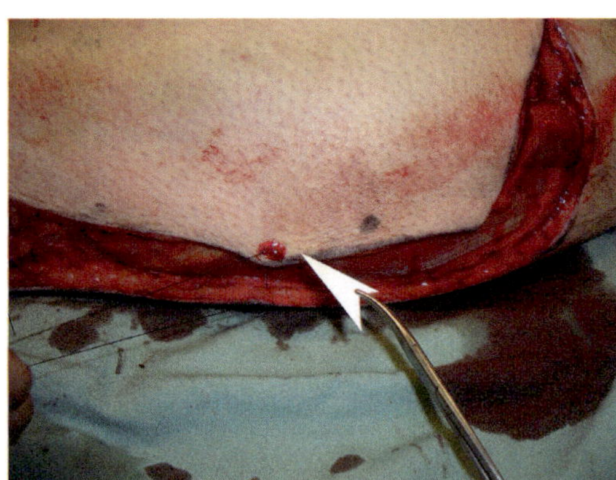

Fig. 3.199 Another reliable sign of viability with the red dot sign on the arrow point. It is a great consolation when doing reconstruction to know these perfusion dynamics are evident and continue to manifest as the procedure continues

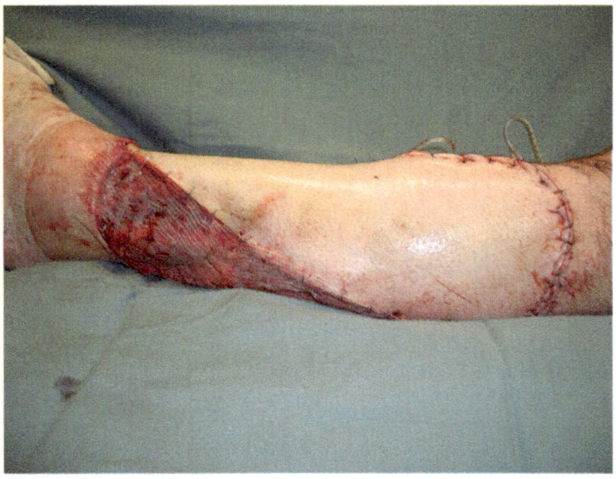

Fig. 3.200 On closure with the secondary defect mesh grafted and the 3-phase single layered suture technique is employed: Locking mattress sutures at the points of maximum tension and spaced throughout the delineations of the flap limit to ensure bony cover. Ordinary locking sutures align the subcutaneous tissue before one attempts the epidermal seal using a continuous nylon technique which creates eversion and a good aesthetic outcome. Vicryl sutures in layered closure are dispensed with as this 3-phase nylon technique provides an alternative for layered closure. In wound management to cut the nylon continuous intermittently is a means of eliminating any transverse suture marks over a 2–3 week period. The tension sutures may need to stay in 3 weeks to prevent margin distraction and possible wound opening

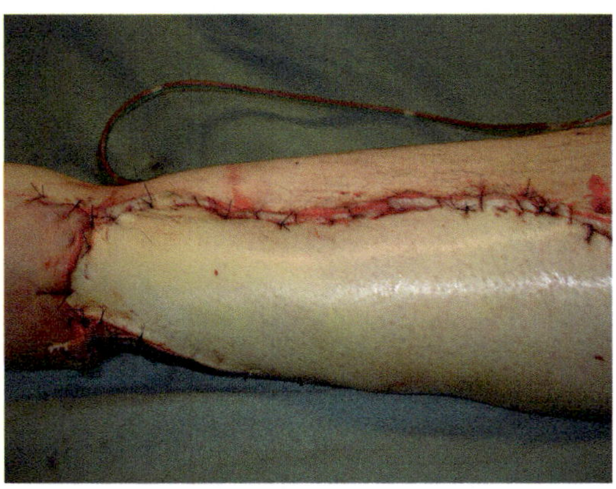

Fig. 3.201 Note the absence of any embarrassment from the point of view of flap vascularity. There is no delineation indicating lines of vascular impedance because the suprafascial and infrafascial perfusion are in continuity contributing to vascular integrity

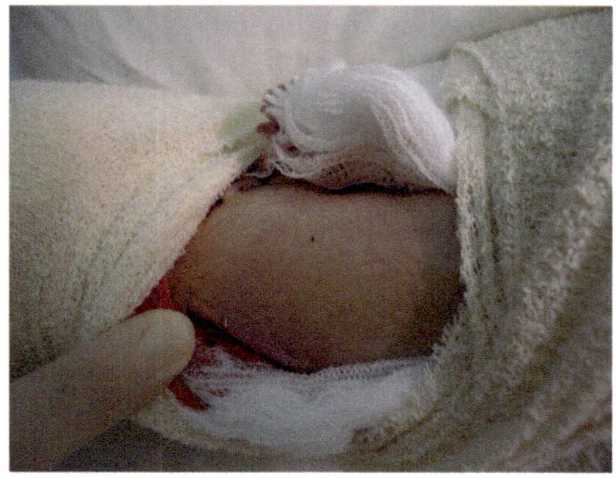

Fig. 3.202 An image of the flap in the postoperative phase

3.1.14 Case 25: Gustilo II B Compound Tibial Fracture (Figs. 3.203, 3.204, 3.205, 3.206, 3.207, 3.208, 3.209, 3.210, 3.211, 3.212, 3.213, and 3.214)

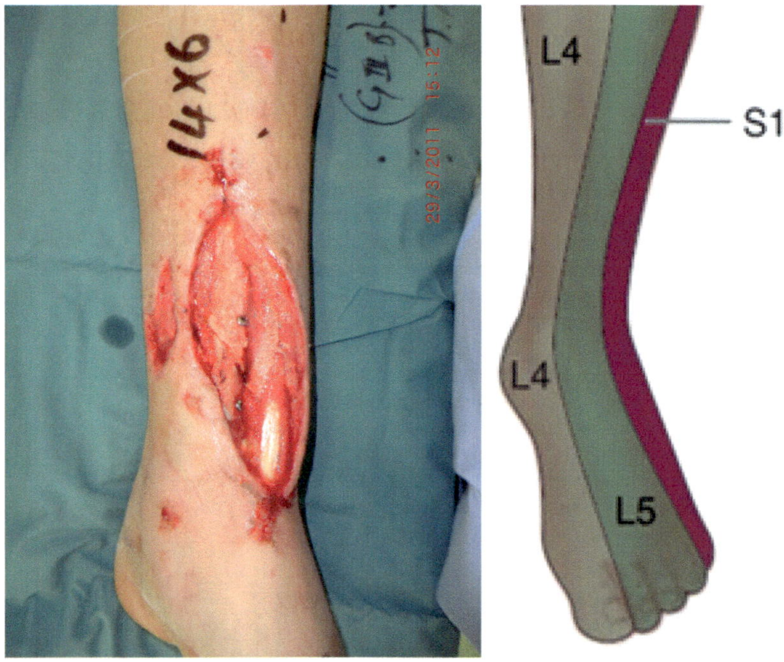

Fig. 3.203 Gustilo classification GRADE II B. Open fracture with wound size 14 × 6 cm with extensive soft tissue loss and periosteal stripping and bone damage after the ORIF. Preoperatively, these wounds usually are associated with massive contamination. Soft tissue coverage using the keystone design but using the principles of a fasciocutaneous island flap reconstruction

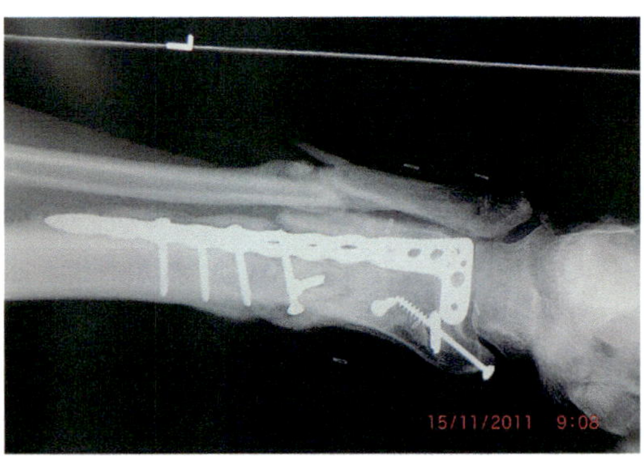

Fig. 3.204 X-ray appearance of the ORIF for the GRADE II B compound fracture of the tibia

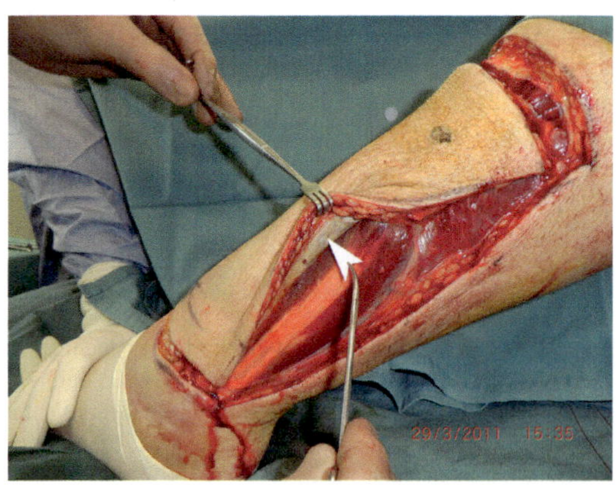

Fig. 3.205 Raising of the fasciocutaneous island flap indicating its fascial base. A total island of the integument which contributes to its hypervascularity possibly due to a sympathectomy effect hypothetically

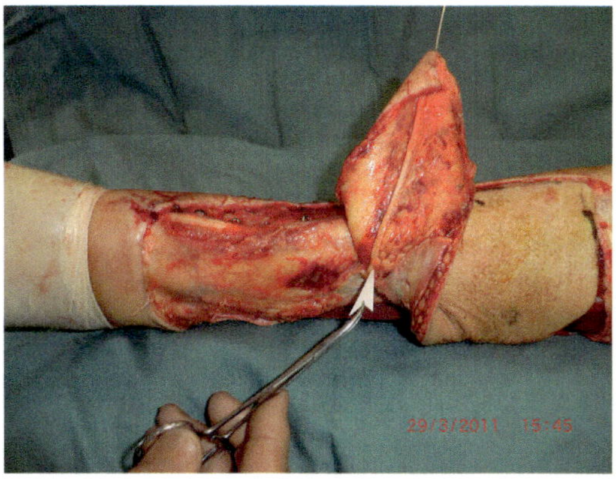

Fig. 3.206 The fasciocutaneous island flap is raised with the neurovascular support indicated by the white arrow marker sitting in the L5 dermatome and employing the superficial peroneal nerve and its neurovascular support axes. All haemostatic points are clipped to prevent vascular necrosis which will always cause extensive obliterative necrosis at the subdermal level

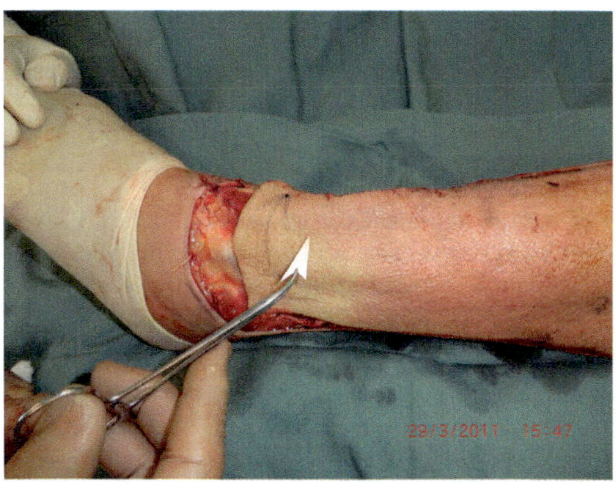

Fig. 3.207 The white arrow points to show the area of developing vascular hyperaemia following the release of the tourniquet indicating the more dominant vascular supply to this flap is proximal rather than distal to ensure the flow is intact. This hyperperfusion stage reflects the hypothetical effect of a sympathectomy which contribute enormously to vascular perfusion ensuring healthy healing and avoids flap necrosis in cases designed under this keystone principle, modifying the fasciocutaneous island flap design

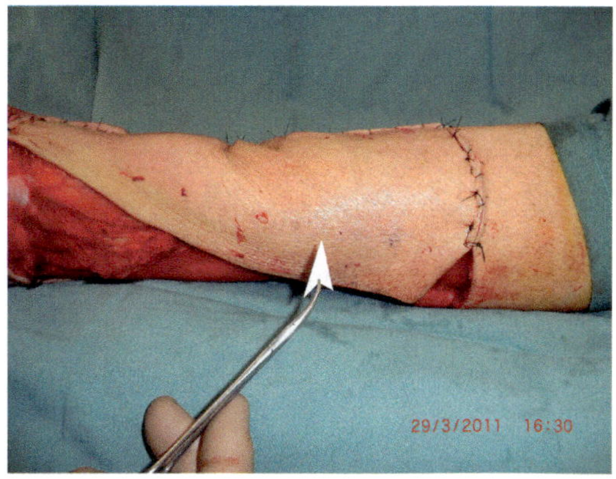

Fig. 3.208 The red flare of the island flap design is indicated by the white arrow marker. The island mark out is quite obvious. The secondary defect is to be closed using a fenestrated graft. Reactive hyperaemia (arrowed) is the basis of the red dot sign where bleeding occurs more on the suture points on the flap than into the surrounding tissue. A sympathectomy effect is the hypothesis behind these vascular dynamics and hyperaemic activity. It takes 15–20 min before this manifestation becomes evident and one can only harken back to ones earlier vascular experiences in training when a lumbar sympathectomy produced the pink foot the following morning, evident on ward rounds

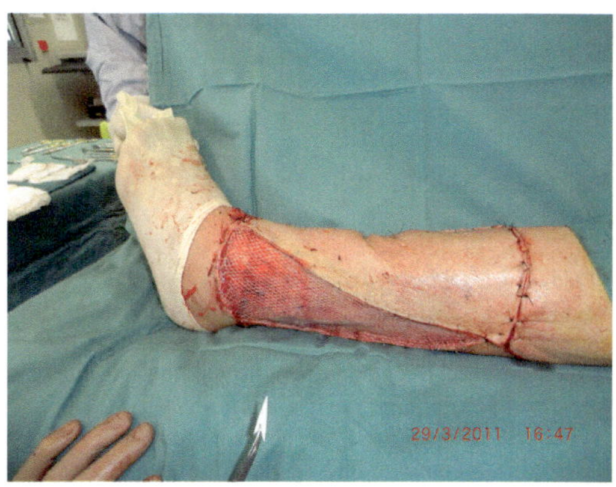

Fig. 3.209 Mesh grafting of the secondary defect completes the procedure in 90 min. The wound repair using the 3-phase nylon suture technique is employed whereby: locking mattress sutures complete the closure at the points of maximum tension which must stay in at least 3 weeks plus. Following this, further wound alignment using locking mattress sutures reduces the size of the secondary defect and helps to complete the closure. A continuous nylon epidermal seal is used where appropriate along the line of the graft. Staples are avoided

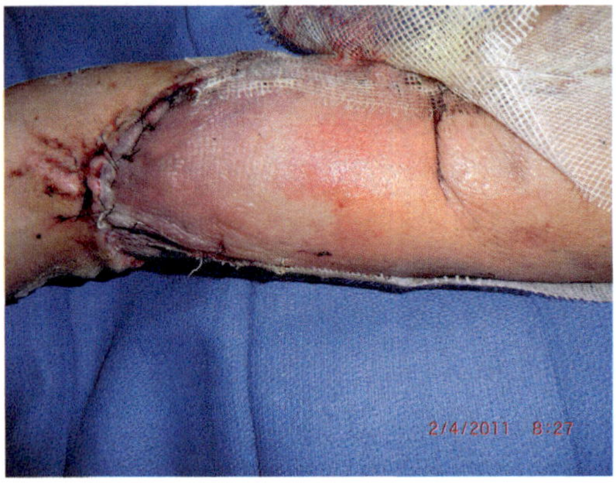

Fig. 3.210 Epidermal venous stasis distally at 5 days. This resolved without complications. One must warn patients about smoking primary or secondary as this will certainly impede the vascular recovery

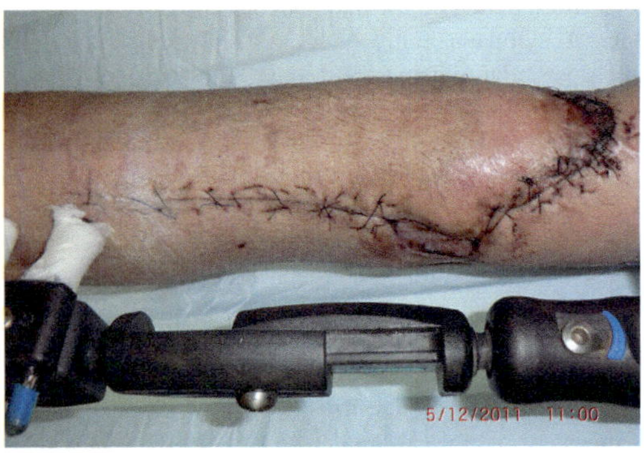

Fig. 3.211 With the ORIF in situ

Fig. 3.212 Appearance at 2 months of the healed wound. The P.A.C.E.S. acronym for the keystone is all exemplified. Fascial lining of the keystone contributes to the resolution of oedema. The fascial lining of the keystone contributes to the healing of the periosteal repair, and this avoids postoperative non-union developing, a common finding in microvascular free flaps. Note the oedema of the flap over the ankle is resolving—compare this with the following 6 month image when the healing is fully completed and oedema resolved and pain free adding to the patient's satisfaction

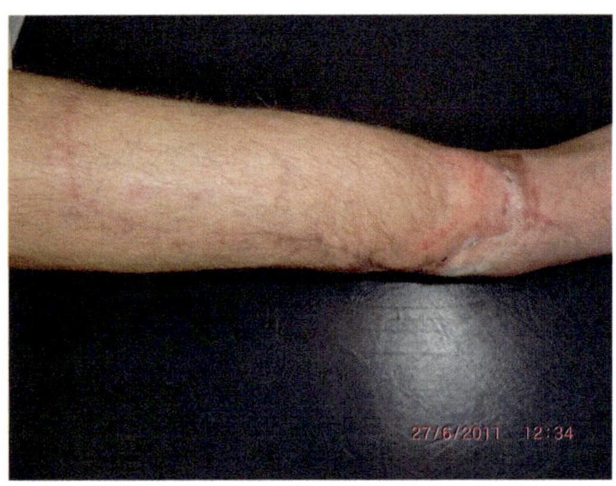

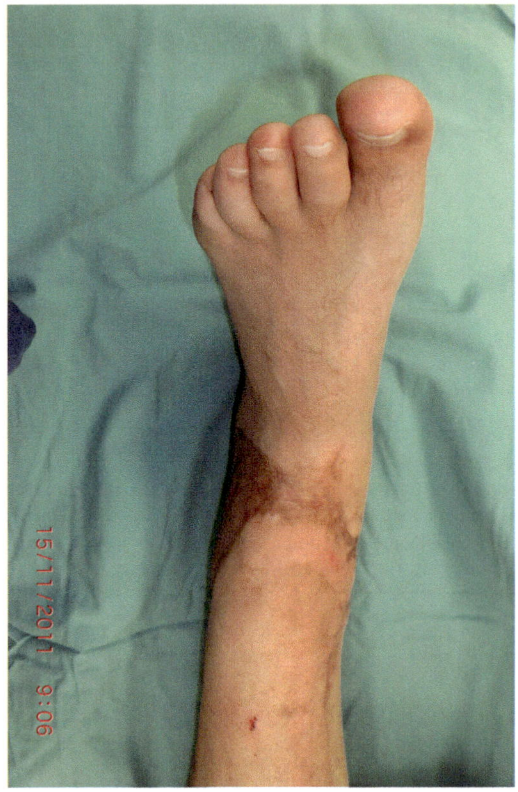

Fig. 3.213 Appearance at 6 months fully healed. Note there is no ring oedema with the wearing of socks which means any peripheral oedema is now subsided

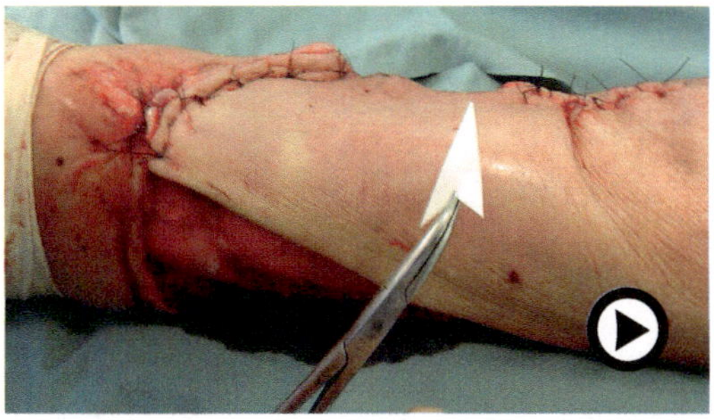

Fig. 3.214 Operative sequence showing the completed insertion and the vascular flare evident in such flaps distally indicating reliable vascular perfusion and consistent with sound healing. No cyanotic lines of tension are evident (Video 3.47 Operative sequence showing the completed insertion and the vascular flare evident in such flaps distally indicating reliable vascular perfusion and consistent with sound healing. No cyanotic lines of tension are evident) (▶ https://doi.org/10.1007/000-d67)

3.1.15 Case 26: Ankle Joint Exposure and Lateral Malleolus Fracture After ORIF (Figs. 3.215, 3.216, 3.217, 3.218, 3.219, 3.220, 3.221, and 3.222)

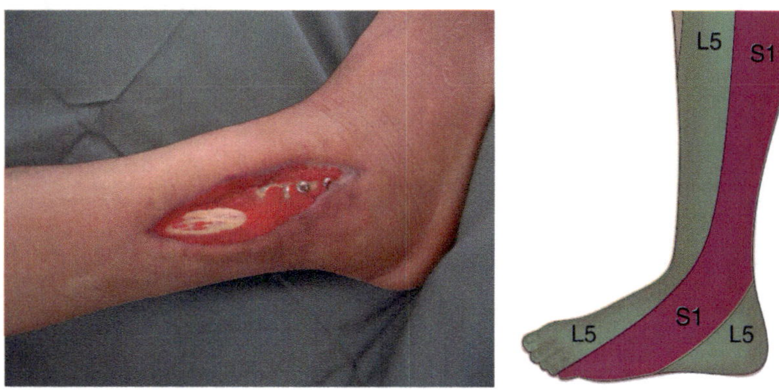

Fig. 3.215 Wound breakdown after ORIF over the lateral malleolus and the bone exposure was solved with the keystone design down the lateral ankle area of the S1 dermatome and its intact sural nerve (reproduced with permission from [2])

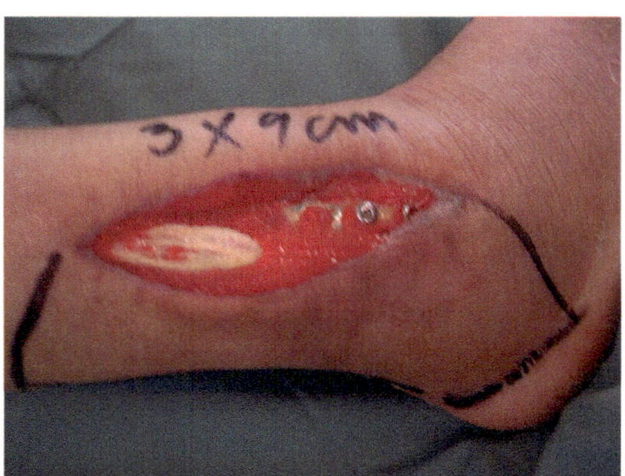

Fig. 3.216 The 3 × 9 cm defect with exposed bone and the keystone flap mark out and dimensions are noted

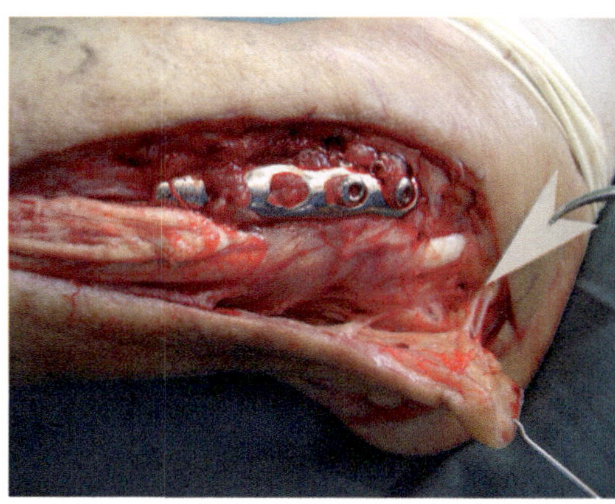

Fig. 3.217 Further debridement around the ankle and malleolus and the fine filamentous perforators are preserved with blunt dissection and teased so that flap mobility is no restricted and the bone and metal are covered. These micro filamentous perforators (white arrowed) are not microscopically defined nor used for microsurgical purposes

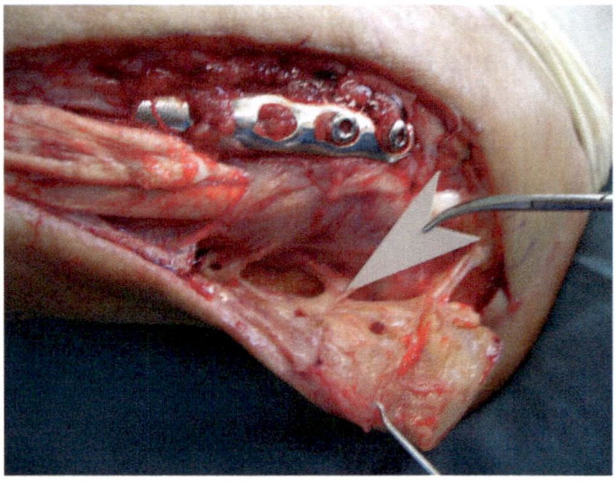

Fig. 3.218 More of the same

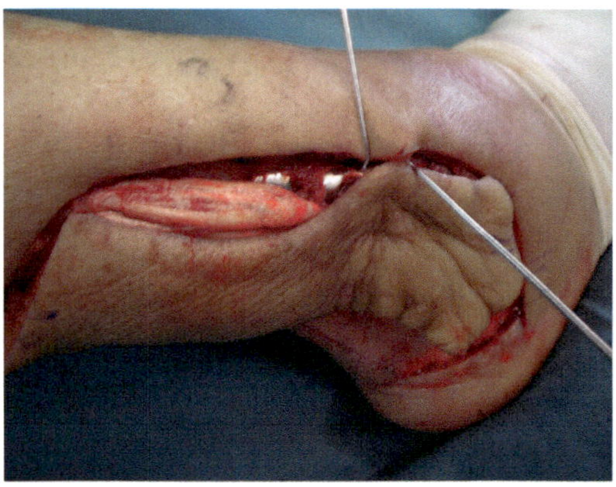

Fig. 3.219 Closure under tension and the locking mattress suture stabilises this definitive position

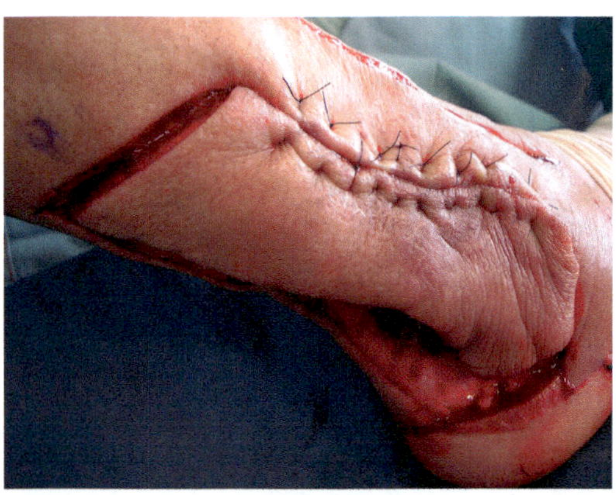

Fig. 3.220 Closing in stages where the interrupted locking mattress suture is arrowed which closes the wound at points of tension. Other mattress sutures complete the alignment of tissue repair before a continuous nylon gives epidermal seal

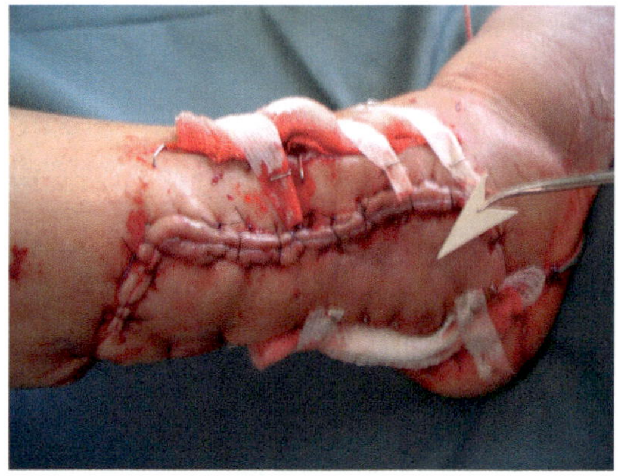

Fig. 3.221 Note the hyperaemia in the flap below the white arrow marker and this was the site of the perforator which was located in the initial blunt dissection in Fig. 3.217

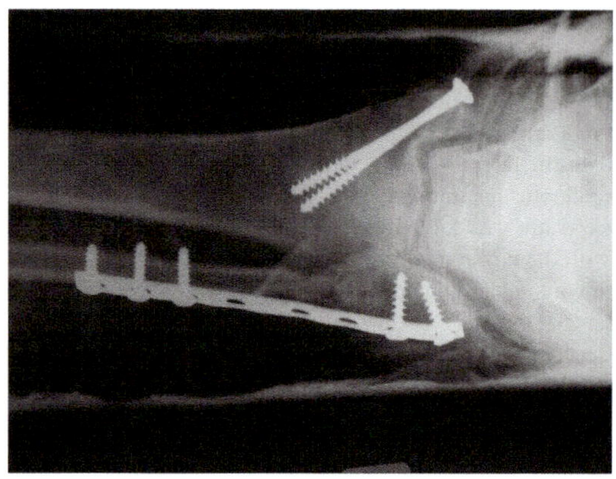

Fig. 3.222 X-ray image of ORIF showing the malleolar stabilisation and the 8 hole plate used to stabilise the fractured fibula

3.1.16 Case 27: Dorsum of the Foot—Soft Tissue Defects Closed with the Keystone in the Same Manner as this Melanoma Defect—the Same Principles Apply for Soft Tissue Closure Over an ORIF of the Metatarsal

This melanoma clinical sequence can be used as the baseline when any metatarsal fractures are closed and stabilised with mini plate procedures and the keystone closure is illustrated for any soft tissue defect and can be applied to both, i.e. closure of soft tissue defects on the dorsum of the foot. Even though K-wires can be used for longitudinal alignment, this provides a more satisfactory alternative without having K-wires protruding through the toes which often lead to inaccurate alignment (Figs. 3.223, 3.224, and 3.225).

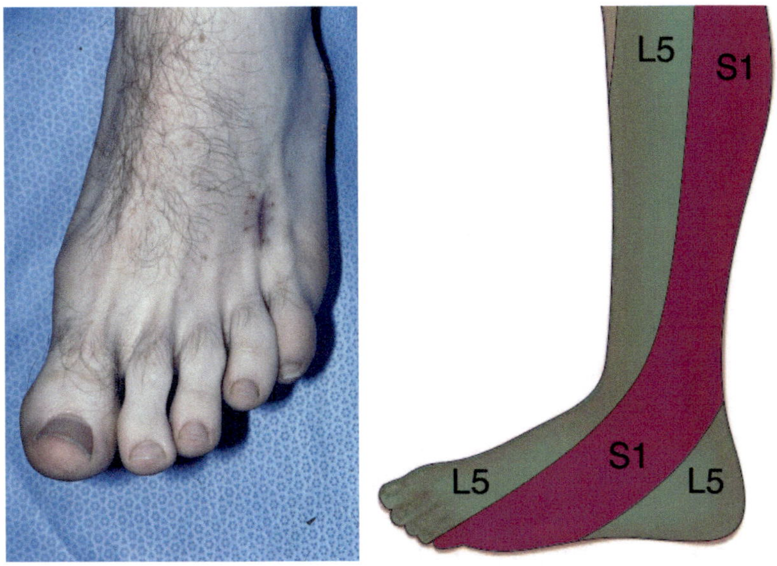

Fig. 3.223 Biopsy site on dorsum of the foot along the alignment of the 5th metatarsal in the L5 dermatome

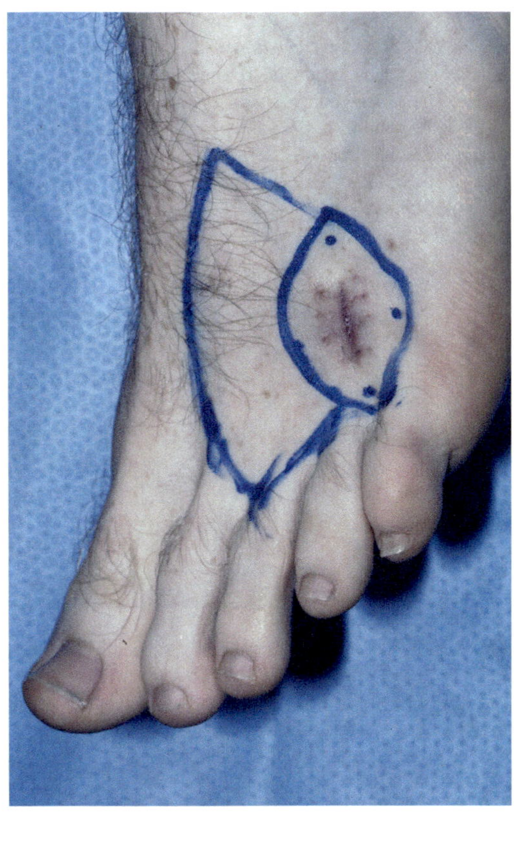

Fig. 3.224 Excisional defect mark out with a 2 cm clearance down to the paratenons down to the extensor tendons. The same principle applies for any ORIF of the metatarsals with metal exposure and closed with a keystone designed on the L5 dermatome on the dorsum of the foot based along metatarsal 1 and preserving the integrity of the distal branches of the superficial peroneal nerve supplying the dorsum. This is not to be implicated in the closure as it may end up with causalgic pain consequences

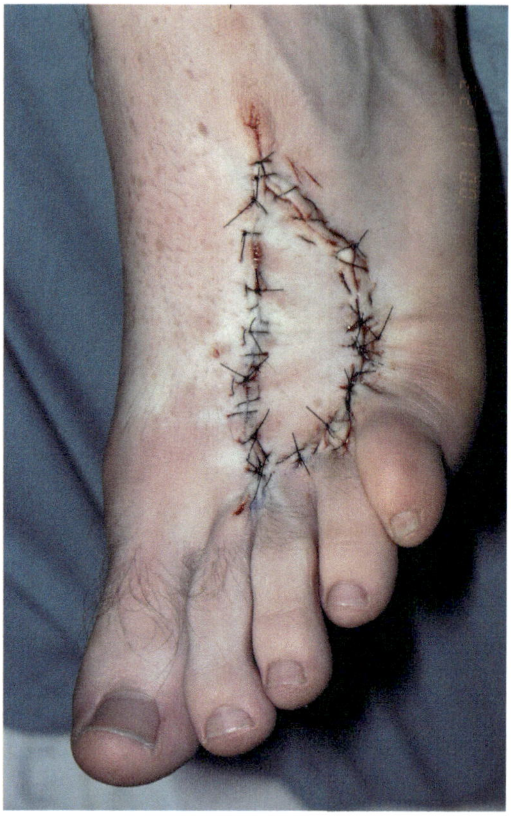

Fig. 3.225 Keystone closure of the melanoma defect, equally applicable to any ORIF for any metatarsal stabilisation. The closure under tension is not a contraindication, as explained above, but certainly the hypervascularisation ensures adequate vascular perfusion to achieve complication free healing in the L5 dermatome as reflected in the keystone characteristic of the acronym P.A.C.E.S.—all exemplified

3.1.17 Case 28: Another Aesthetic Outcome on a Female Foot

Another keystone outcome to meet the patient's satisfaction exemplifying the P.A.C.E.S. acronym for characteristics of the keystone along the lateral side of the foot. The keystone scar which is barely discernible is outlined with blue dots. The Clarke level II 0.55 mm melanoma, avoiding skin grafting on the dorsum of the foot which has an aesthetic restriction, particularly relevant in ladies with tight footwear (Figs. 3.226 and 3.227).

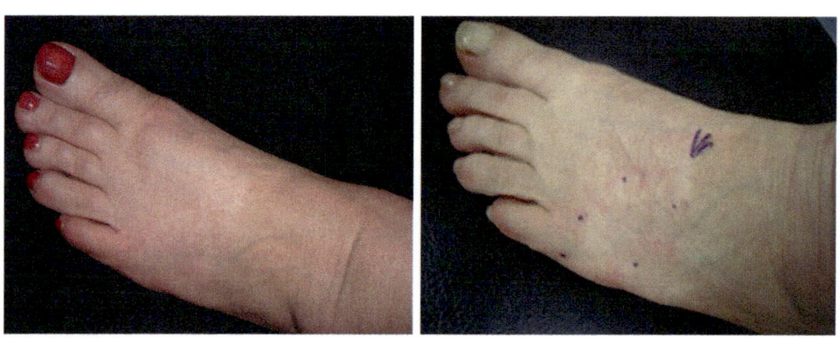

Fig. 3.226 The postoperative appearance of keystone scars on the dorsum of the foot. This scar is barely discernible. The 3-phase single layer closure technique was used as well as the dressing technique for removal to achieve this aesthetic outcome. The wear and tear factor of normal sensate tissue has practical applications on this site, particularly when wearing tightly fitting footwear

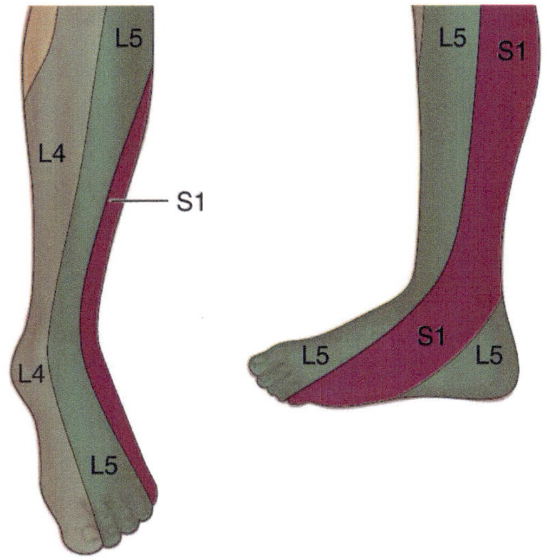

Fig. 3.227 The dermatomal mark out is the guide for the location of the random perforators coming through the dorsal fascia

3.1.18 Case 29: Toe Amputations Covered with Keystones with a Design Similarity to that Used for Melanoma Defects

The melanoma keystone technique on the dorsum of the foot is an excellent alternative for wound closure following toe amuptation/s. Pathology Level I melanoma in a superficial naevus in this 53-year-old female is a clinical case illustrated. As in the previous illustrations where orthopaedic ORIF procedures may be necessary but this keystone cover becomes a simple alternative over any ORIF procedure. Any amputation of toes can be covered in a similar manner (Figs. 3.228, 3.229, 3.230, 3.231, 3.232, 3.233, 3.234, 3.235, 3.236, 3.237, 3.238, 3.239, 3.240, 3.241, and 3.242).

In summary the P.A.C.E.S. characteristics of the keystone were all exemplified and the patient's satisfaction is noted as well.

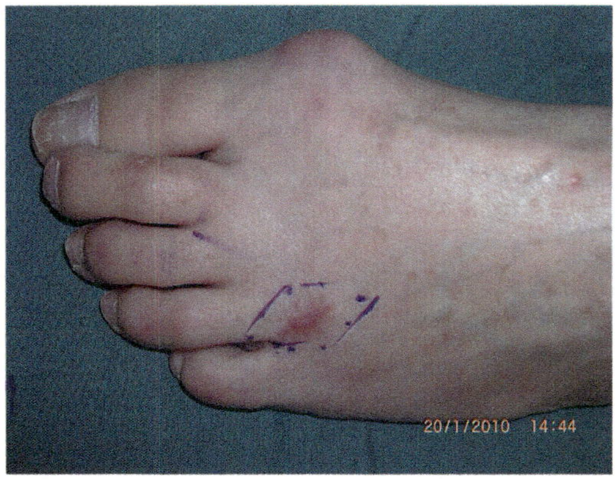

Fig. 3.228 The presenting melanoma following biopsy before excision

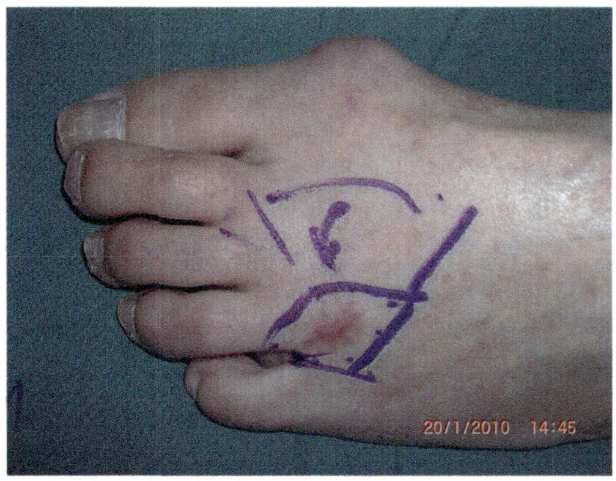

Fig. 3.229 The mark out and the design prior to insertion for the melanoma defect or even a bony remnant if toe amputation is necessary

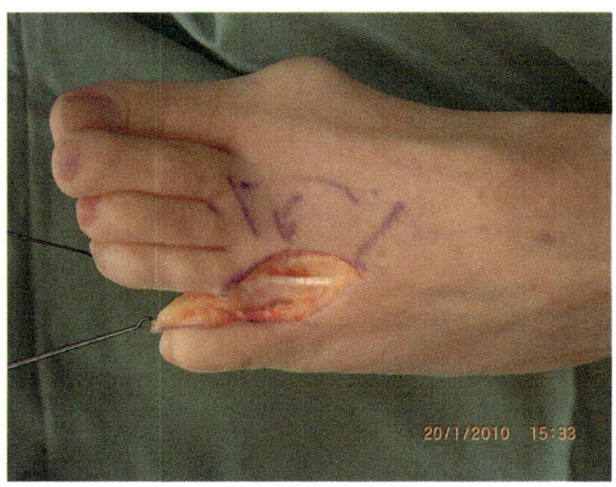

Fig. 3.230 The excision of the lesion at the head of the 4th and 5th metatarsals down to the paratenon of the extensor complex to the 4th toe. The closure of this soft tissue defect with the associated keystone mark out to cover exposed tendons is illustrated

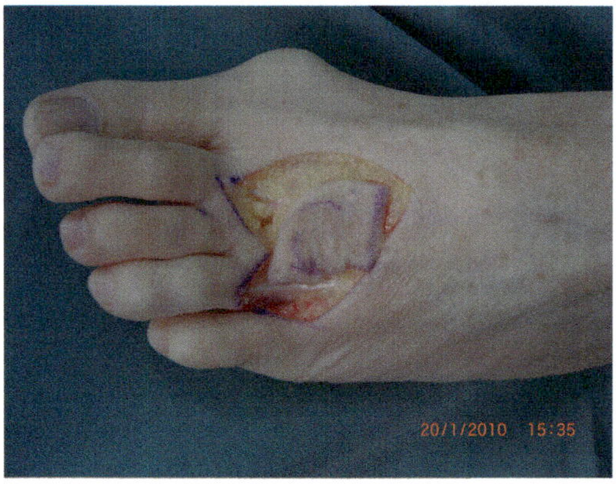

Fig. 3.231 The outline of the keystone on random perforators in the vicinity of the 3rd and 4th metatarsal heads

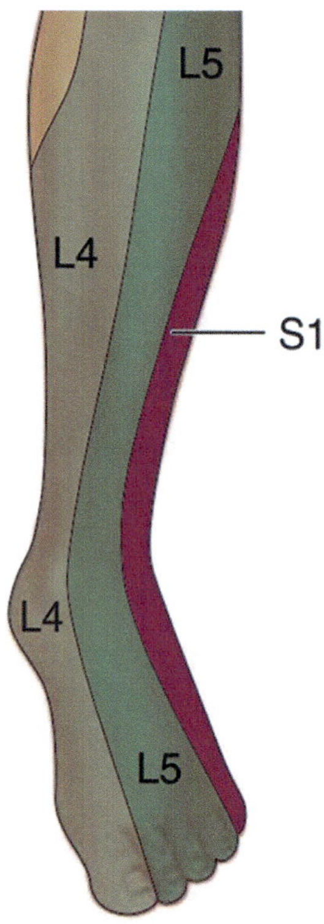

Fig. 3.232 The dermatomal mark out is the guide for the location of the random perforators coming through the fascia

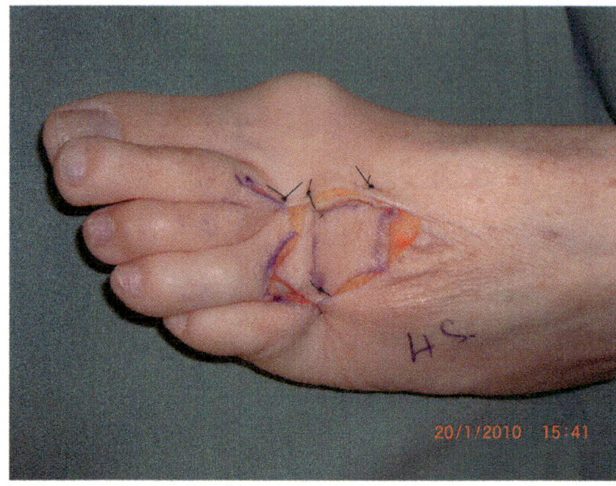

Fig. 3.233 Closure under tension and no embarrassment to the vascular supply which is all perforator based and not subdermal. No undermining of the subdermal complex just direct tensional closure over MTP 4 and 5

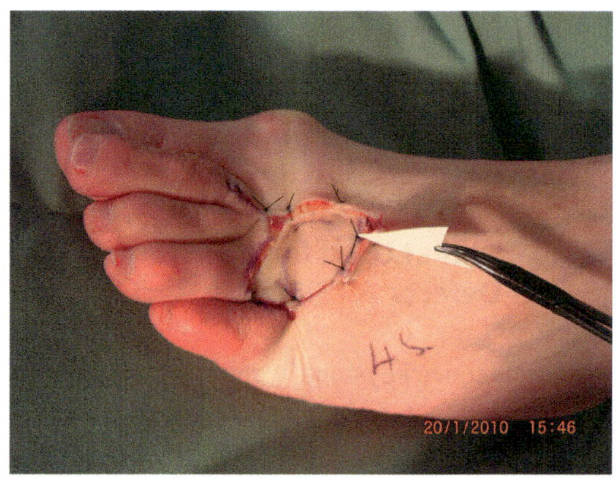

Fig. 3.234 The Red Dot Sign is evident on the arrowhead

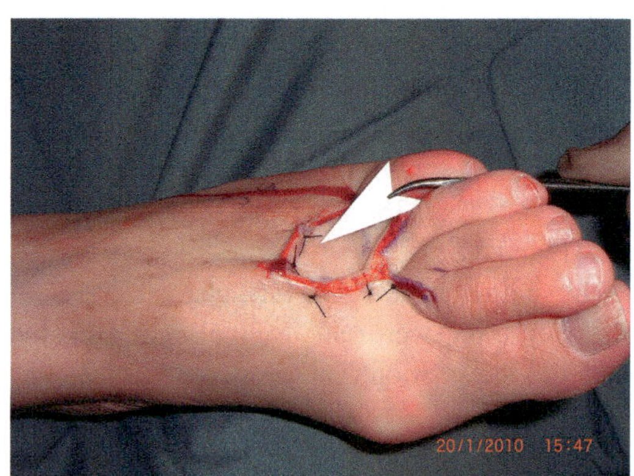

Fig. 3.235 Staged closure and the pink flare in the flap is noted based on subdermal perforators in spite of epidermal closure under tension. This confirms vascular viability

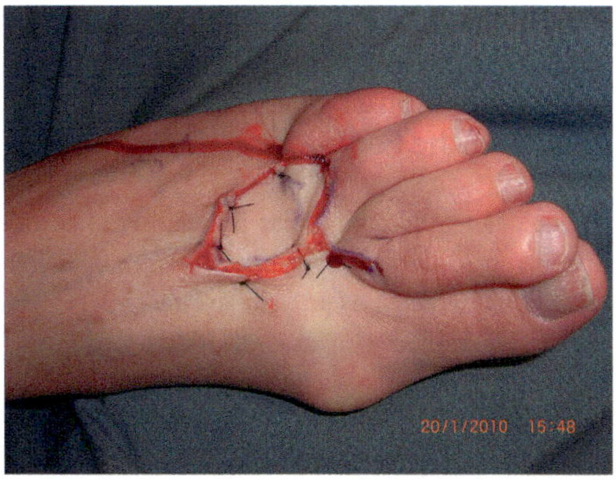

Fig. 3.236 Closure prior to completion

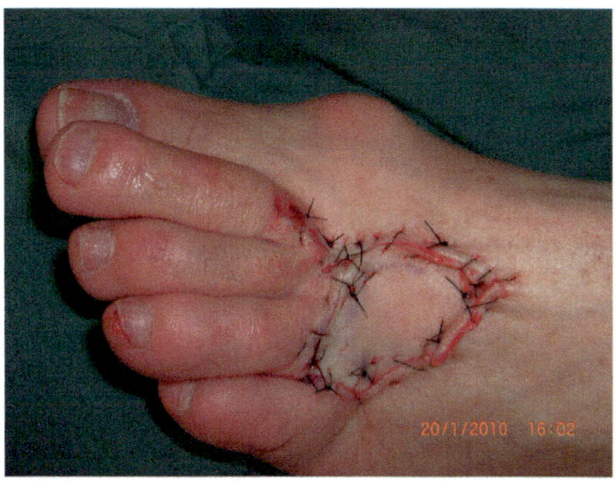

Fig. 3.237 Completed in an economic timeframe of 45 min, and the 3-phase locking mattress surgical suture technique is used

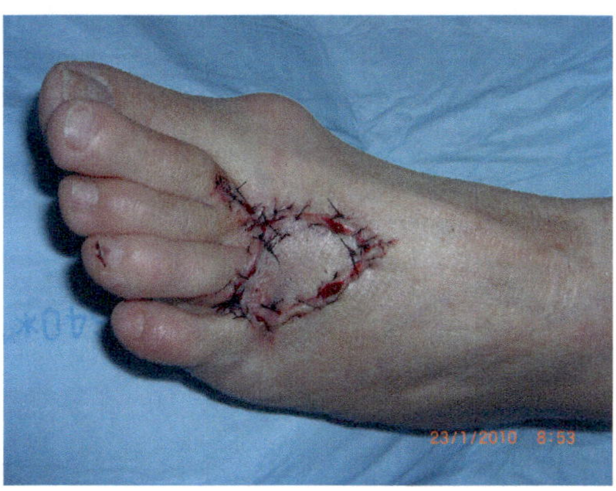

Fig. 3.238 Postoperative appearance at 3 days with no elements of demarcation of necrosis

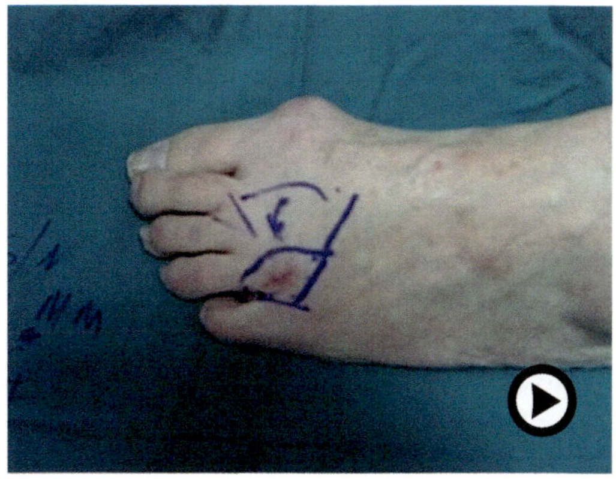

Fig. 3.239 Video of planned keystone repair. It is easy to visualise how one of the V–Y points on the keystone can be used to cover bony remnants if there are associated toe amputation/s (Video 3.48 Video of planned keystone repair. It is easy to visualise how one of the V–Y points on the keystone can be used to cover bony remnants if there are associated toe amputation/s) (▶ https://doi.org/10.1007/000-d68)

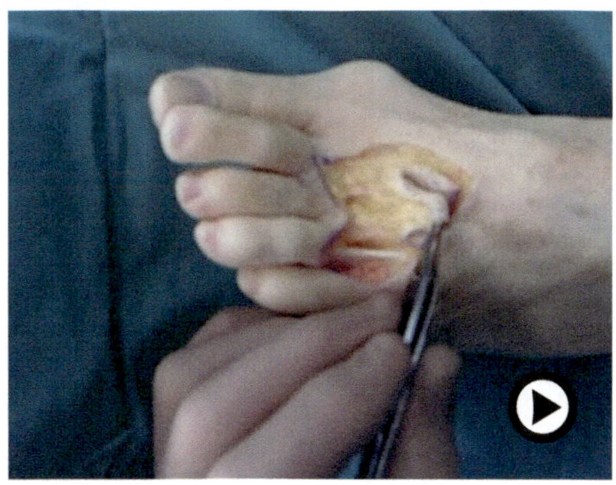

Fig. 3.240 Operative sequence (Video 3.49 Operative sequence) (▶ https://doi.org/10.1007/000-d69)

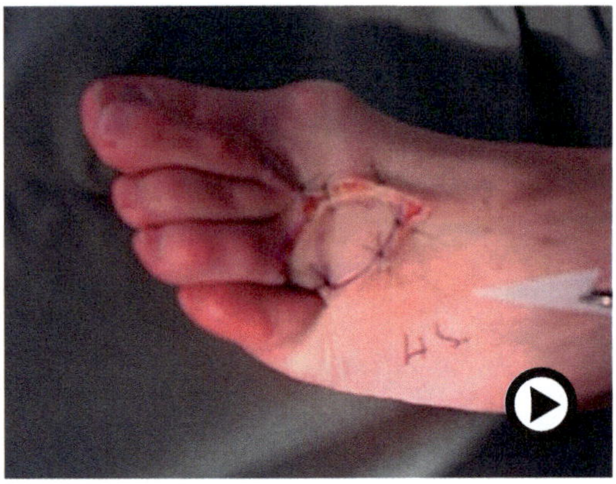

Fig. 3.241 Operative sequence (Video 3.50 Operative sequence) (▶ https://doi.org/10.1007/000-d6a)

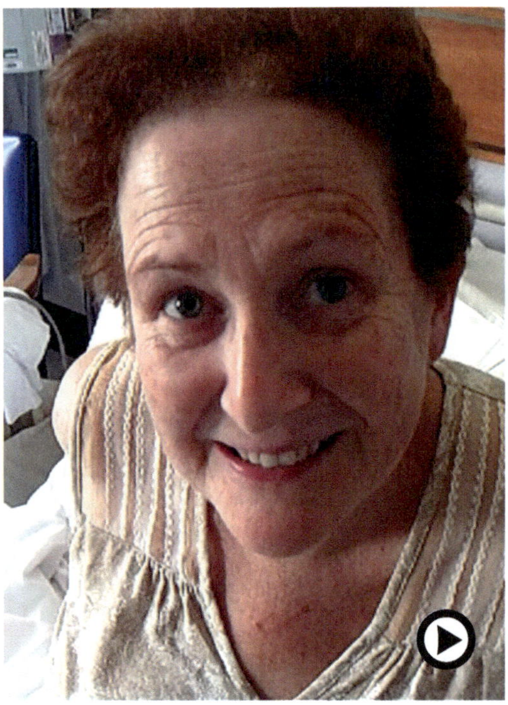

Fig. 3.242 Postoperative in hospital—patient perspective, pain free giving an in-reality confirmation of the operative success (Video 3.51 Postoperative in hospital—patient perspective, pain free giving an in reality confirmation of the operative success) (▶ https://doi.org/10.1007/000-d6b)

3.1.19 Case 30: Covering a Calcaneal Defect with a Plantar Keystone from the Arch of the Foot

This calcaneal excision and planned reconstruction using a plantar surface keystone island flap rotated, advanced and transposed over the exposed calcaneal site. It is designed to have the plantar fascia as the basis for the rotation of the keystone reaching to cover the calcaneal defect. Hence, the integrity of the weight bearing surface with sensate tissue is retained in this 80 year old patient (Figs. 3.243, 3.244, 3.245, 3.246, 3.247, 3.248, 3.249, 3.250, and 3.251).

In summary, this simple plantar keystone supplying sensate tissue to the heel from the medial plantar keystone is superior to any sural nerve reversal for plantar innervation with its vascular embarrassment a regular finding [8].

All the P.A.C.E.S. characteristics were again exemplified.

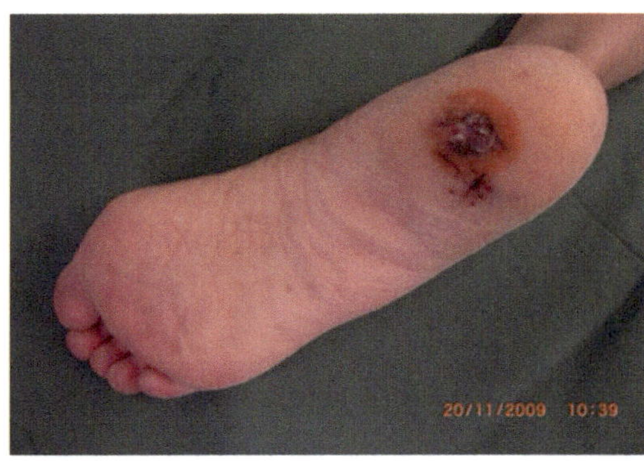

Fig. 3.243 The preoperative appearance of an acral lentiginous melanoma on the weight bearing surface of the heal

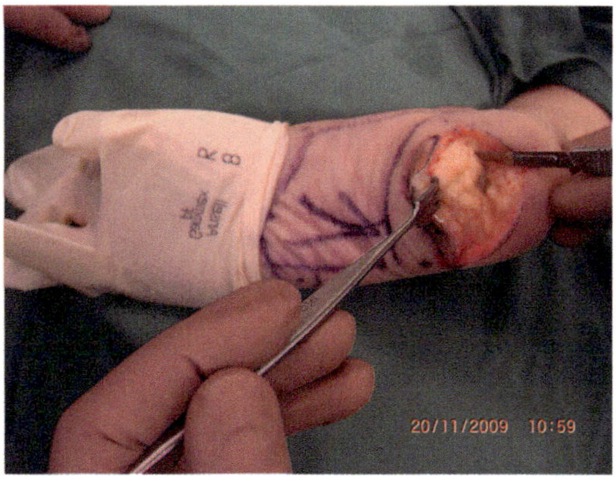

Fig. 3.244 Staged excision of the lesion down to and including periosteum of the calcaneum. The keystone reconstruction of this weight bearing surface over the calcaneum is designed from the skin, fat and fascia of the plantar arch. Division of the medial and lateral sides allows rotation over the calcaneal defect. The plantar fascia renders support and sensate tissue to this weight bearing surface of the heel. The surgical manoeuvre to enclose the distal half of the foot within a sterile surgical glove ensures a sterile surgical field

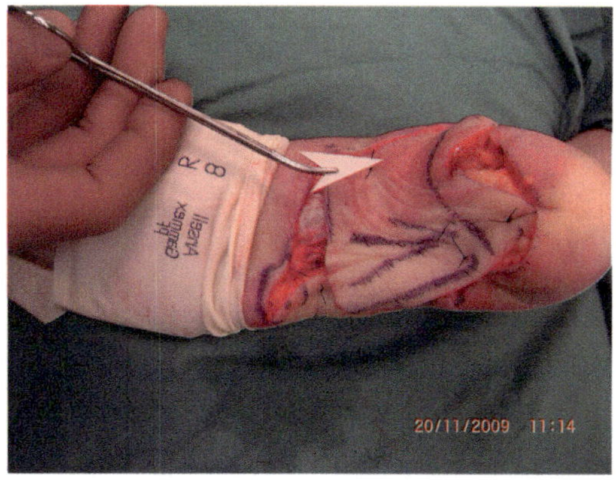

Fig. 3.246 A later stage of the reconstruction and the release of tourniquet confirms its viability in situ. Note the reactive hyperaemia evident through the medial side of the keystone indicating the medial plantar arterial supply is the predominant input and on the lateral side the lateral plantar input would have been divided to allow rotation, advancement and transposition of the keystone over the calcaneum. It is based on a single perforator support from the medial side, away from the axis of rotation

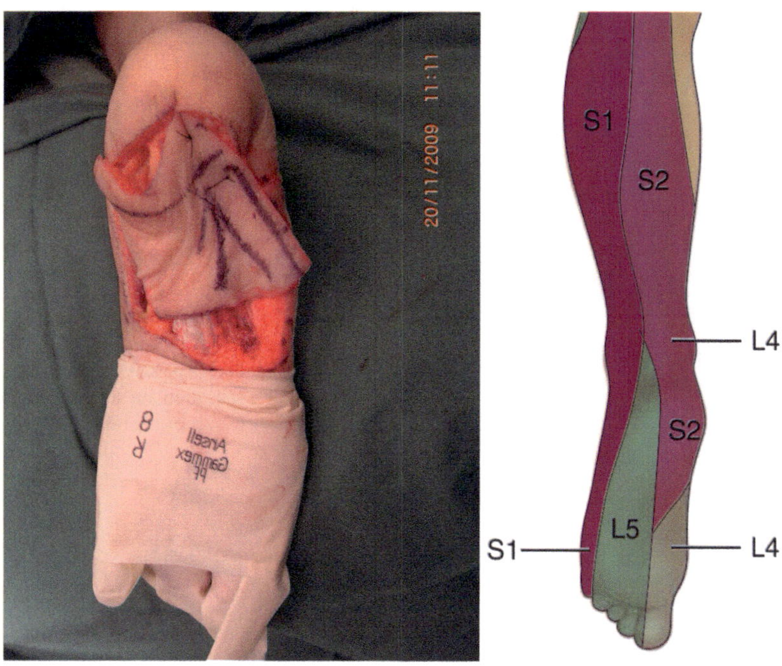

Fig. 3.245 The keystone island flap is designed to include the total plantar surface based on the plantar fascia for random vascular support. This is mainly overlying the L5 dermatome and is delineated along the lateral and medial margins. The plantar fascia is released distally enough to ensure cover of the weight bearing surface of the heel (reproduced with permission from [2])

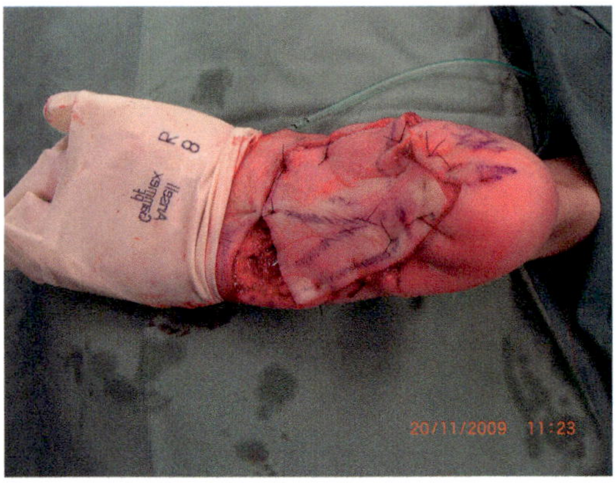

Fig. 3.247 Staged repair closing under tension with mattress locking sutures. The arrow indicates the site of planned skin grafting closure for the secondary defect. However, it was found unnecessary as loco-regional closure provided wound apposition, without the need for any graft which was a backup line if necessary. The wound was closed directly avoiding any vascular impedance. The hyperaemic appearance at 20 min (timestamp on image) is unchanged

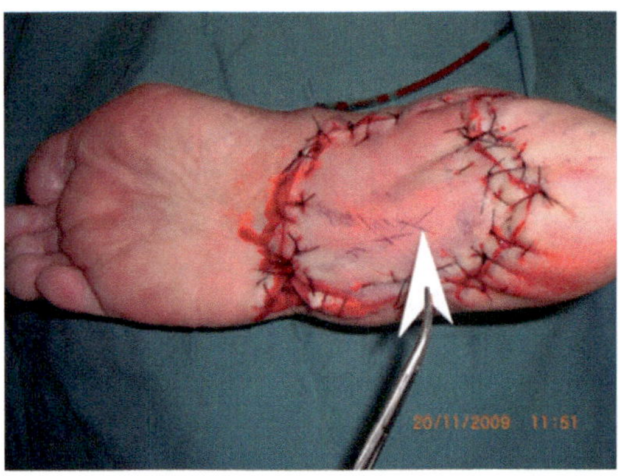

Fig. 3.248 Further staged closure and reactive hyperaemia (arrowed) is quite noticeable, and the secondary defect at the base of the 5th metatarsal has been closed directly without any vascular embarrassment

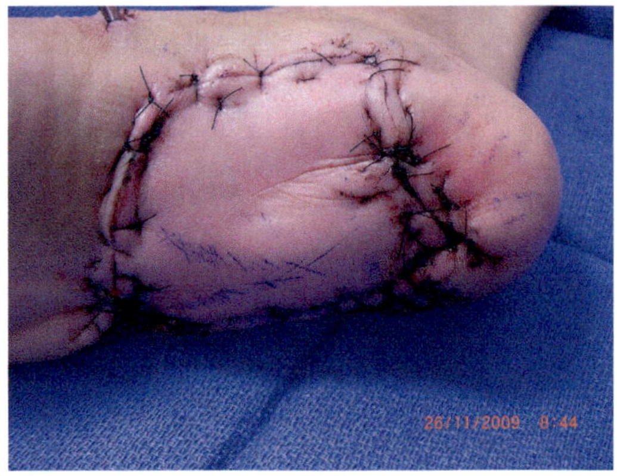

Fig. 3.249 Postoperative appearance at 5 days with no evidence of any vascular impedance, avoiding necrosis. The suture technique enclosure uses a 3-phase surgical technique of locking mattress sutures at the points of maximum tension and then further mattress sutures to gain wound closure and finally a continuous nylon throughout to achieve epidermal seal

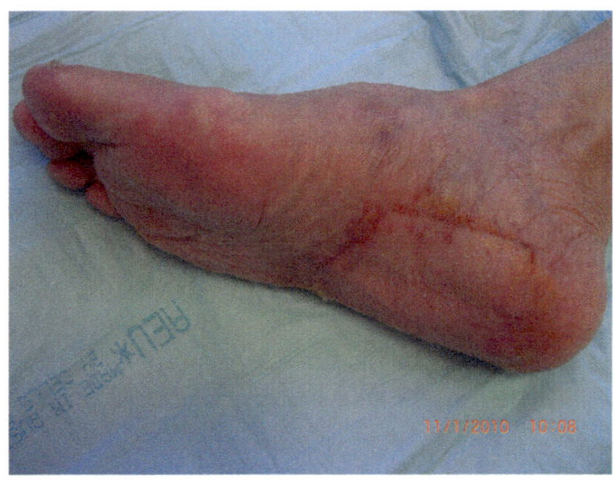

Fig. 3.250 The appearance at 1 month following staged removal of sutures with intact sensation obvious when the heel is palpated (see video) showing the retention of intact sensation on the weight bearing surface on the plantar aspect of the heel

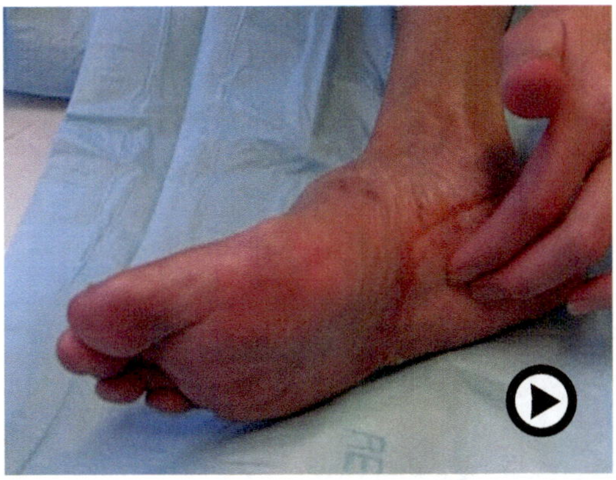

Fig. 3.251 Video illustrating sensory recovery and thus protective sensation facilitates mobilisation (Video 3.52 Video illustrating sensory recovery and thus protective sensation facilitates mobilisation) (▶ https://doi.org/10.1007/000-d6c)

3.1.20 Case 31: Closure of Soft Tissue Calf Defects Using the Yin Yang Keystone Design (Figs. 3.252, 3.253, 3.254, 3.255, 3.256, 3.257, 3.258, 3.259, and 3.260)

All the characteristics of the keystone thus are exemplified, including aesthetic appearance.

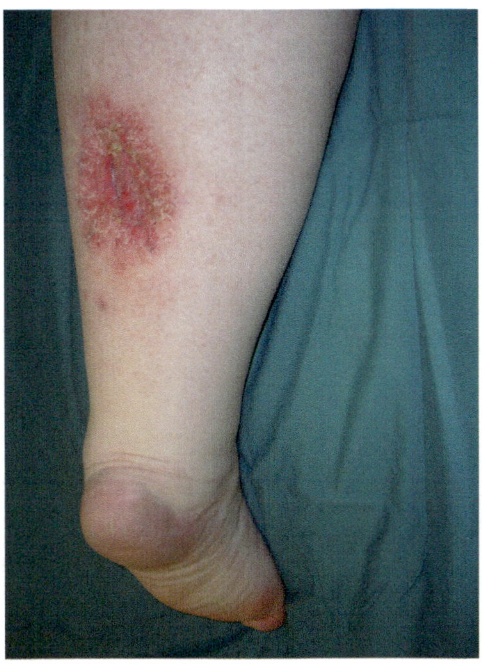

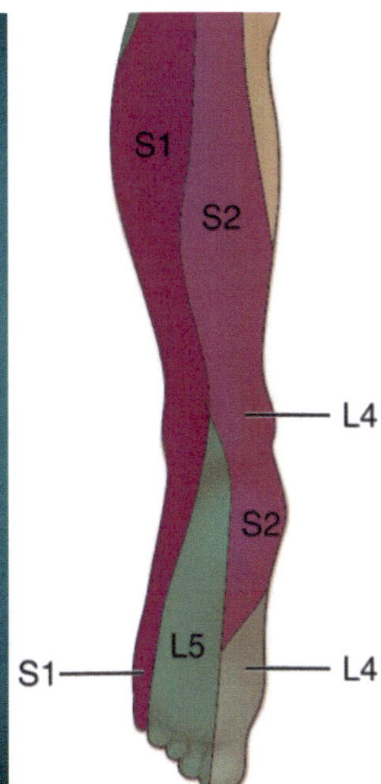

Fig. 3.252 Recurrent melanoma of the lower limb over the muscle bulk of the gastrocnemius complex. This muscle element in the wound facilitates closure under tension by compressing the muscle bulk for this 11 × 8 cm defect of the calf

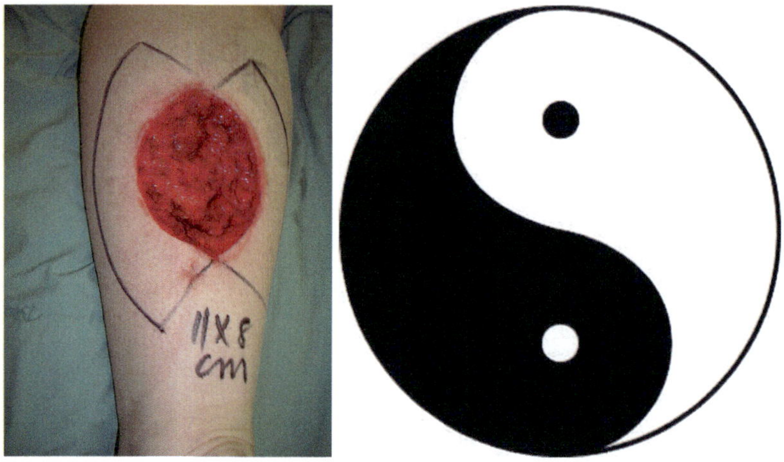

Fig. 3.253 To avoid tension under direct closure, the bilateral keystones can then be described and developed in a Yin Yang arrangement to facilitate this manouevre when tissues were tight on closure with the top part of one side and the bottom part of the other which gives a Yin Yang appearance. This overcomes the tension restriction and the period of delayed healing, or delayed removal of sutures is thus avoided

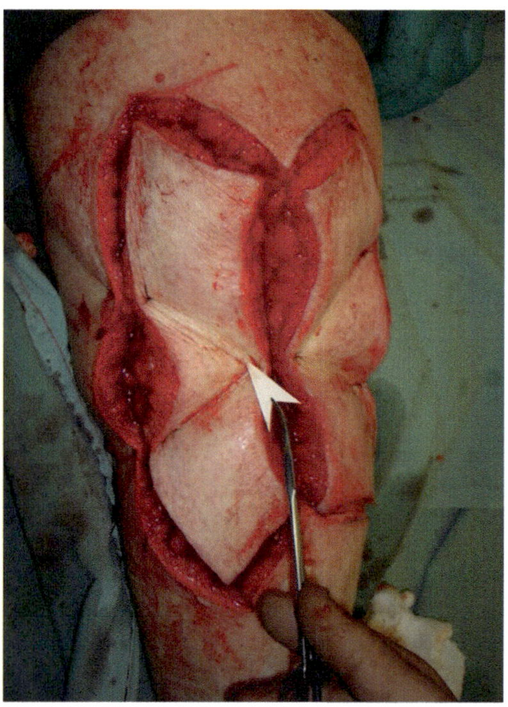

Fig. 3.254 Lines of tension are obvious but perfusion is not restricted and the hyperaemic phase allows full vascularity to return to achieve pain free healing representing one of the keystone characteristics

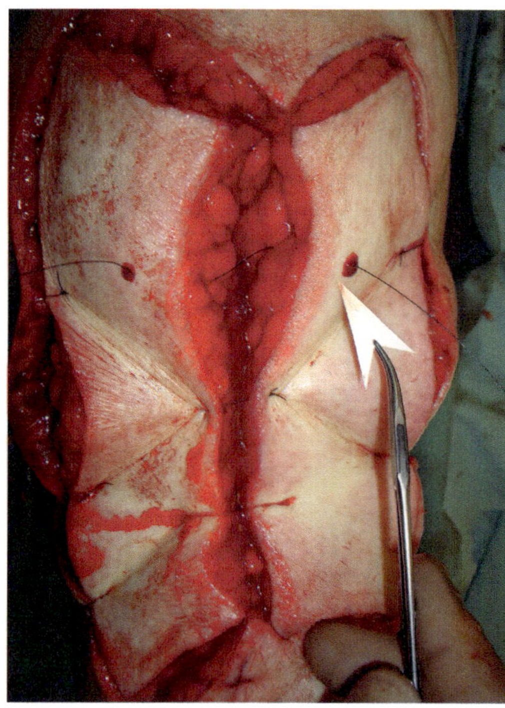

Fig. 3.255 The red dot signs indicate there is not vascular impedance and full vascular flow is present in spite of closure under tension and the Yin Yang design minimises the tension factor while the red dot sign is the comfortable indicator of intact vascular supply without evidence of any cyanosis, another observational finding

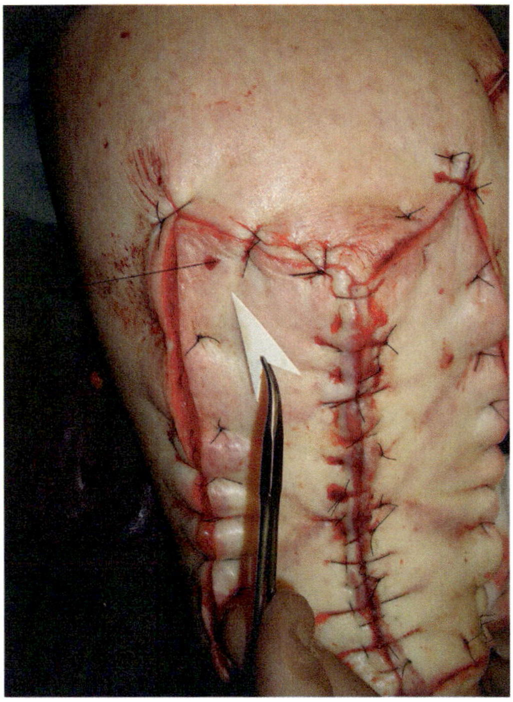

Fig. 3.256 The red dot sign is evident throughout (arrowed) indicating the hypervascularity stage and sound vascular perfusion with closure under tension

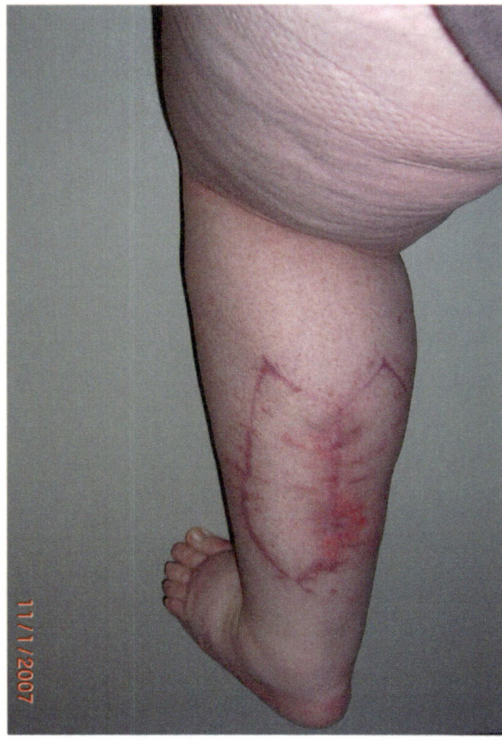

Fig. 3.258 Tensional closure of a bilateral keystone took some weeks to settle before it was appropriate to remove finally all the tension sutures needing regular dressings as a backup. The patient's compression stocking has left residual indentaion around the thigh while oedema continues to resolve taking some weeks to settle back to normal to the patient's satisfaction

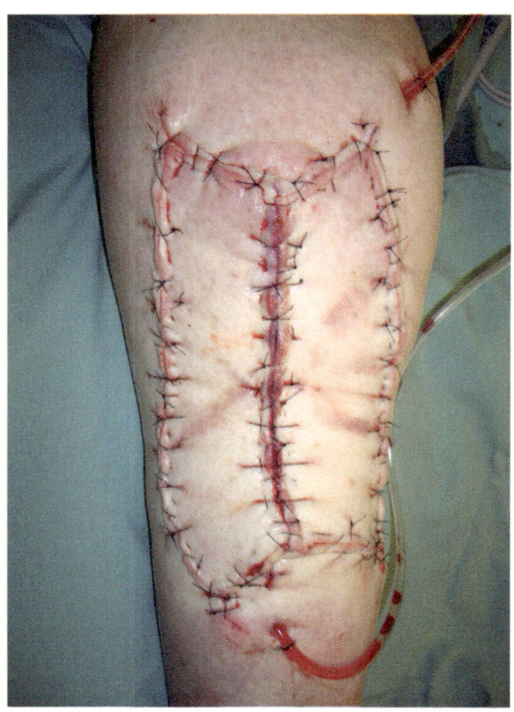

Fig. 3.257 The wound is closed using the 3-phase locking mattress suture technique with the continuous nylon achieving epidermal seal. Note the bilateral Redi-vac drainage achieving function while aligned along the keystone defect as well as the operative defect and there was no demarcation line of potential necrosis

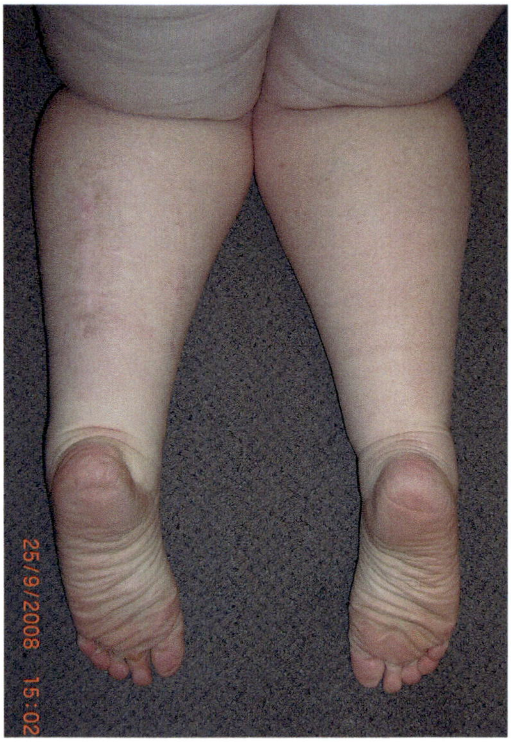

Fig. 3.259 The final aesthetic outcome to close a defect 11 × 8 cm and this will have orthopaedic indications for any access through the gastrocnemious complex, even associated with ORIF procedures

Fig. 3.260 A closeup of the final aesthetic outcome and the patient indicated that her satisfaction in the outcome allows her to avoid using trousers to disguise her deformity as she had done for years

3.1.21 Case 32: Lower Limb Amputation Repair Reflecting Complications in Tissue Cover Solved with the Keystone Principle

A referral case of a previous unsuccessful flap repair and ongoing trophic ulceration in an amputation stump with prosthesis. The keystone provides sensate soft tissue cover over the amputation prominence (Figs. 3.261, 3.262, 3.263, 3.264, 3.265, 3.266, 3.267, and 3.268).

All P.A.C.E.S. characteristics of the keystone are evident, again to the patient's satisfaction, avoiding the need for ongoing dressings.

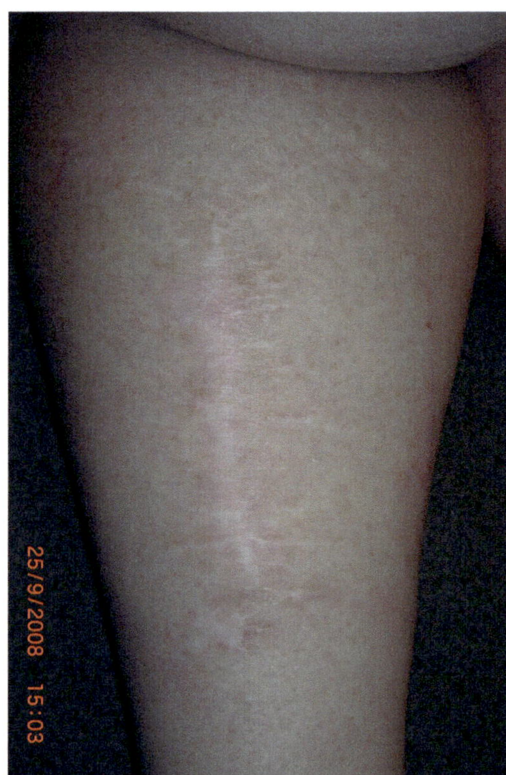

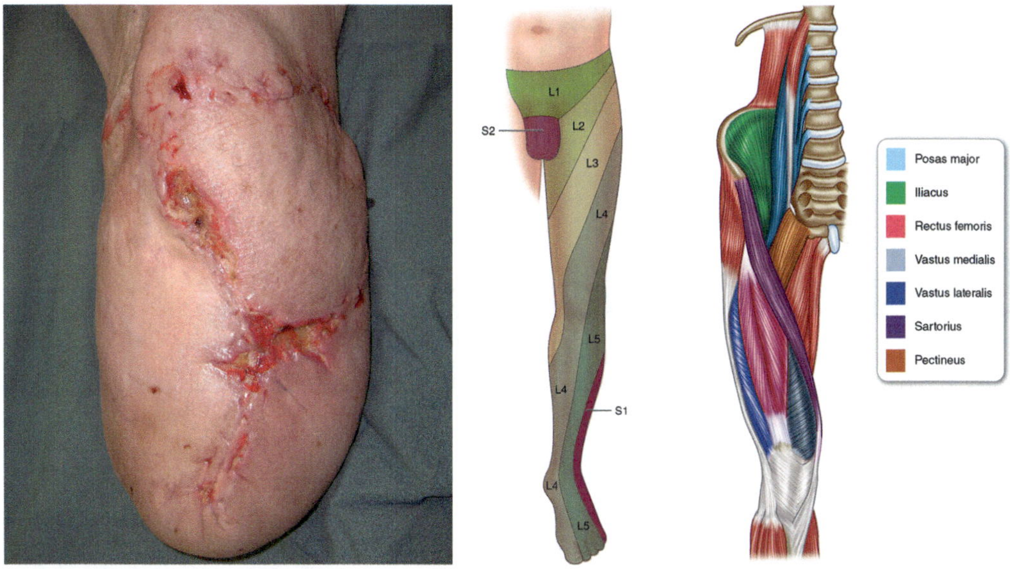

Fig. 3.261 The various muscles that have been used to date for wound closure would have employed parts of rectus femoris, vastus medialis and vastus lateralis. However, when the areas of sensory change within the dermatomes are a compass guide for the keystone reconstruction and preoperatively areas of intact sensation are defined as the basis for the keystone repair leading to its sensate recovery (reproduced with permission from [2])

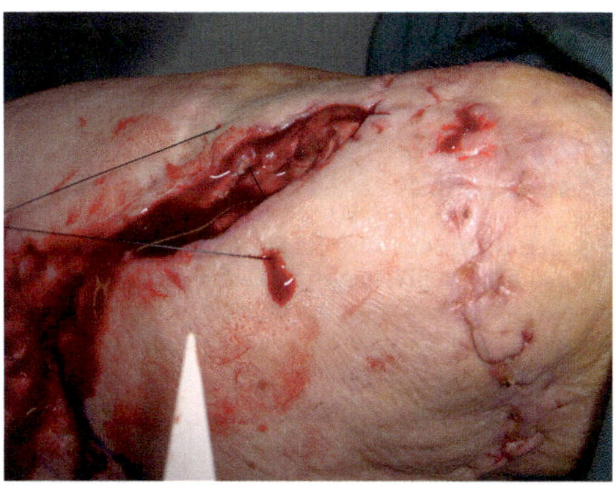

Fig. 3.262 A progress repair of the fasciocutaneous island flap of loose tissue around the stump. The keystone red dot sign is a single indicator of what has clinically supposed to be a sympathectomy effect because of the cutaneous division but retaining an intact fascial base with its suprafascial and infrafascial intact circulation [7]. If the red dot sign is indicated that the circulation will allow me to close under tension and the sensate tissue covering the amputation stump is a safeguard against future prosthetic applications—simply weight bearing is a possible outcome without the potential for trophic ulceration which must occur in non-sensate flap closures of the free flap variety

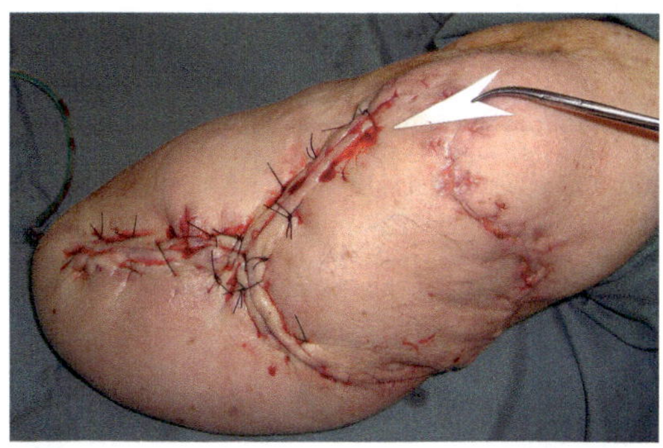

Fig. 3.263 The repair completed and the white arrow indicates the area of the subdermal vascular perfusion

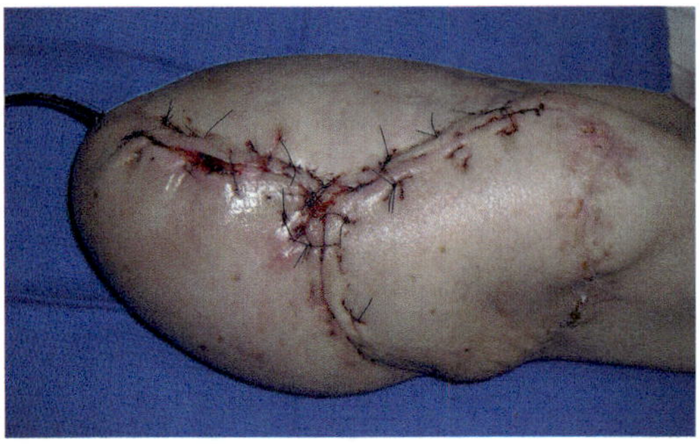

Fig. 3.264 The wound closure with Redi-vac drainage using our 3-phase locking mattress suture technique at the dermal epidermal level which retains a fascial component in the base of the myocutaneous flap

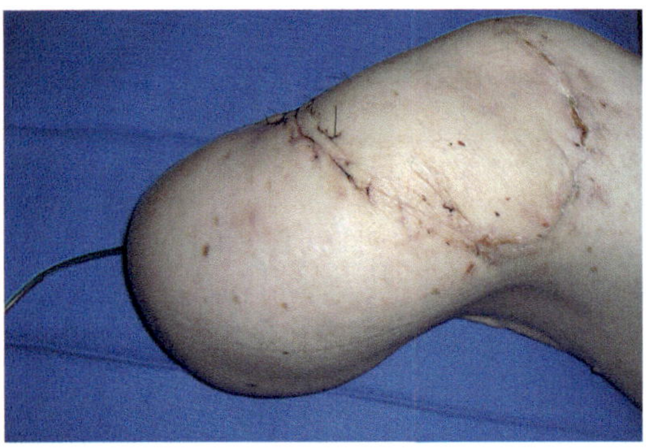

Fig. 3.265 The end result with staged removal of the epidermal seal continuous nylon which achieves a sound wound closure. Whereas the V–Y tension points, again using locking mattress sutures may need to stay in situ for up to 3 weeks for security

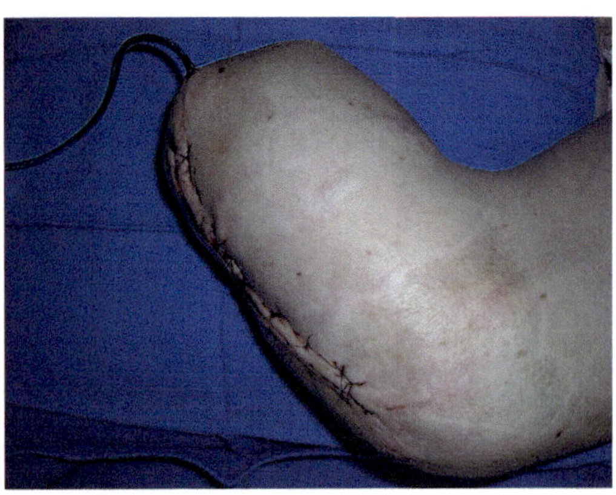

Fig. 3.266 Another view of the staged removal of sutures

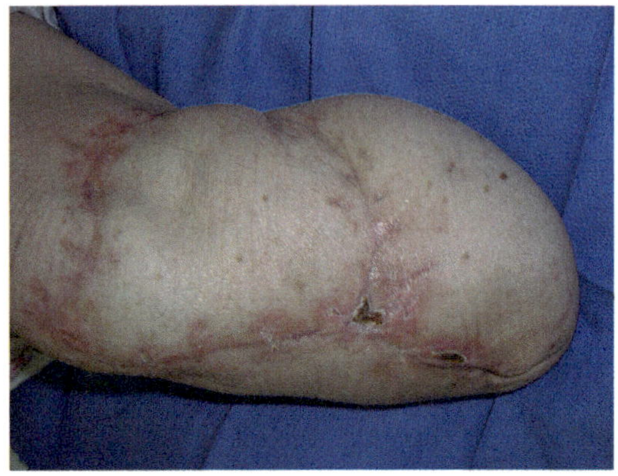

Fig. 3.267 Another site of the V–Y tension closing points

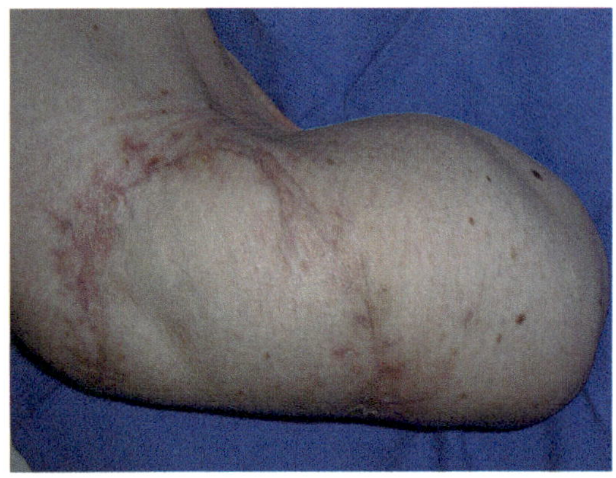

Fig. 3.268 Another view of the resolution of the scar tissue and incidentally, staples have no place in wound closure of these lower limbs because of their lack of refinement and potential for wound breakdown. Note the resolution of trophic ulceration and the resolution of oedema

3.1.22 Case 33: Amputation Reconstruction with a Keystone

Another referral case for amputation scar revision because of trophic ulceration (Figs. 3.269, 3.270, 3.271, 3.272, and 3.273).

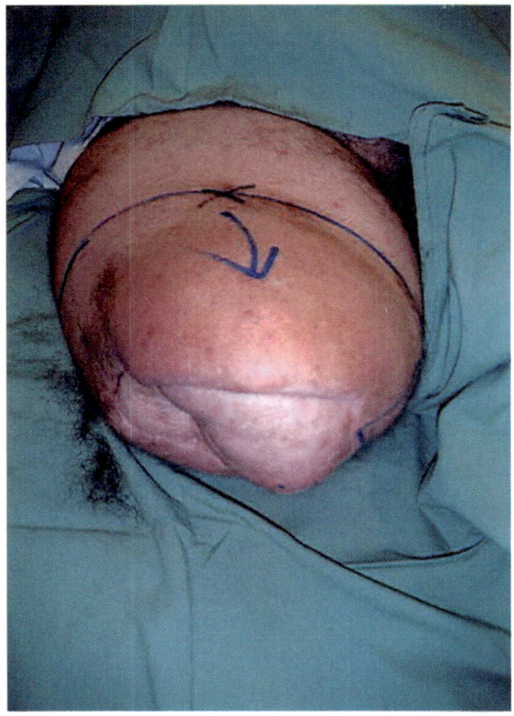

Fig. 3.269 The preoperative mark out of the myocutaneous flap for rotation advancement over the amputation level

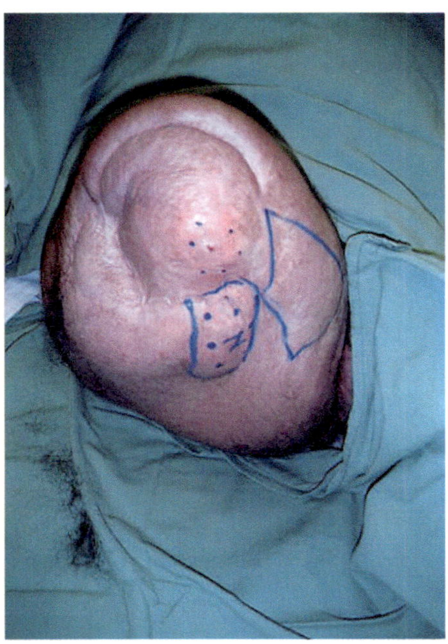

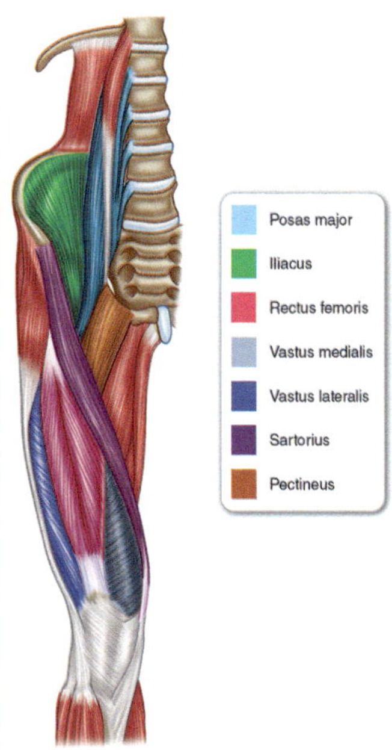

Fig. 3.270 Removal of ongoing scar tissue with deep attachment to the bone in the vicinity of the reconstruction, indicating possibly the healed site of former trophic ulceration. The vastus medialis muscle has been part of the keystone design from the point of view of delineation and the hypervascularity that so results allows us to close under tension with red dot signs indicating sound perfusion of the integument

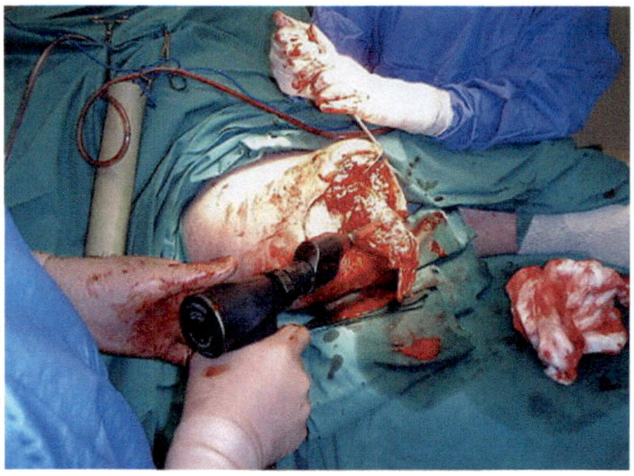

Fig. 3.271 Further mechanical refinement of the bony amputation site

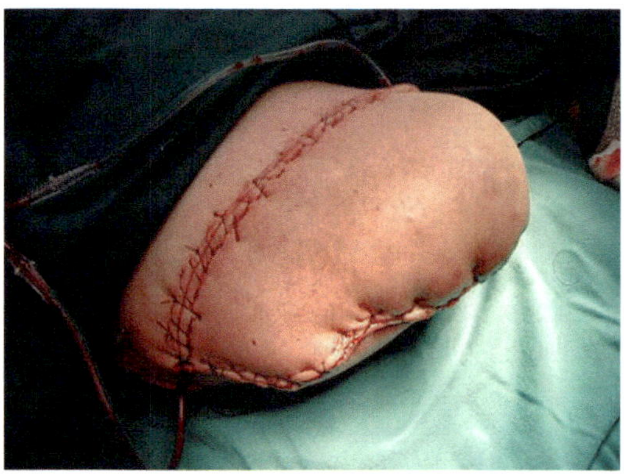

Fig. 3.272 Note the hyperaemic flare in the flap consistent with its sympathetic effect of hypervascularity in spite of closure under tension

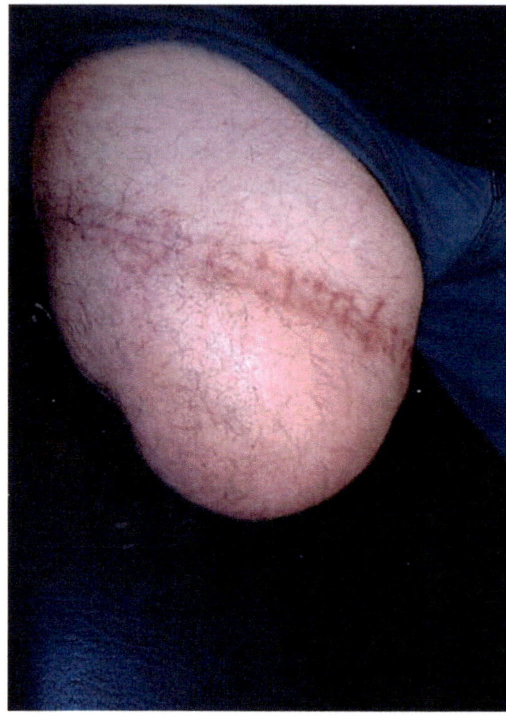

Fig. 3.273 Further images of the healed wound after removal of the locking mattress sutures and the continuous nylon for epidermal seal. Protective sensate tissue offers an additional cover to the amputated femoral stump to facilitate the subsequent application of the prosthesis

3.1.23 Case 34: Anterior Thigh Keystone to Close Groin Defect of a Mitotic Lesion

This case example of closure of the large groin defect and the surgical mark out of the anterior thigh keystone for closure (Figs. 3.274, 3.275, 3.276, 3.277, 3.278, 3.279, 3.280, 3.281, and 3.282).

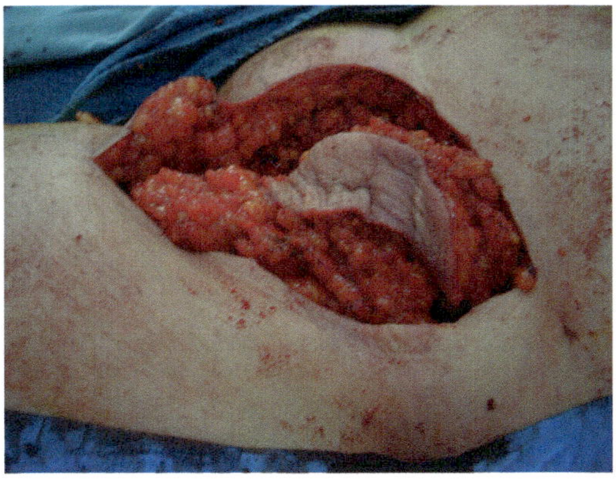

Fig. 3.274 The anterior thigh keystone

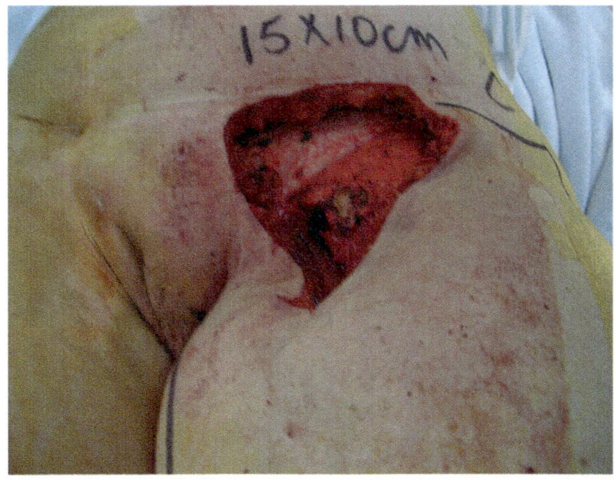

Fig. 3.276 The anterior thigh keystone flap on mark out in preparation for closure of the groin defect

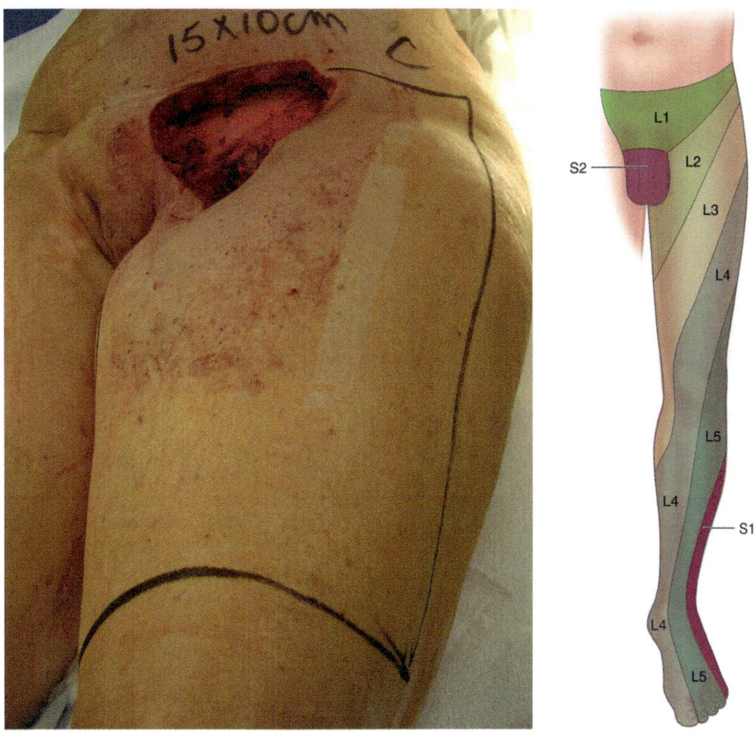

Fig. 3.275 On completion of the groin clearance 15 × 10 cm defect along the inguinal ligament and the anterior thigh keystone L2–L3 dermatomes is demarcated

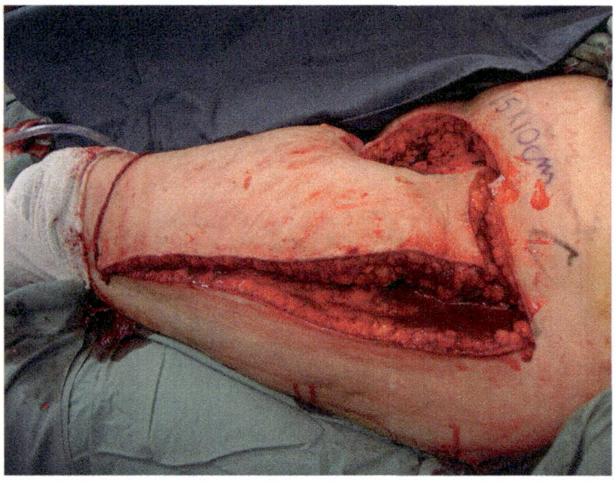

Fig. 3.277 Dissection is completed an essential prerequisite that there is no undermining and there must be at least 1/3 deep attachment for random perforators along the muscle of the rectus femoris

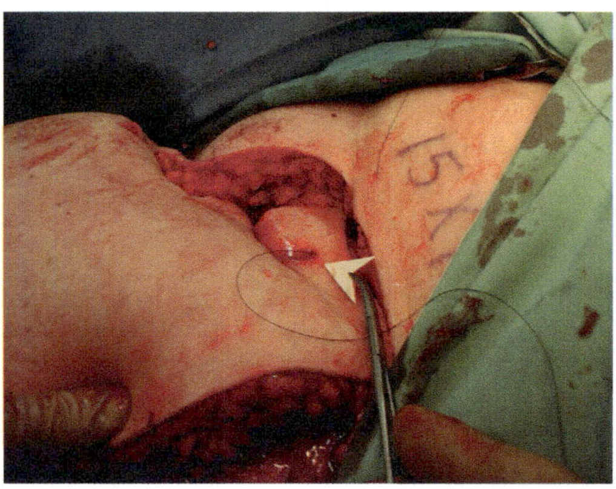

Fig. 3.278 The red dot sign is a confirmation of the hypervascularity—query a sympathectomy effect—usually an indicator of a sound vascular support. This is one of the characteristic signs of a successful keystone on a fascial-based island with dilatation of the suprafascial and infrafascial vascular support [7]

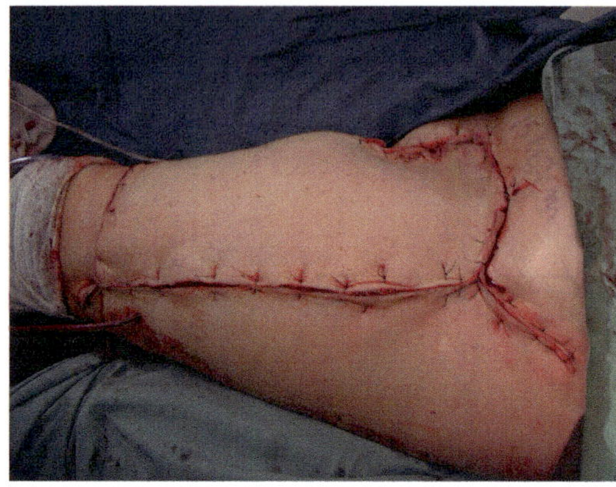

Fig. 3.279 The repair of the anterior thigh keystone and closure of groin defects indicating the hypervascularity contributing to its successful healing without necrosis

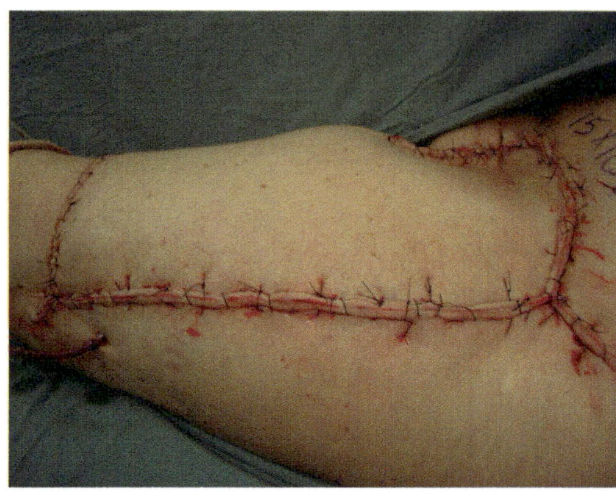

Fig. 3.280 The lateral thigh drain tube is an essential precaution as the tissues tend to drain excessively along the line of tensor fascia lata laterally along the thigh. This usually stays in 10 days to prevent any haematoma, one of the potential rare complications of thigh keystone

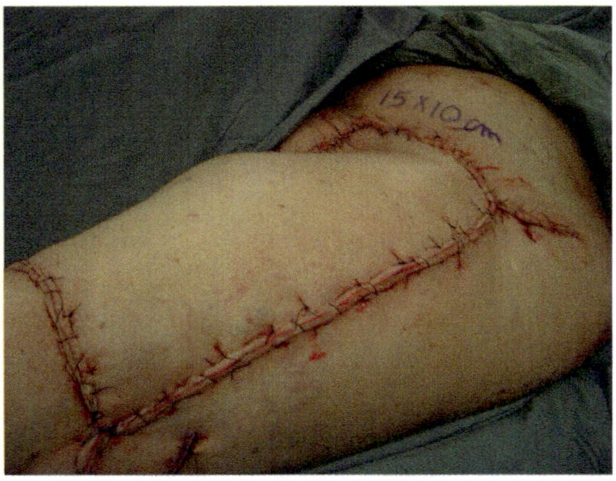

Fig. 3.281 Note the tension locking sutures at prime positions of maximum tension

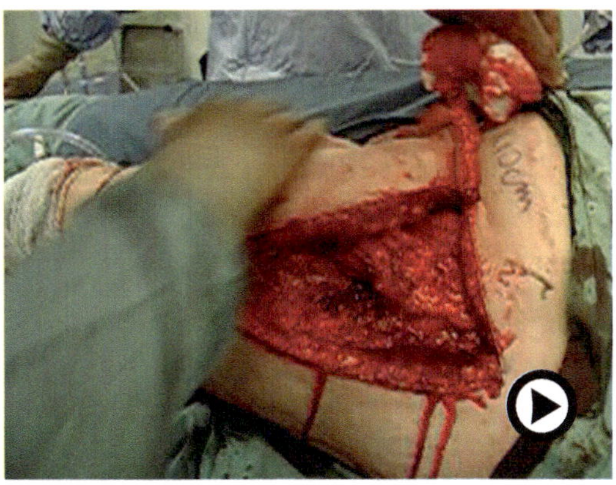

Fig. 3.282 After division of the tensor fascia lata down the lateral compartment (Video 3.53 After division of the tensor fascia lata down the lateral compartment) (▶ https://doi.org/10.1007/000-d6d)

3.1.24 Case 35: Another Clinical Version of the Anterior Thigh Keystone (Figs. 3.283, 3.284, 3.285, 3.286, and 3.287)

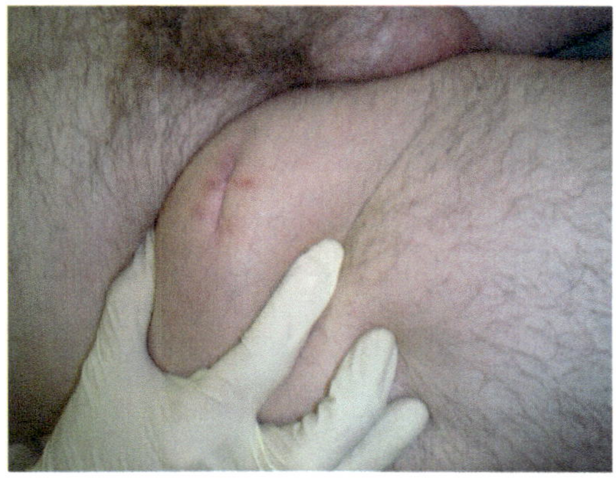

Fig. 3.283 The tumour mass of the groin before excision and the orthopaedic link is if there is any need to have a closure of a groin defect, the anterior thigh keystone will help solve the problem

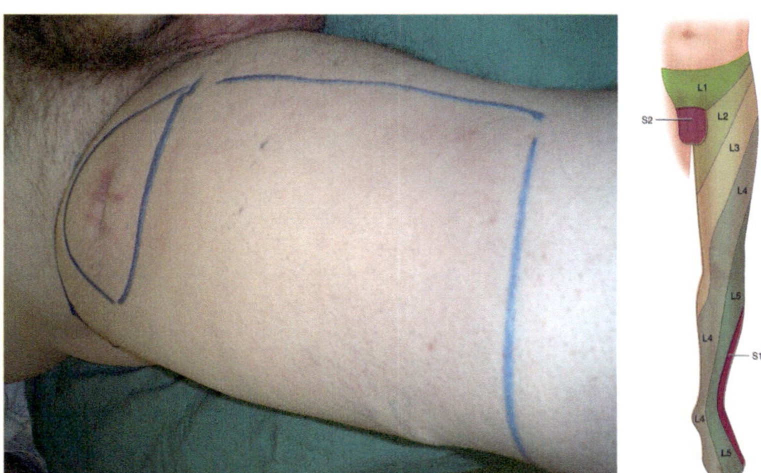

Fig. 3.284 Delineation of the anterior thigh keystone. This can be undermined in the distal 1/3 to close any amputation site for a femoral amputation with sensate tissue

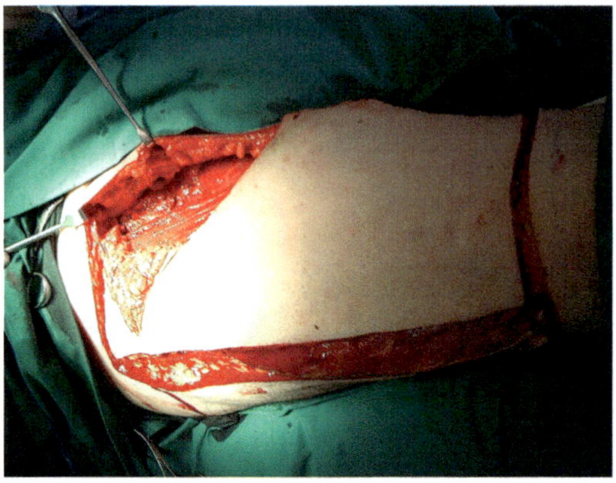

Fig. 3.285 Stages of the repair for closure of the groin defect

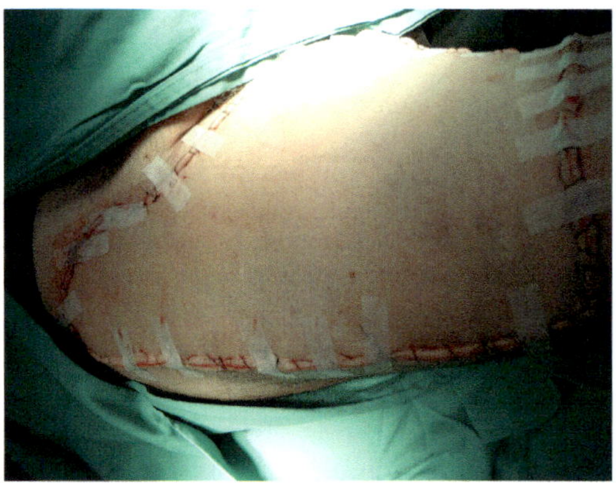

Fig. 3.286 Closure completed using the 3-phase single layer locking mattress suture technique positioned at the key points of tension

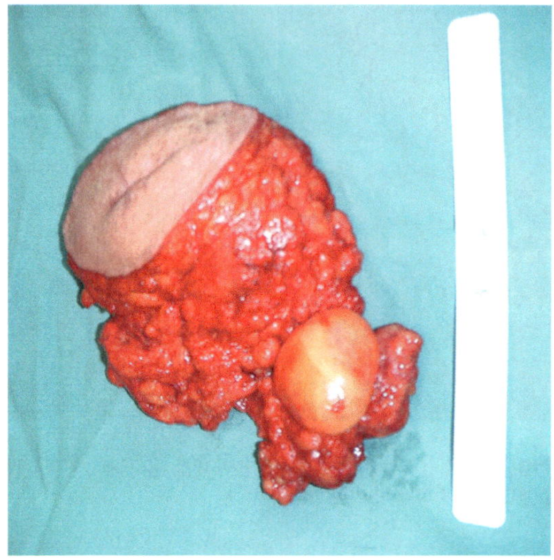

Fig. 3.287 The tumour mass

3.1.25 Case 36: Bunion Closure Complication Solved with a Keystone Based on the L5 Plantar Dermatome

This lady had a complication from an unsuccessful bunion surgery with a failure to get wound closure that needed a second-stage reconstruction when the wound broke down. Whether or not she was a smoker is not recorded but such wound breakdowns are consistent with people who smoke. Review also the images of Case 29 and the text (Figs. 3.288, 3.289, 3.290, 3.291, 3.292, 3.293, and 3.294).

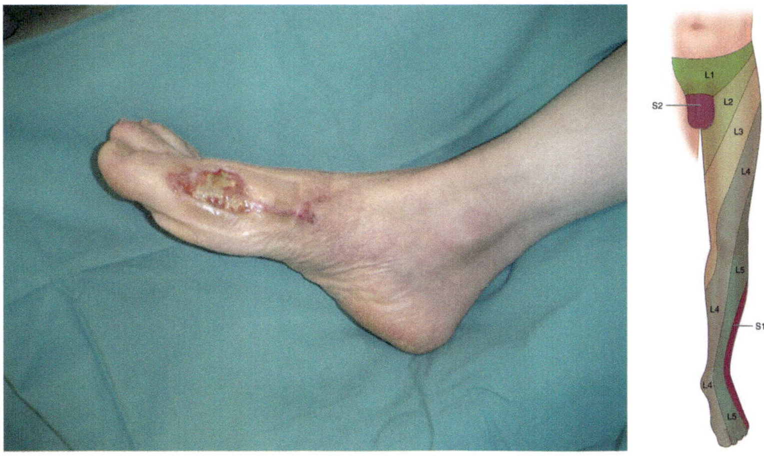

Fig. 3.288 The L5 plantar dermatome for closure of a bunion defect on the dorsal surface following wound breakdown

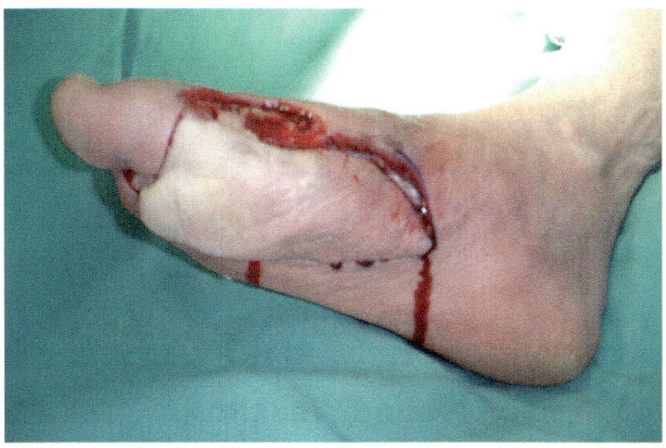

Fig. 3.289 The slow recovery of perfusion and the proximal 1/3 is fully vascularised before it spreads distally to the limits of the MTP area of the big toe

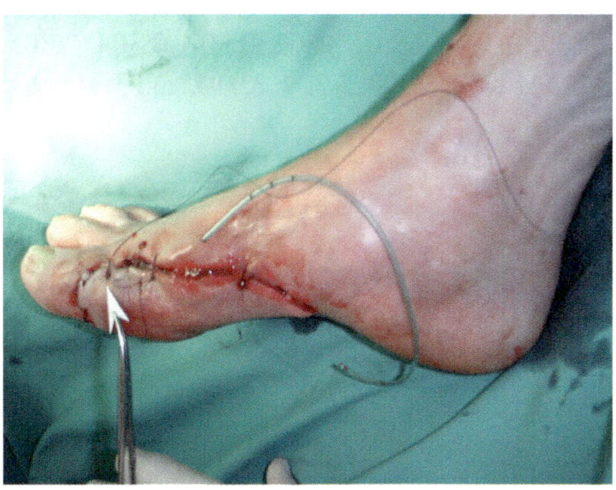

Fig. 3.290 The arrow indicates the slow recovery phase of hypervascularisation in the L5 plantar dermatome with the Redi-vac drain installed

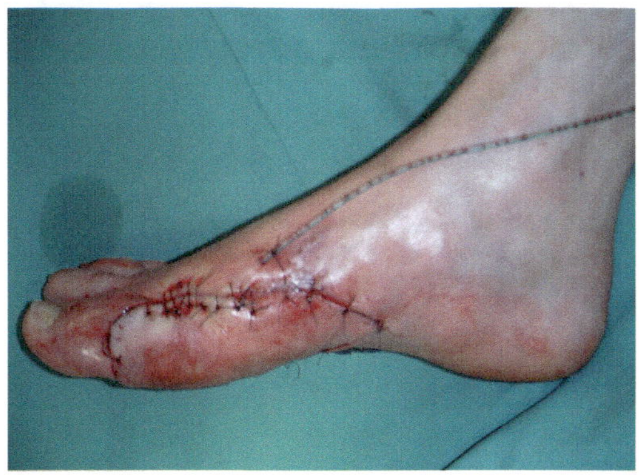

Fig. 3.291 Staged healing and the distal limit shows an element of sluggish recovery but of no consequence

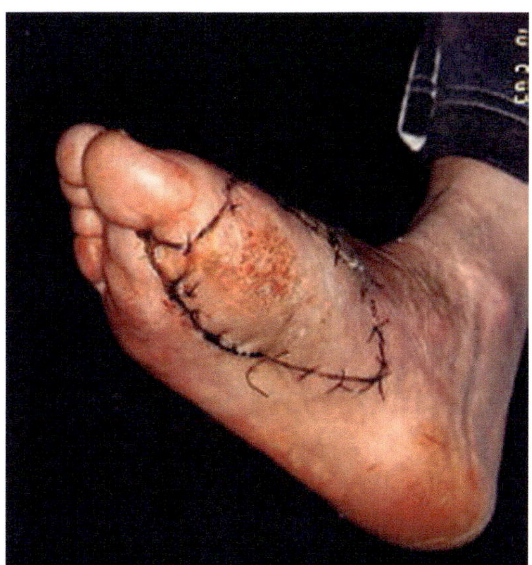

Fig. 3.292 The healed wound showing full perfusion to the MTP area and no element of any vascular impedance and the hyperdynamic flow is consistent with the sympathectomy effect observed which expedites healing

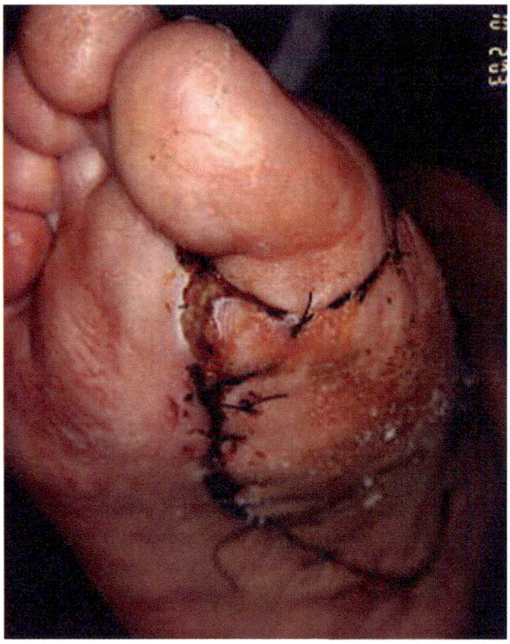

Fig. 3.293 Flexing the toe and the locking mattress suture at the MTP crease stays in 3 weeks

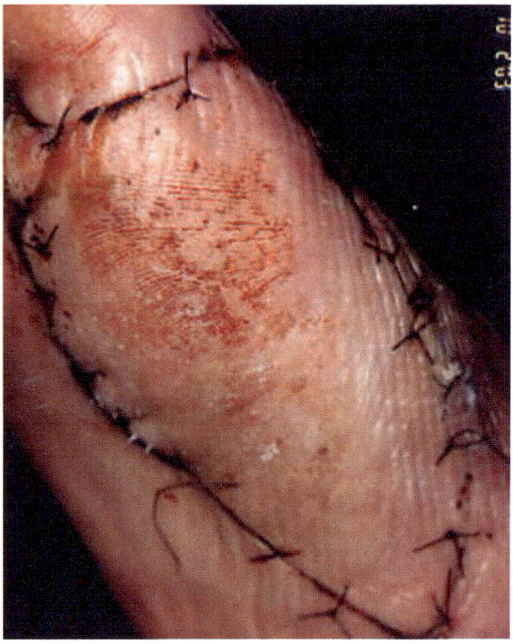

Fig. 3.294 The healing wound

3.1.26 Case 37: A Diabetic Ankle Following an ORIF Procedure and Wound Breakdown

This diabetic ankle with a defect size of 9 × 5 cm was closed with a keystone aligned along the L5 dermatome—fasciocutaneous island of the keystone variety (Figs. 3.295, 3.296, 3.297, 3.298, 3.299, 3.300, 3.301, 3.302, 3.303, 3.304, 3.305, 3.306, 3.307, 3.308, 3.309, 3.310, and 3.311)

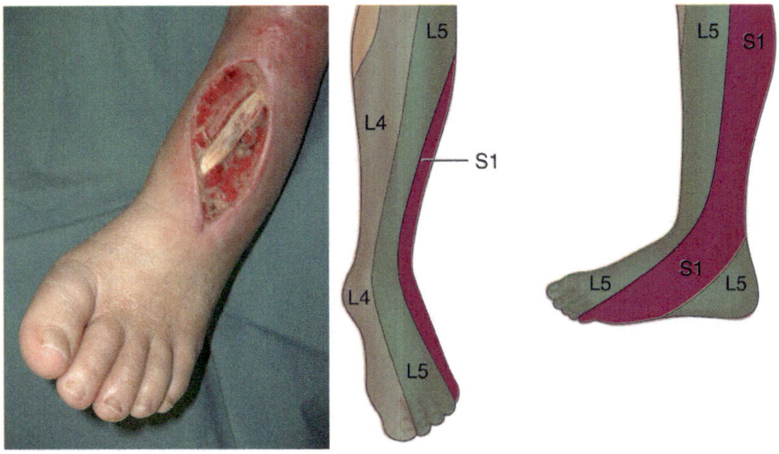

Fig. 3.295 Case on presentation of an ORIF of the ankle in a diabetic with exposure of the tibialis anterior and the swelling reflects its chronicity

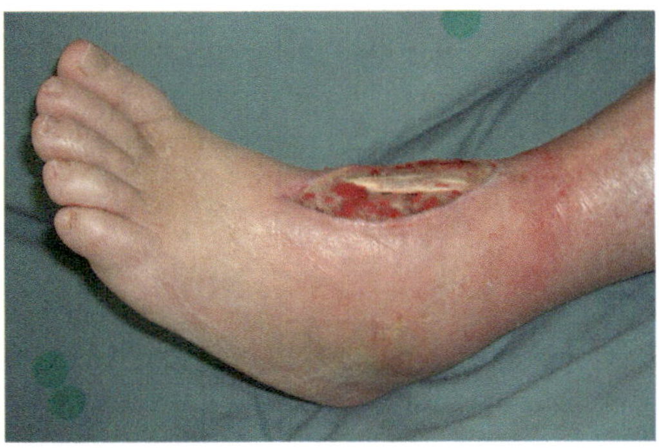

Fig. 3.296 A lateral view of the same problem reflecting oedema

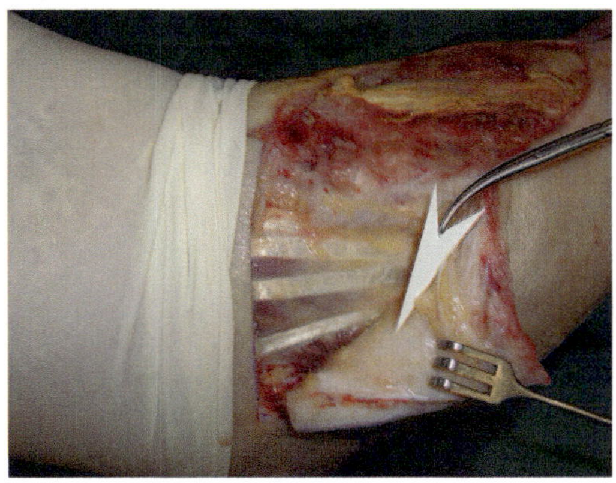

Fig. 3.298 Raising the fascial lined flap as an island on the superficial peroneal nerve distribution

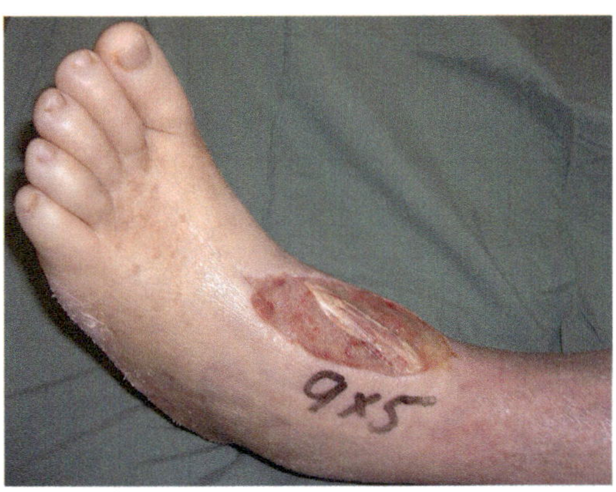

Fig. 3.297 A referral from the orthopaedic department of this 9 × 5 cm defect which should have been referred intraoperatively to prevent this complication and oedema is a consequence of delayed healing

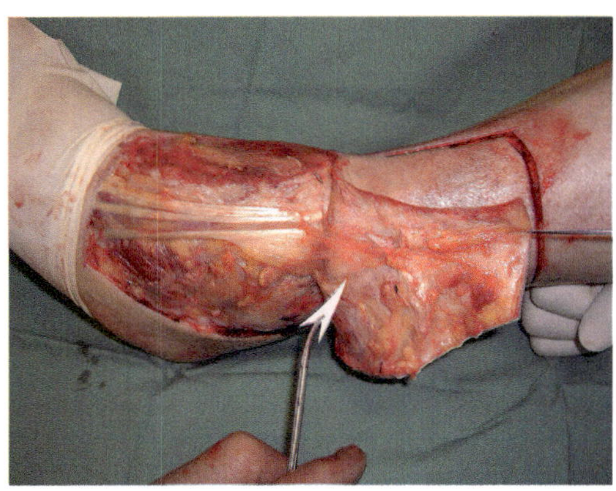

Fig. 3.299 The deep surface showing the suprafascial and infrafascial vascular network and the arrow points to the fine bleeding points of the suprafascial circulation and haemostasis is achieved using Weck vascular clamps, not diathermy to minimise any points of focal necrosis

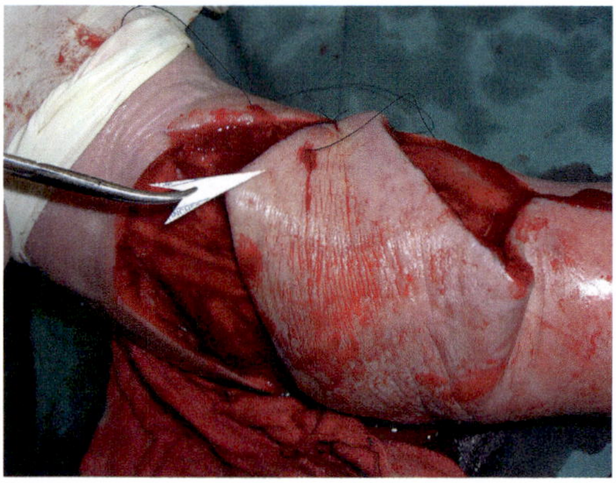

Fig. 3.300 Tourniquet release and the red dot sign confirming its vascular integrity and safety, i.e. it bleeds more on the flap side rather than the receiving site at the exit point of the locking mattress suture

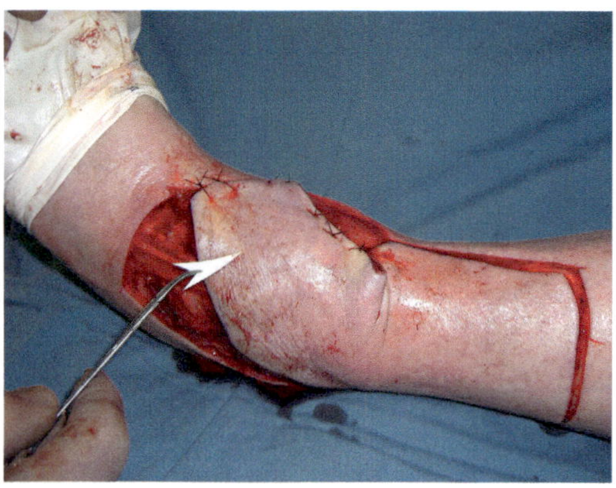

Fig. 3.301 Progress in the reconstruction with full vascular perfusion and the secondary defect sites are prepared for mesh grafting. Note there is a resolution of oedema even at this early stage, another characteristic of the keystone repair

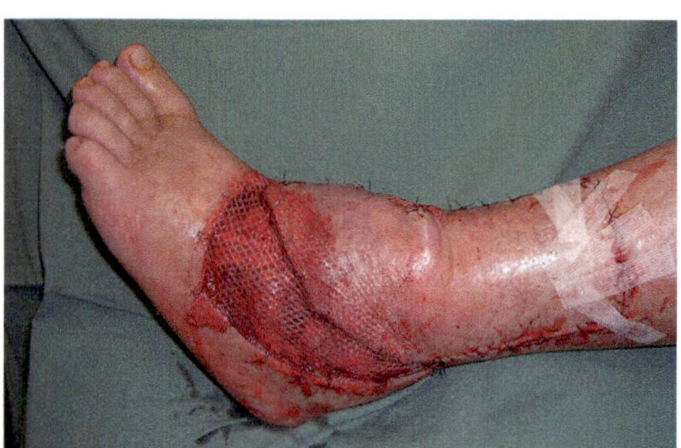

Fig. 3.302 Mesh grafting for the secondary defects

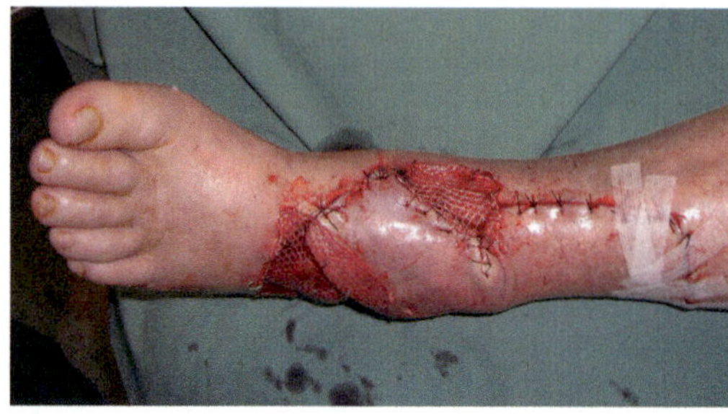

Fig. 3.303 Another site of the mesh grafting above the medial malleolus of the (L) ankle. The oedema of the foot is noted, and the keystone contributes to the resolution of this oedema, even at this early stage. The excision of dog ear along the anterior line reflects the reliability of the vascular perfusion

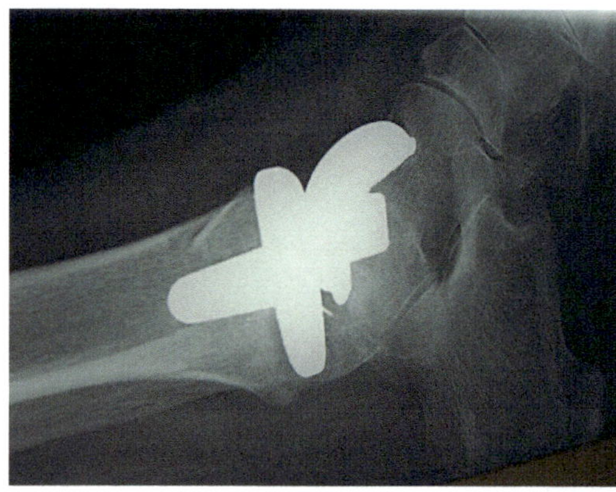

Fig. 3.304 Image of the ORIF component stabilising the joint

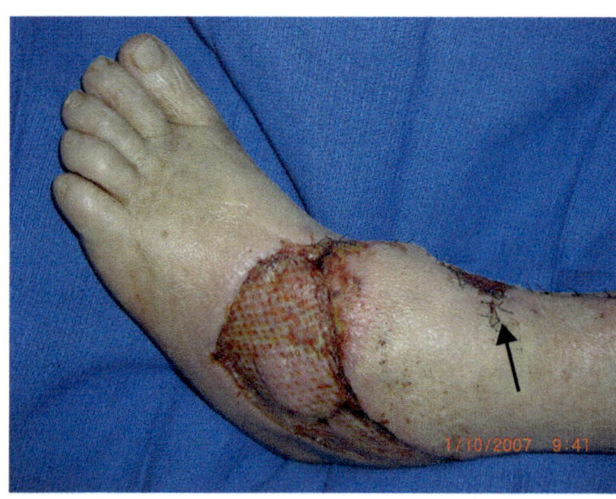

Fig. 3.305 Progress healing and note the dog ear excision without necrosis

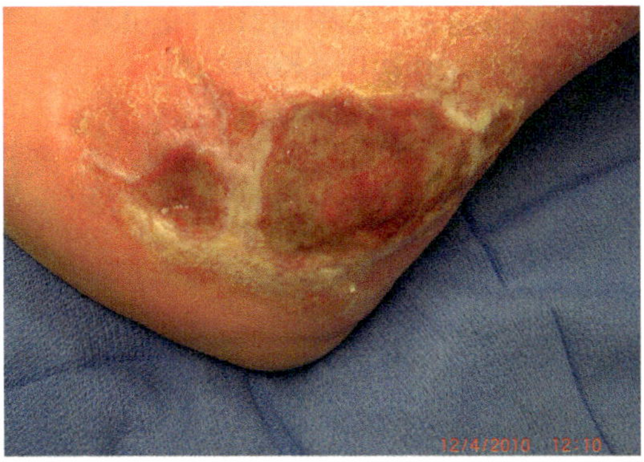

Fig. 3.306 Three-year appearance and the diabetic background would contribute to the delayed healing in this 80 year old where compliance may be a contributing factor to the delayed healing

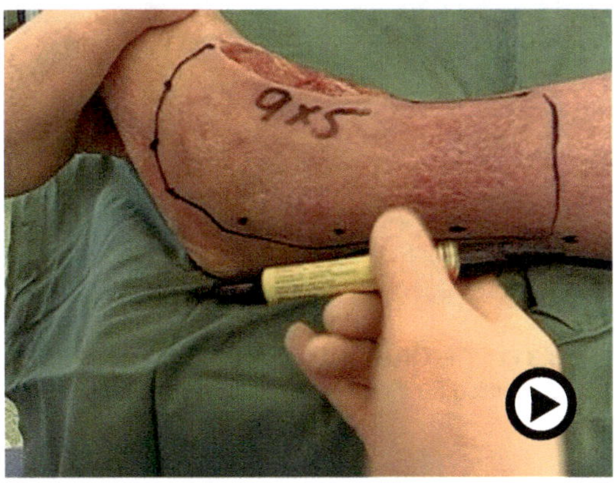

Fig. 3.307 Operative plan (Video 3.54 Operative plan) (▶ https://doi.org/10.1007/000-d6e)

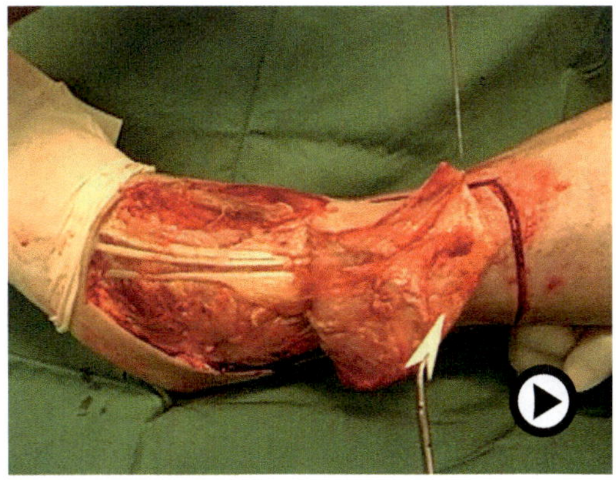

Fig. 3.308 Operative sequence showing the plane of dissection to show the suprafascial and infrafascial circulation—the lifeline for the viability of this fascial island flap. Haemostasis is secured using Weck clips to eliminate any topical necrosis from coagulative morbidity. The dynamic flow in the proximal part of the flap must be associated with a more prominent perforator (Video 3.55 Operative sequence showing the plane of dissection to show the suprafascial and infrafascial circulation—the lifeline for the viability of this fascial island flap. Haemostasis is secured using weck clips to eliminate any topical necrosis from coagulative morbidity. The dynamic flow in the proximal part of the flap must be associated with a more prominent perforator) (▶ https://doi.org/10.1007/000-d6f)

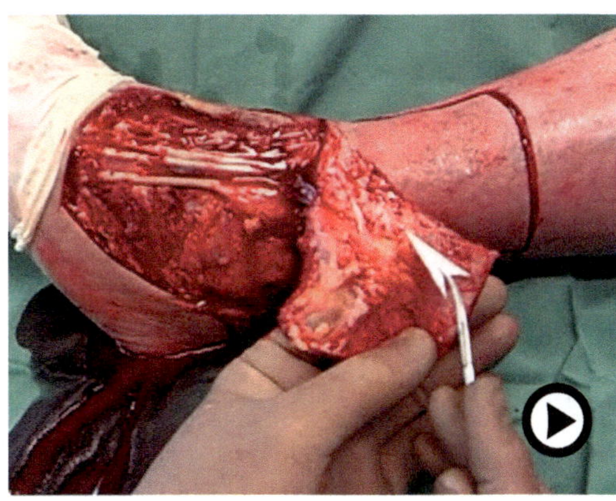

Fig. 3.309 More microcirculatory ooze points awaiting haemostasis. Note the plane of dissection is above the level of the paratenons of the extensor complex adjacent to the lateral malleolus, again best achieved by blunt dissection using the digit otherwise sharp dissection may cause a penetration (Video 3.56 More microcirculatory ooze points awaiting haemostasis. Note the plane of dissection is above the level of the paratenons of the extensor complex adjacent to the lateral malleolus, again best achieved by blunt dissection using the digit otherwise sharp dissection may cause a penetration) (▶ https://doi.org/10.1007/000-d6g)

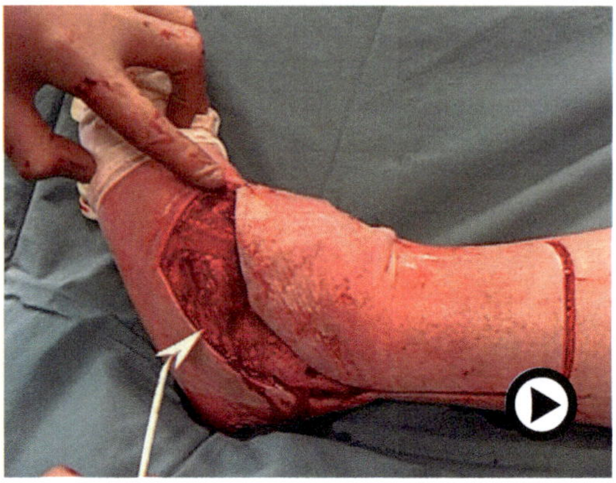

Fig. 3.310 On closure, awaiting grafting for secondary defect and direct closure here is totally contraindicated which would otherwise imperil the flap (Video 3.57 On closure, awaiting grafting for secondary defect and direct closure here is totally contraindicated which would otherwise imperil the flap) (▶ https://doi.org/10.1007/000-d6h)

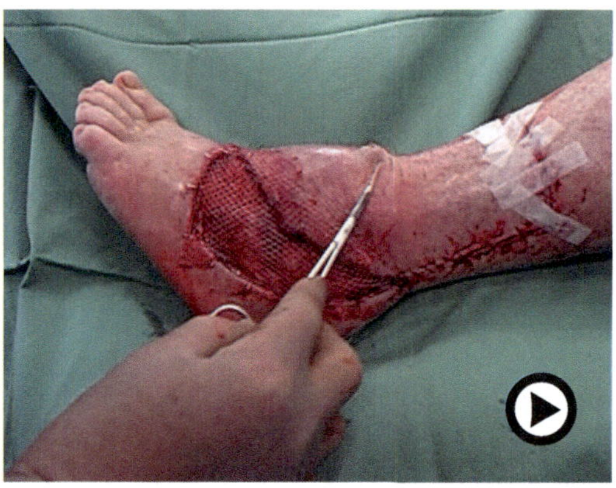

Fig. 3.311 Mesh grafting completed and the instrument indicates, with pressure, vascular perfusional recovery on pressure, again confirming vascular reliability (Video 3.58 Mesh grafting completed and the instrument indicates, with pressure, vascular perfusional recovery on pressure, again confirming vascular reliability) (▶ https://doi.org/10.1007/000-d6j)

3.1.27 Case 38: ORIF of the Fibular Closed with a Keystone

This ORIF of the fibular has created tension which will only cause wound breakdown if closed directly. The keystone design from the posterior orientated along the direction of the sural nerve neurovascular supply which incorporates neurovascular and somatic sensory factors and provides cover (Figs. 3.312, 3.313, 3.314, 3.315, 3.316, 3.317, 3.318, 3.319, and 3.320).

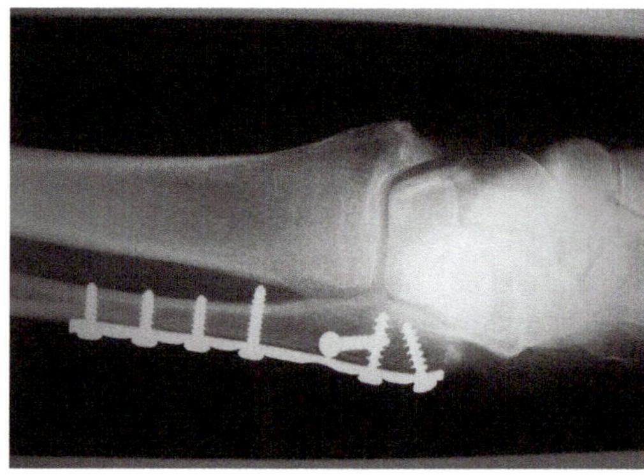

Fig. 3.312 The ORIF metal on view, a little protuberant hence the need for closure under tension

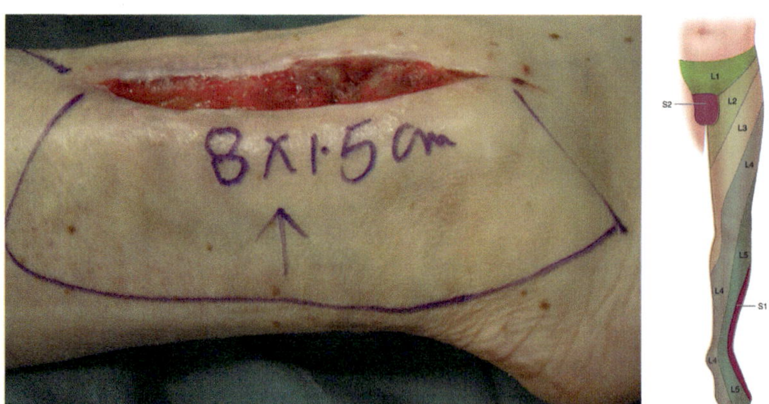

Fig. 3.313 The 8 × 1.5 cm operative defect and the mark out of the keystone design creating an arc flap incorporating both L5 and S1 dermatomes

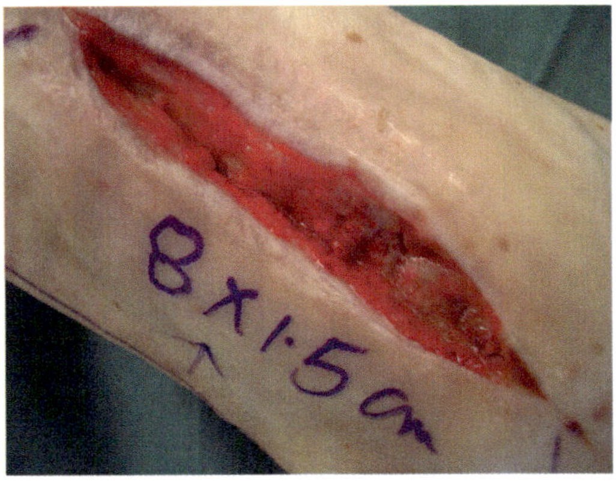

Fig. 3.314 Closeup of the wound in depth approximately 2 cm

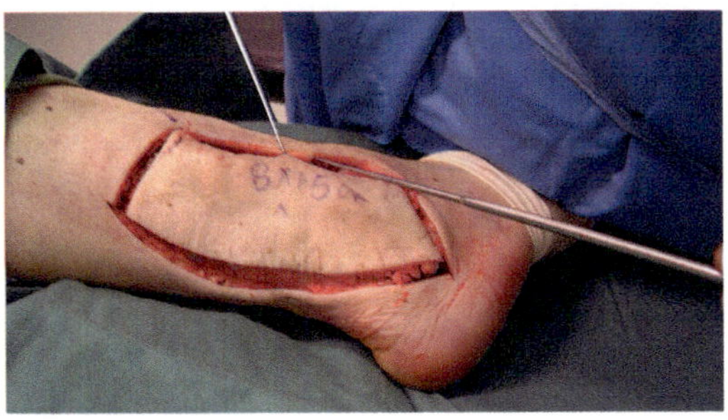

Fig. 3.315 The flap straddling both surgical defects anteriorly over the ORIF and posteriorly the sural nerve site has to be cautiously closed to avoid needle damage to the perineural structures

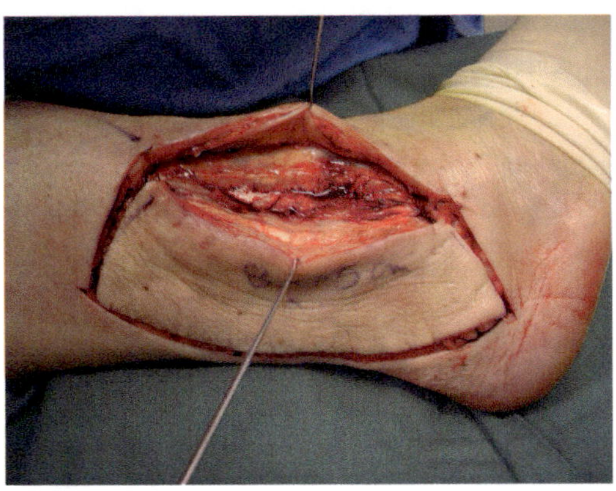

Fig. 3.316 Part of the staged closure before the release of tourniquet

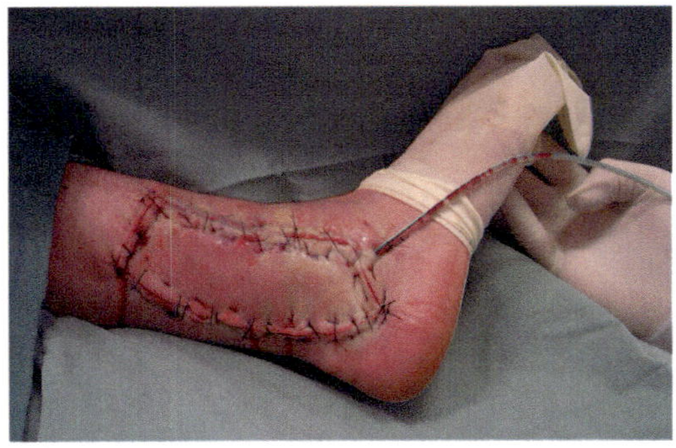

Fig. 3.317 The 3-phase locking mattress sutures create a single layer of wound apposition. The fascia is not repaired and Redi-vac drainage is in situ to drain both sites (bending the Red-vac drain into a U-shape provides access and drainage to both surgical sites with a single tube and the open end beneath the flap)

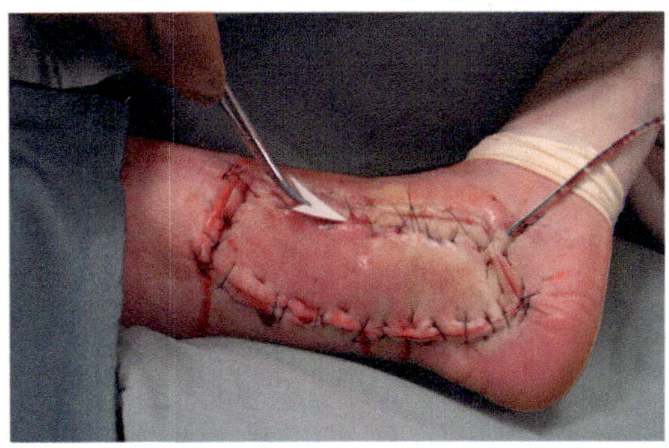

Fig. 3.318 The white arrow indicates the red dot sign (arterialised blood not cyanotic) indicating the hypervascularity now extending to the limits of the flap with the release of tourniquet

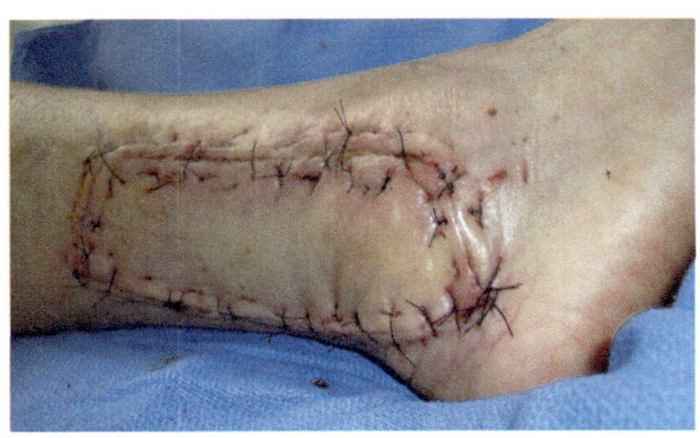

Fig. 3.319 Seven days postoperative image, no necrosis and the 3-phase locking mattress suture technique can be visualised staying in situ 3 weeks, reflecting an element of tension in the closure of the epidermis

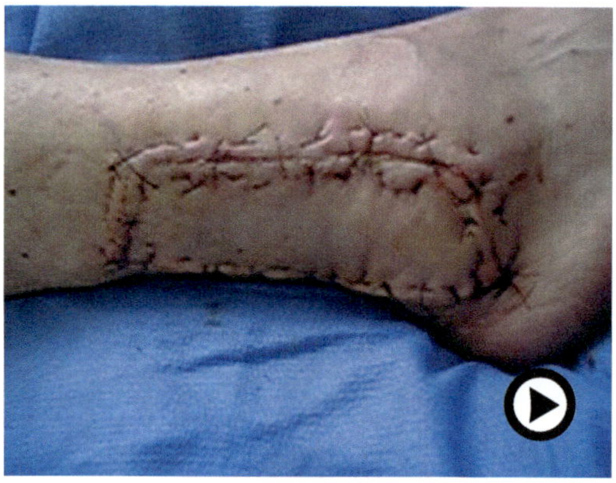

Fig. 3.320 The completed wound closure and the keystone insertion using the standard 3-phase locking mattress suture technique staying in situ for at least 3 weeks. If on release of any sutures the wound bleeds, delay further removals for another week (Video 3.59 The completed wound closure and the keystone insertion using the standard 3-phase locking mattress suture technique staying insitu for at least 3 weeks. If on release of any sutures the wound bleeds, delay further removals for another week) (▶ https://doi.org/10.1007/000-d4s)

3.1.28 Case 39: Providing Sensate Tissue to the Plantar Surface for Weight Bearing Protection Thus Avoiding Callosities

Providing sensate tissue on the weight bearing plantar surface of the foot previously grafted and toe amputation (Figs. 3.321, 3.322, 3.323, 3.324, 3.325, 3.326, 3.327, 3.328, and 3.329).

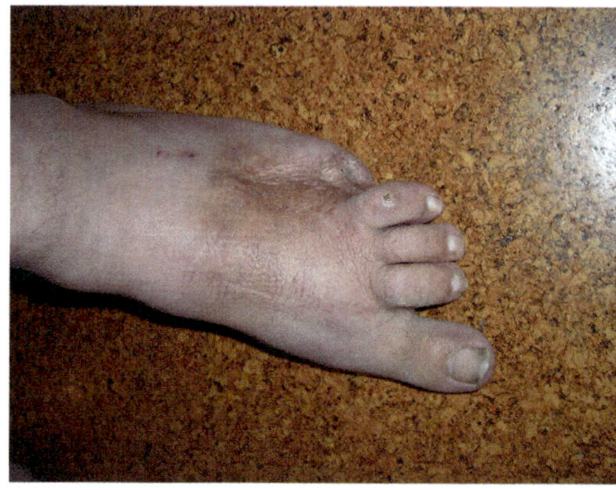

Fig. 3.321 The patient on presentation and the potential for trophic ulceration when wearing industrial footwear

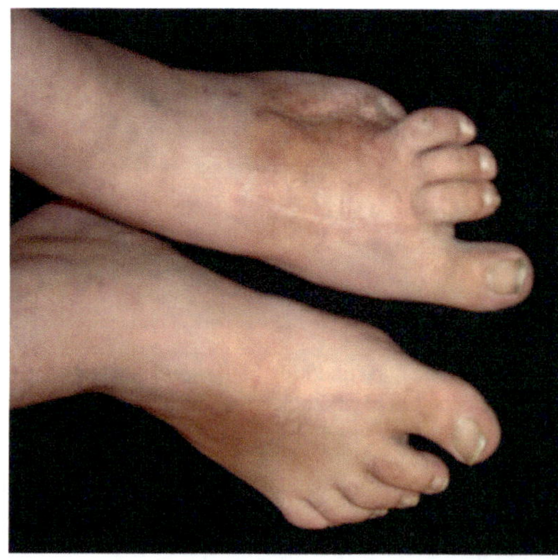

Fig. 3.322 Comparison dorsal appearance of both feet

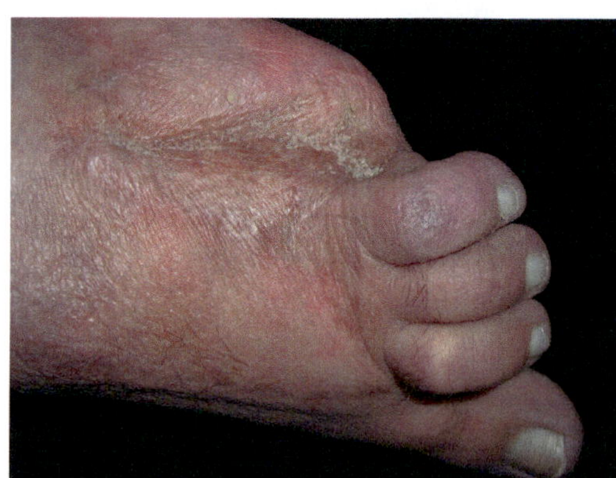

Fig. 3.323 Close of up scar tissue formation over the little toe amputation site. The clawed toes can be attended to at the same time by dividing the superficial flexor tendons to each digit, allowing extension and avoiding the hammer toe appearance

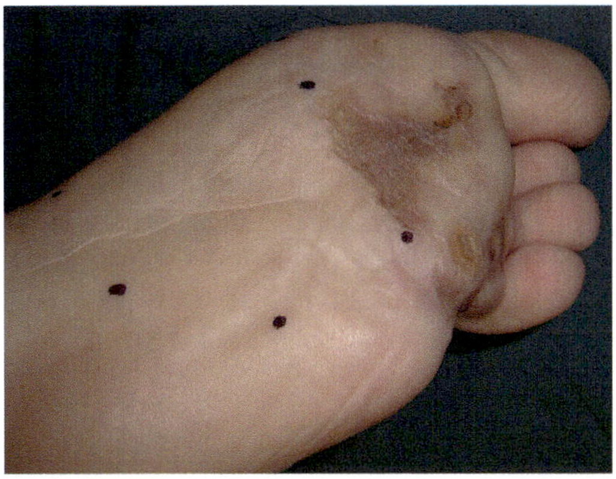

Fig. 3.324 The grafted surface, the site of repetitive trophic ulceration and the black dots outline the keystone mark out design planned to provide sensate tissue to the base of the toes

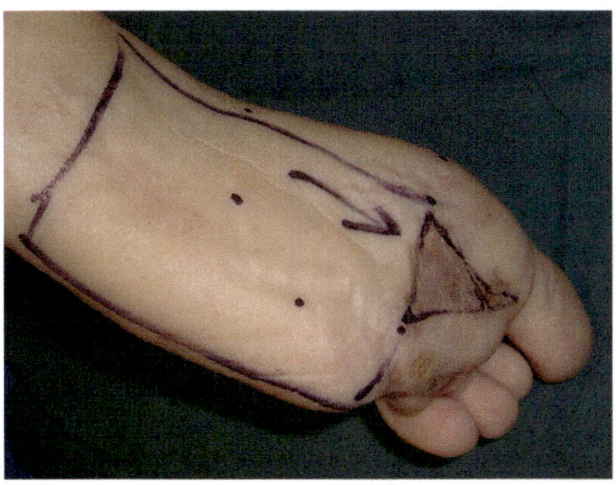

Fig. 3.325 The keystone mark out, the direction of movement and prior to excision of the old skin graft site

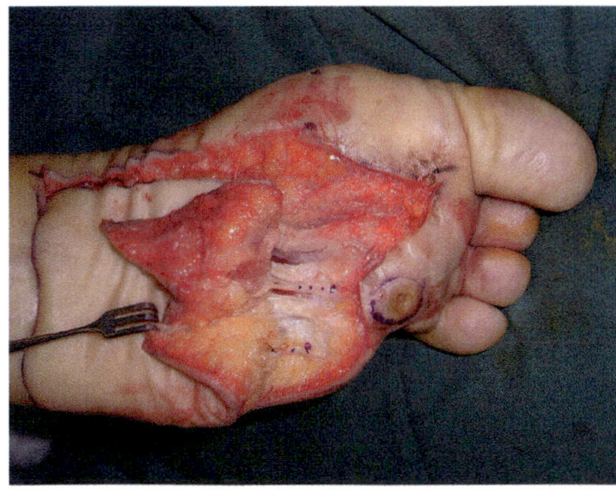

Fig. 3.326 The size of the plantar defect approximately 10 × 6 cm

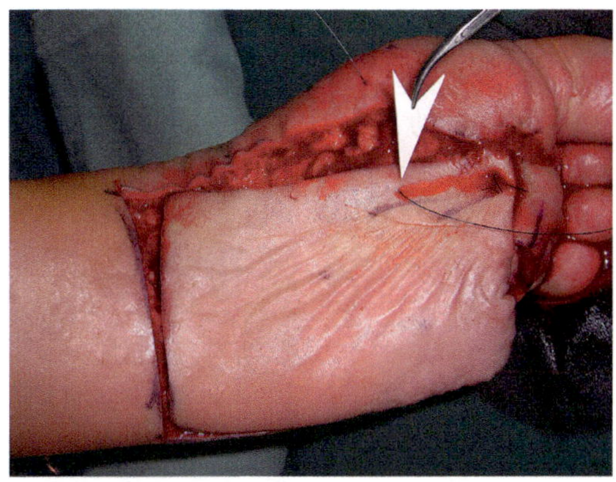

Fig. 3.327 The advancement, rotation and transposition of the keystone. Note the vascular flare and the red dot sign (arrowed). This is based on the plantar fascia ensuring its vascular reliability

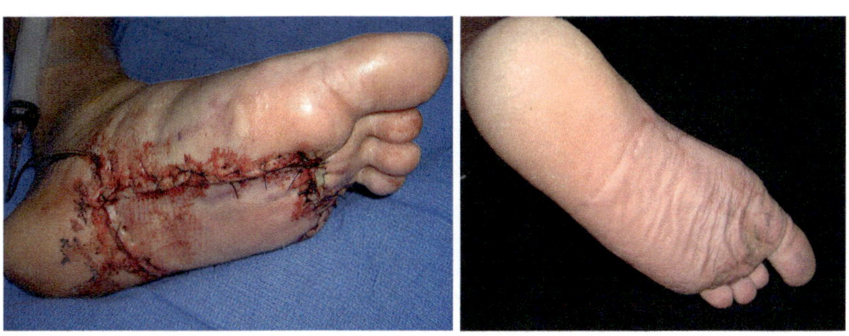

Fig. 3.328 On completion under tension, no lines of demarcation to indicate any element of any vascular impedance. The flap healed without complication, sensate tissue was supplied and the scars with the standard 3-phase locking mattress suture technique are barely discernible

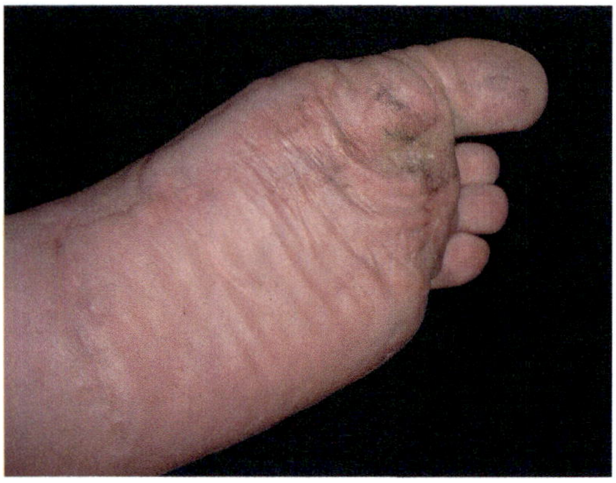

Fig. 3.329 After a 3-week staged removal of sutures at the appropriate times and the 3-phase locking mattress suture technique ensures stability and sensate tissue to cover the metatarsal heads with a well healed wound, eliminating another factor of potential trophic ulceration over metatarsals 3, 4, 5. The scar outline of the keystone flap is barely discernible if this 3-phase technique in suturing is utilised. Non-weight bearing is continued for 2–3 months

3.1.29 Case 40: Excisions of Mitotic or Nodular Lesions on the Plantar Surface

This excision of a mitotic/nodular lesion on the plantar surface and the keystone mark out for excision and closure (Figs. 3.330, 3.331, 3.332, 3.333, 3.334, and 3.335).

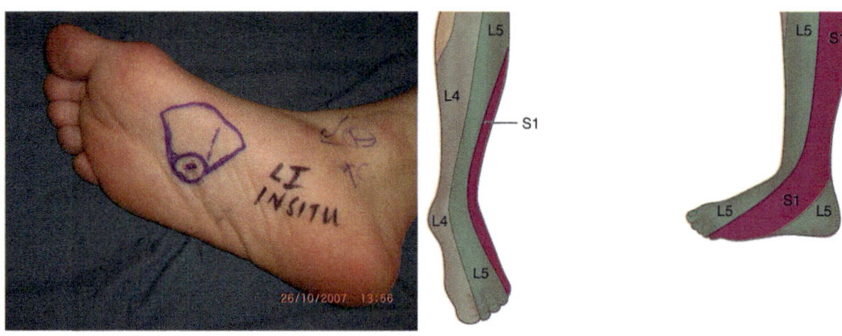

Fig. 3.330 The planned excision and the keystone solution

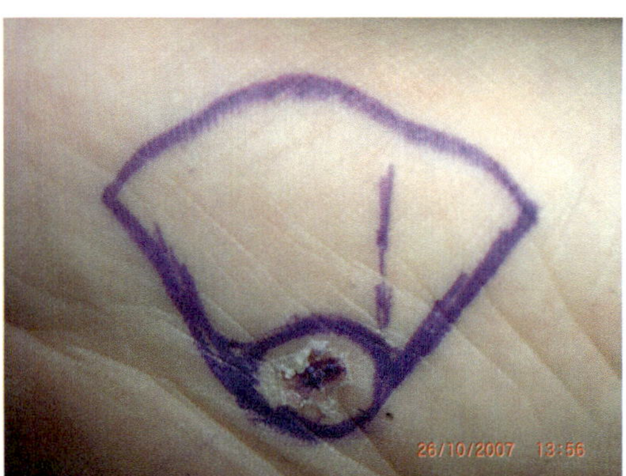

Fig. 3.331 Another view of the mitotic lesion after biopsy

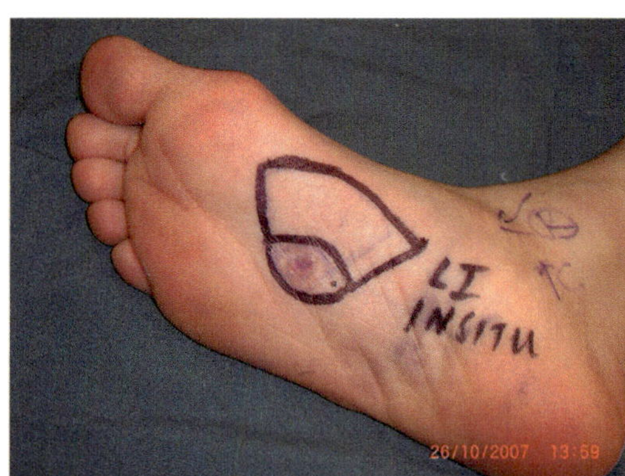

Fig. 3.332 The lesion and the keystone mark out for repair

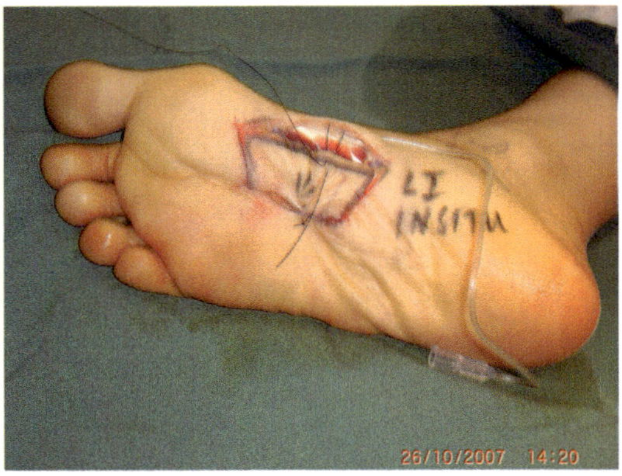

Fig. 3.333 The appearance during reconstruction when tension closure across the plantar surface is used to close the defect under Redi-vac drainage

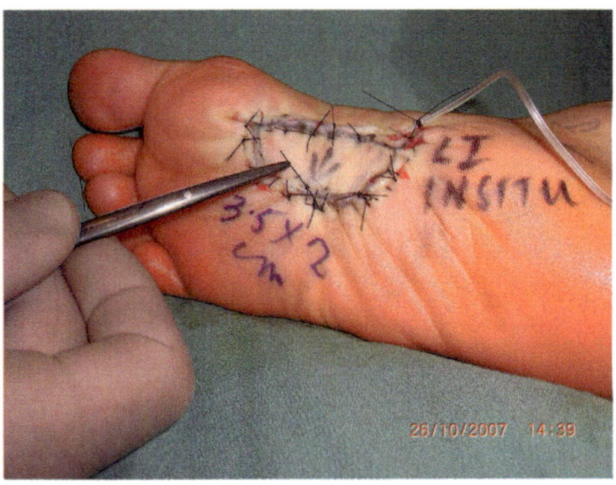

Fig. 3.334 The appearance after excision of a 3.5 × 2 cm lesion, and the keystone cover and the vascular recovery in the flap are indicated with a pointer

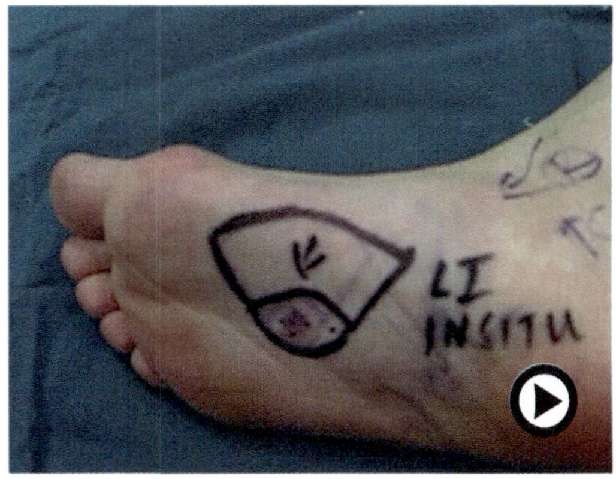

Fig. 3.335 Planned procedure for excision of the melanoma on the plantar grade surface and the looseness of the arch of the foot, when manually gripped, shows the degree of laxity present in the plantar integument confirming how it works, i.e. there is enough lax tissue to close this under tension based on subdermal perforators along the plantar line (Video 3.60 Planned procedure for excision of the melanoma on the plantar grade surface and the looseness of the arch of the foot, when manually gripped, shows the degree of laxity present in the plantar integument confirming how it works i.e. there is enough lax tissue to close this under tension based on subdermal perforators along the plantar line) (▶ https://doi.org/10.1007/000-d6m)

References

1. Aggarwala S, Cheung MY, Hsieh F. Profunda artery perforator flap—a novel approach to soft tissue reconstruction post lower limb amputation: a case report. AJOPS. 2024;7(1):89290. https://doi.org/10.34239/ajops.89290.
2. Behan F. Lower limb defects using the keystone technique. In: Atlas of keystone reconstructive technique in melanoma management. Cham: Springer; 2023. https://doi.org/10.1007/978-3-031-39868-1_5.
3. Gravvanis A, Kyriakopoulos A, et al. Flap reconstruction of the knee: a review of current concepts and a proposed algorithm. World J Orthop Surg. 2014;5(5):603–13.
4. Kamath JB, Shantaram Shetty M, et al. Soft tissue coverage in open fractures of tibia. Indian J Orthop. 2012;46(4):462–9.
5. McCraw JB, Fishman JH, Sharzer LA. The versatile gastrocnemius myocutaneous flap. Plast Reconstr Surg. 1978;62(1):15–23.
6. Alonso JE, Regazzoni P. Bridging bone gaps with the Ilizarov technique: biologic principles. Clin Plast Surg. 1991;18(3):497–504.
7. Rodriguez-Unda N, Abraham J, Saint-Cyr M. Keystone and perforator flaps in reconstruction. Clin Plast Surg. 2020;47(4):635–48.
8. Almeida MF, da Costa PR, Okawa RY. Reverse-flow island sural flap. Plast Reconstr Surg. 2002;109(2):583–91.

Further Reading

Robbins TH. Rectus abdominis myocutaneous flap for breast reconstruction. Aust N Z J Surg. 1979;49(5):527–30.

Potential Complicating Circumstances

4

Contents

4.1 Case Presentations

4.1.1 Case 41: Chronic Osteomyelitis of L Medial Malleolus in a Diabetic (Figs. 4.1, 4.2, 4.3, 4.4, 4.5, 4.6, 4.7, 4.8, 4.9, and 4.10)

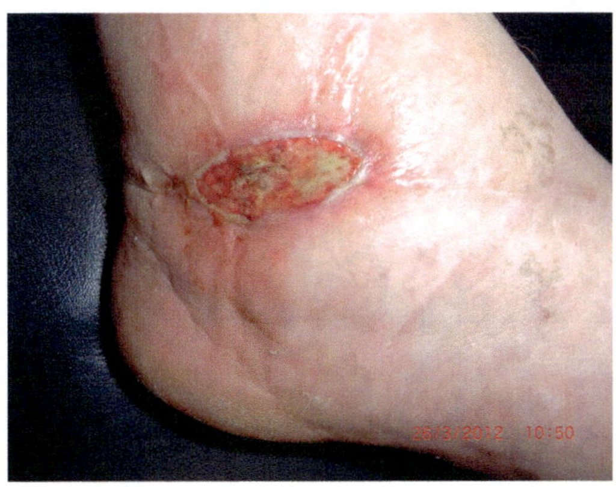

Fig. 4.1 Chronic osteopmyelitis apperance in a diabetic after a failed skin graft and the trophic ulceration is aggravated by wearing of shoes in non-sensate tissue characteristic of a diabetic

Supplementary Information The online version contains supplementary material available at https://doi.org/10.1007/978-3-031-76702-9_4. The videos can be accessed individually by clicking the DOI link in the accompanying figure caption or by scanning this link with the SN More Media App.

F. Behan, *Keystone Flap for Complex Orthopaedic Problems*,
https://doi.org/10.1007/978-3-031-76702-9_4

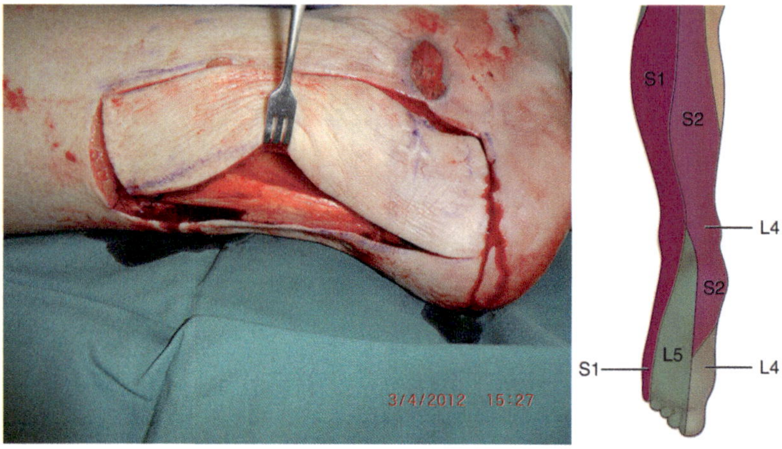

Fig. 4.2 Longitudinal fasciocutaneous island flap of ~4 × 10 cm is raised down to the level of the tendoachilles with blunt dissection leaving all microperforators from the fascia to the skin intact. The dissection is in the fascial plane preserving lining for the Keystone flap. The saphenous nerve in the S1 dermatome must be totally preserved to preserve the neurovascular axes and provide protective sensation over the heel—the site of the present trophic ulceration in a diabetic foot (Reproduced with permission from [1])

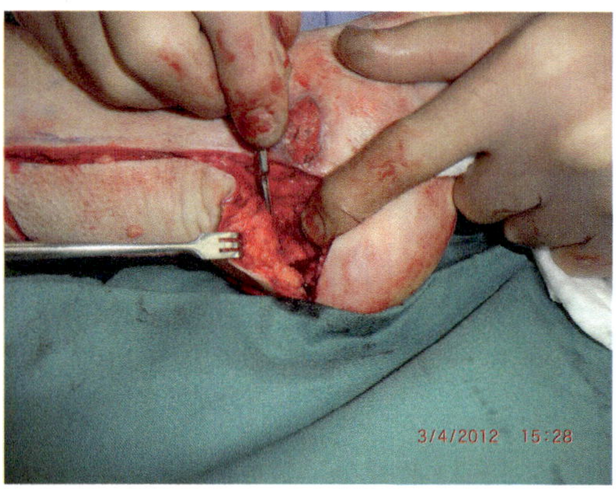

Fig. 4.3 Raising the flap retaining the fascial base

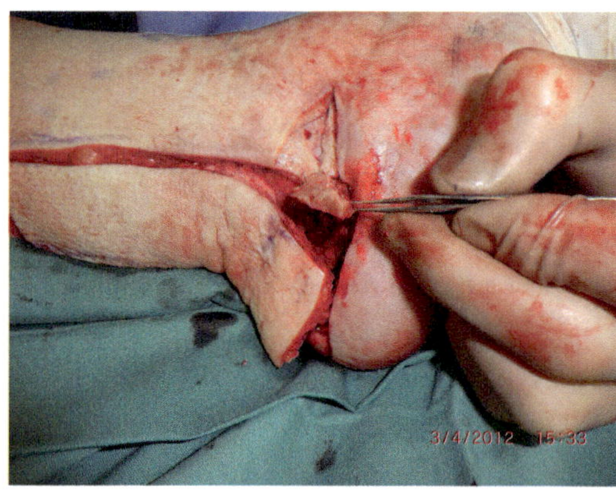

Fig. 4.5 Removal of part of the underlying bony prominence of the lateral malleolus

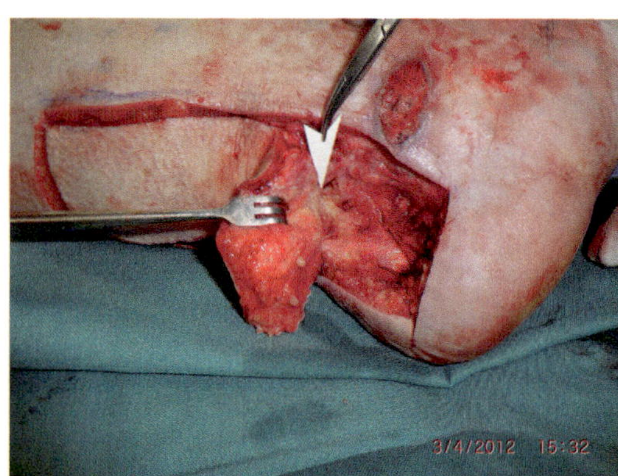

Fig. 4.4 The white arrow points indicate random perforators and the perfusional dynamics auger well for future healing indicating vascular integrity. Note the island of the flap at the proximal limits is just incised to create the island, and no undermining is necessary and the wound is just closed directly. The islanding creates the hyperaemia to guarantee vascular perfusion in this Keystone concept as indicated on the white arrow

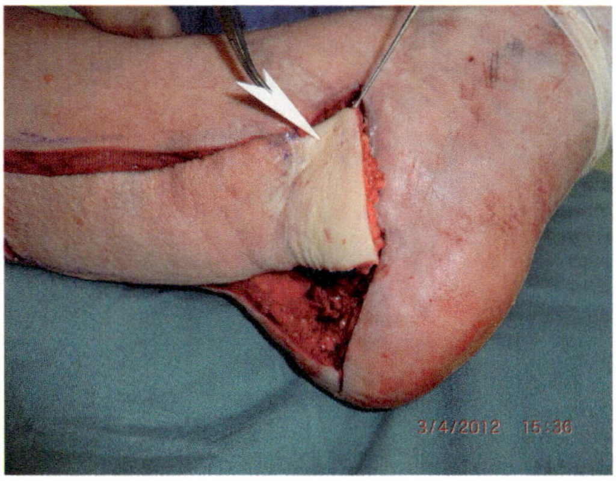

Fig. 4.6 Hyperaemic flare is developing towards the limits of the flap which are sometimes slow in the ankle joint area and are all based on random suprafascial perforator circulation input. Distally the suprafascial lining has microsurgical perfusion as evidenced by the dots. Secondly, the chronic inflammation would have an impedance effect on vascular perfusion—of a temporary nature

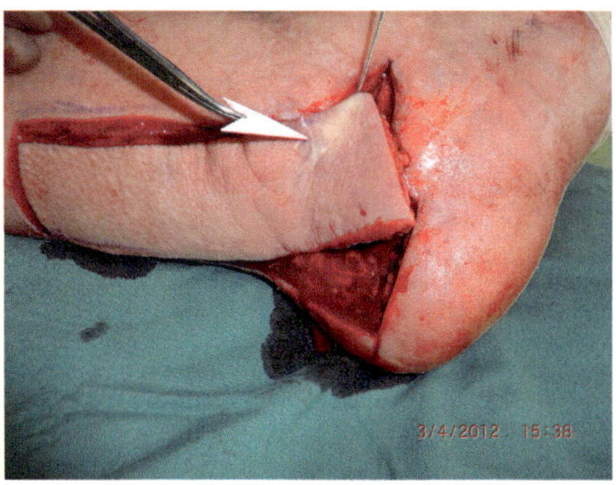

Fig. 4.7 A line of tension on the skin hook may occur with the V–Y suture. Note the distal pink flare is complete

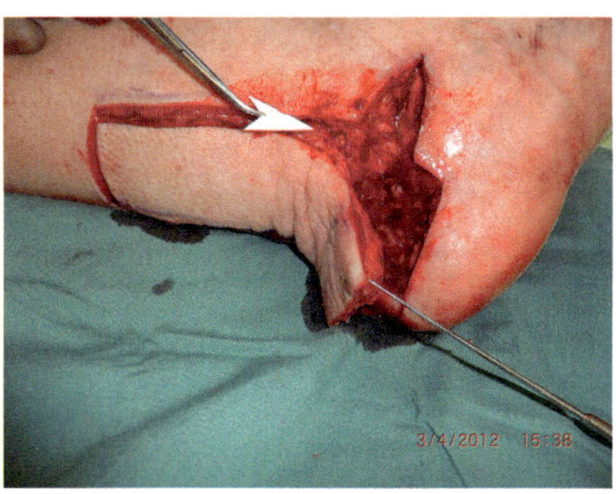

Fig. 4.8 Part of the staged repair before complete wound closure with the 3-phase nylon locking mattress suture technique

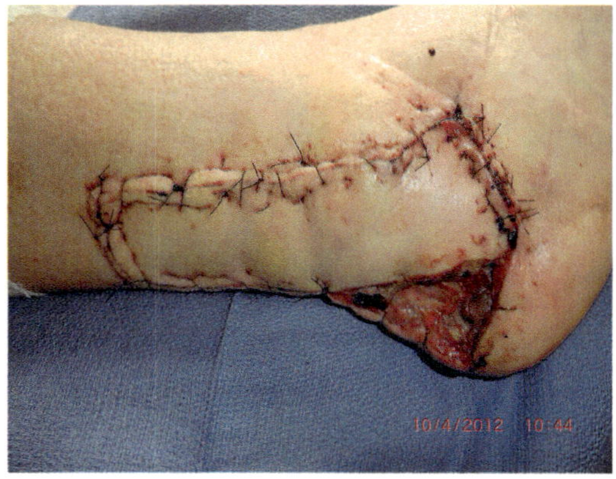

Fig. 4.9 Wound closure with the standard 3-phase nylon locking mattress suture technique. Locking mattress sutures at the points of tension. These stay in 3 weeks. Ordinary mattress sutures around periphery of the flap may stay in 10 days to 2 weeks for security. The continuous epidermal suture has the loops cut at 7 days to overcome cross hatching. The posterior secondary defect ~4 × 3 × 3 cm is grafted

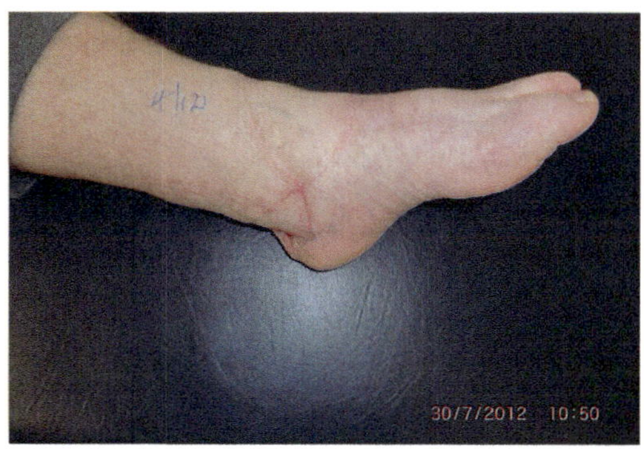

Fig. 4.10 Appearance at 4 months with the oedema resolving. Normal footwear possible following multiple microvascular procedures, the resultant chronic wound breakdown extended over 2 years before it was solved by the keystone technique

4.1.2 Case 42: Flap Necrosis Complication in a Smoker for Popliteal Fossa Repair Solved by Debridement and Re-suture with a Fasciocutaneous Keystone

Keystones are not exempt from vascular complications in smokers, and this advice is mandatory in the postoperative phase (Figs. 4.11, 4.12, 4.13, 4.14, 4.15, 4.16, 4.17, 4.18, 4.19, 4.20, and 4.21).

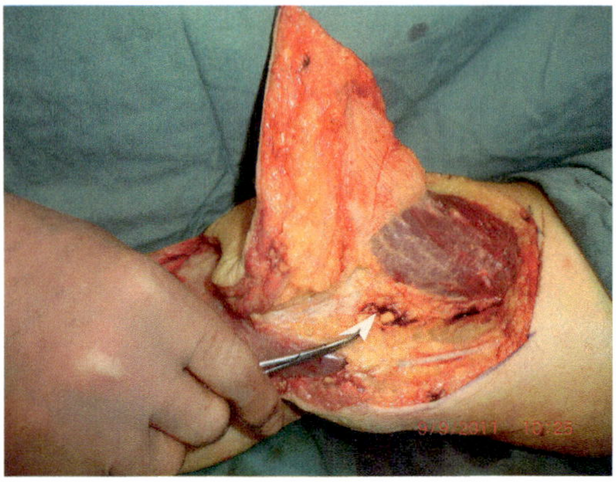

Fig. 4.11 Double keystones based on random perforators over the gastrocnemius muscle

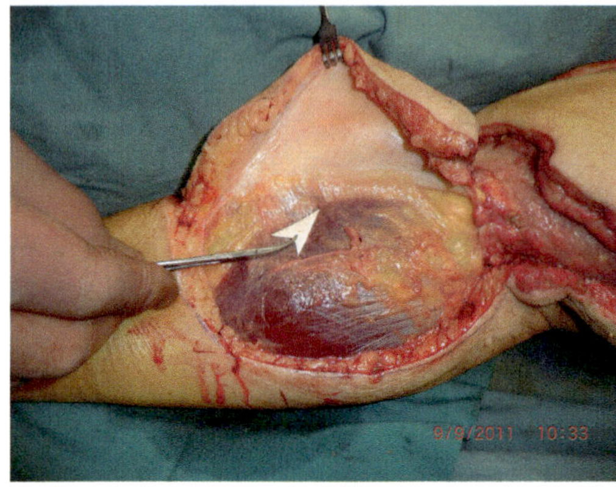

Fig. 4.14 Another perforator site randomly found with the blunt dissection technique otherwise it may have been divided

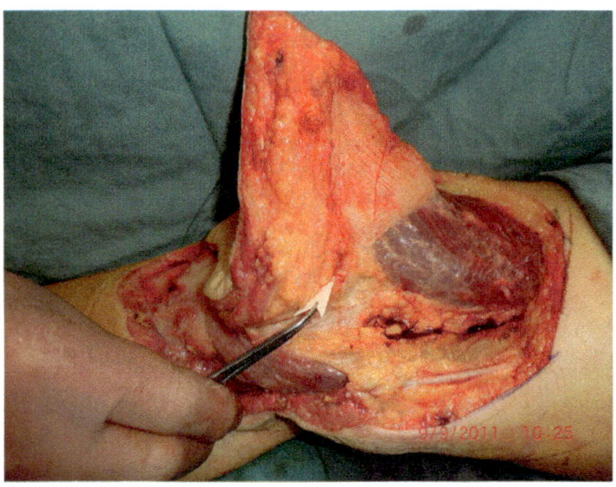

Fig. 4.12 The arrow indicates the perforator site from the muscle belly through the gastronemius fascia

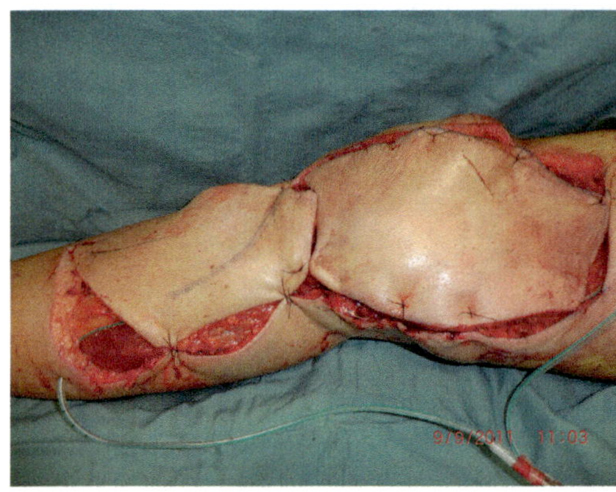

Fig. 4.15 Flap duplication above facilitates the closure with the second FCIF of the keystone design. The skin graft site below avoids undue tension in the closure inferiorally

Fig. 4.13 The blunt dissection is earsily mastered and is used to protect any random perforators in this L4 dermatome site. The dissecting index finger is in the plane between the fascial lining of the FCIF, and the gastrocnemius layer is visualised next to the arrow

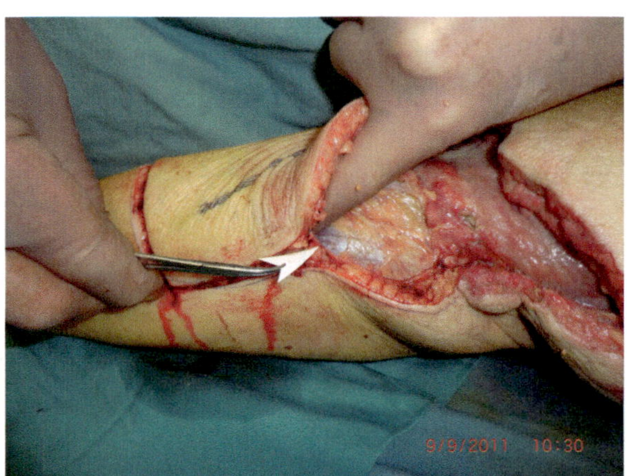

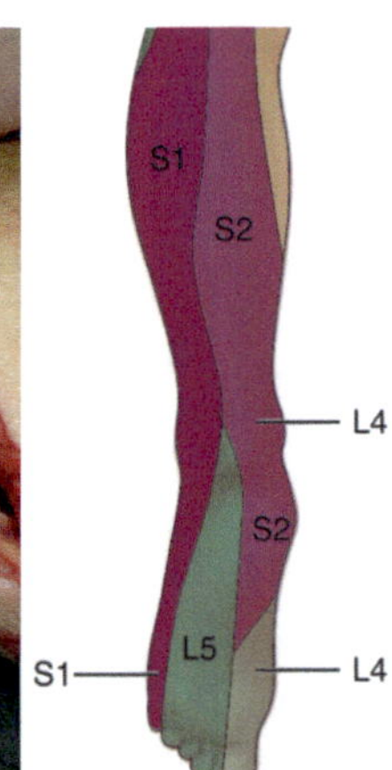

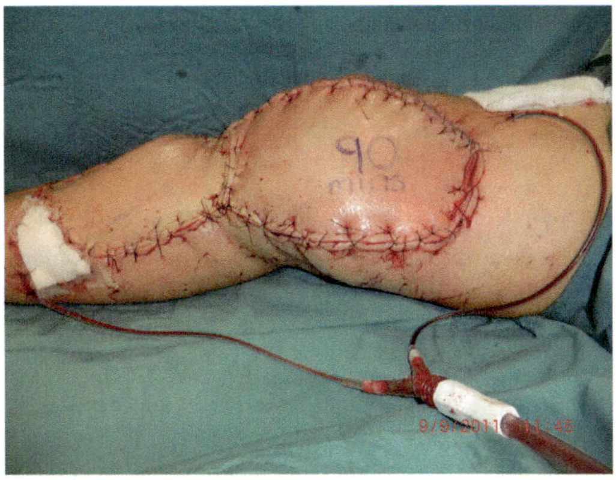

Fig. 4.16 The wound closed and the skin graft distally was completed in 90 min, and the skin graft was a means of minimising tension and the oedema present some 6 weeks since the initial accident. It was referred down from the country because of the chronic nature and site of this popliteal defect

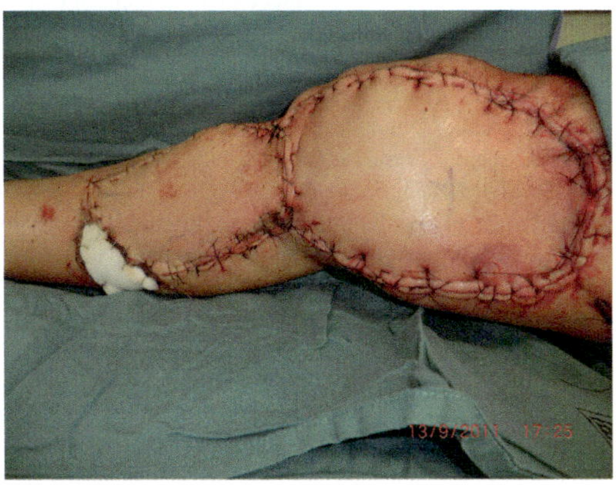

Fig. 4.17 Seven days postoperative showing the elements of hyperaemic reaction in this smoker, the cause of the mild margin wound necrosis

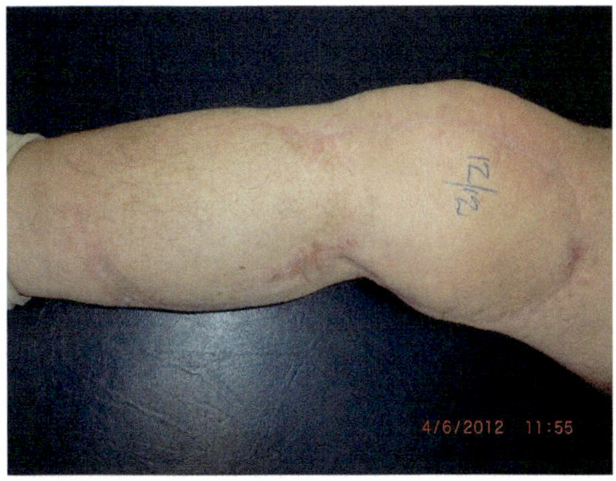

Fig. 4.18 Twelve month appearance with a functional R lower limb and patient returned to work. Delayed healing in this heavy smoker did not impede his return to work. The flaps have retained protective sensation. Full range of pain free movement in the R knee retained

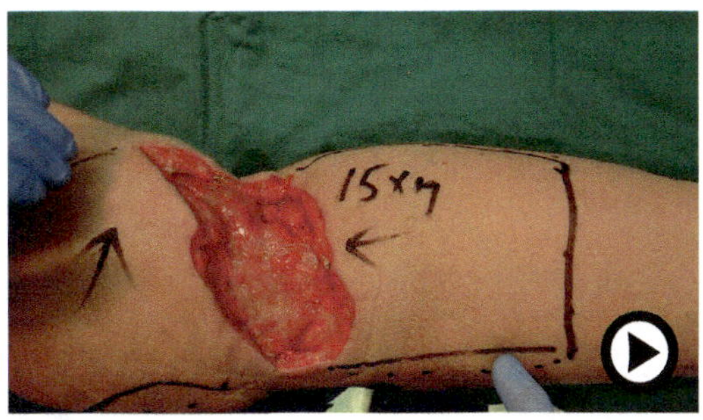

Fig. 4.19 The popliteal fossa defect after a second debridement and failure of an initial closure under direct pressure in a patient who continued to smoke. Like microvascular procedures, smoking is contraindicated so also for Keystone island flaps. Avoiding grafting in the popliteal fossa will obviate any subsequent scar contracture, a consequence of slow healing across the flexion joint (Video 4.1 The popliteal fossa defect after a second debridement and failure of an initial closure under direct pressure in a patient who continued to smoke. Like microvascular) (▶ https://doi.org/10.1007/000-d6p)

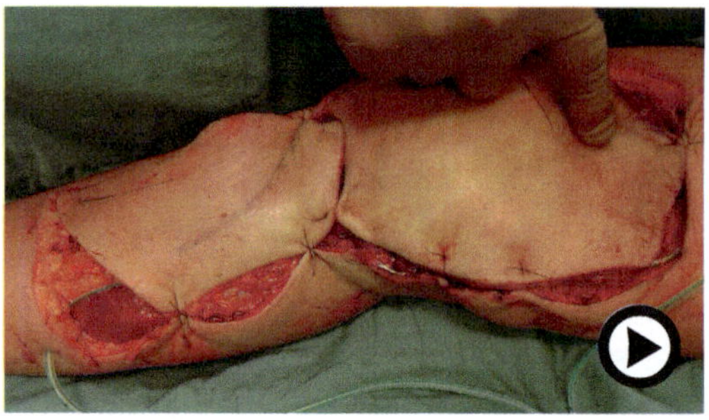

Fig. 4.20 Note the vascular flare in the major Keystone from the calf confirming its vascular integrity with its possible sympathectomy effect because it has been islanded and the autonomic circulation reacts by this obvious sign, a characteristic of the keystone concept (Video 4.2 Note the vascular flare in the major keystone from the calf confirming its vascular integrity with its possible sympathectomy effect because it has been islanded and the autonomic circulation reacts by this obvious sign, a characteristic of the keystone concept) (▶ https://doi.org/10.1007/000-d6n)

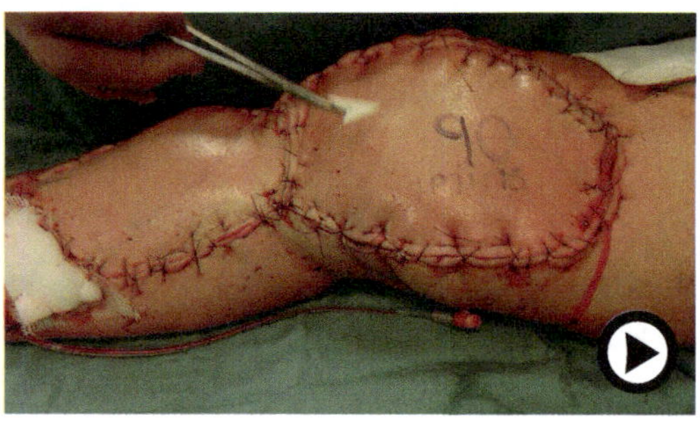

Fig. 4.21 Timeframe of 90 min for completion with an SSG to the secondary defect inferiorly to avoid tensional closure and eliminates any lines of demarcation where skin necrosis may surface and this eliminates this problem (Video 4.3 Timeframe of 90 min for completion with an SSG to the secondary defect inferiorly to avoid tensional closure and eliminates any lines of demarcation where skin necrosis may surface and this eliminates this problem) (▶ https://doi.org/10.1007/000-d6q)

Further Reading

1. Behan F. Lower limb defects using the keystone technique. In: Atlas of keystone reconstructive technique in melanoma management. Cham: Springer; 2023. https://doi.org/10.1007/978-3-031-39868-1_5.
2. Behan F, et al. Vascular basis of laterally based forehead island flaps and their clinical applications. Transactions of the 2nd Congress of the European Section of the International Confederation of Plastic and Reconstructive Surgery; 1973.
3. Behan F. Dashboard dislocations. Br J Hosp Med. 1973;1(9):363.
4. Behan F, et al. Reconstruction of plantar pad after degloving injury of foot. Surg Gynecol Obstet. 1973;137(65):971.
5. Behan F, et al. Subungual malignant melanoma difficulty in diagnosis. Br Med J. 1974;1:310–2.
6. Behan F, JS Wilson. The principle of the angiotome a system of linked axial pattern flaps. Transactions of the 6th International Congress on Plastic and Reconstructive Surgery, Paris; 1975.
7. Behan F. The fascio-cutaneous island flap: an extension of the angiotome concept. Aust N Z J Surg. 1992;62:874–86.
8. Behan F, et al. Fasciocutaneous island flaps for orthopaedic management in lower limb reconstruction using dermatomal precincts. ANZ J Surg. 1994;64(3):155–66.
9. Behan F, et al. Island flaps, including the Bezier type in the treatment of malignant melanoma. ANZ J Surg. 1995;65(12):870–80.
10. Behan F. The venous island conduit (VIC) flap for ring avulsion injuries. J Hand Surg. 1998;23(4):465–71.
11. Behan F. The keystone design perforator island flap in reconstructive surgery. ANZ J Surg. 2003;73:112–20.
12. Behan F, Sizeland A, Porcedu S, Somia N, Wilson J. Keystone island flap; an alternative reconstructive option to free flaps in irradiated tissue. ANZ J Surg. 2006;76:407–13.
13. Pelissier P, Santoul M, Pinsolle V, Casoli V, Behan F. The keystone design perforator island flap: part I. Anatomic study. J Plast Reconstr Aesthet Surg. 2007;60:883–7.

14. Behan F. Evolution of the fascio-cutaneous island flap leading to the keystone flap principle in lower limb reconstruction. ANZ J Surg. 2008;78:116–7.
15. Behan FC, Lo CH, Ramin S. Perforator territory of the keystone flap – use of the dermatomal roadmap. J Plast Reconstr Aesthet Surg. 2008;62(4):551–3. https://doi.org/10.1016/j.bjps.2008.08.078.
16. Behan FC, Lo CH, Shayan R. Perforator territory of the keystone flap: use of the dermatomal roadmap. J Plast Reconstr Aesthet Surg. 2009;62:551–3.
17. Behan F, Sizeland A, Gilmour F, Hui A, Seel M, Lo CH. Use of the keystone island flap for advanced head and neck cancer in the elderly. J Plast Reconstr Aesthet Surg. 2010;63:739–45.
18. Behan FC, Rozen WM, Tan S. Yin-Yang flaps: the mathematics of two keystone island flaps for reconstructing increasingly large defects. ANZ J Surg. 2011;81:574–5.
19. Behan FC, Rozen WM, Lo CH, Findlay M. The omega-variant designs (types A and B) of the keystone perforator island flap. ANZ J Surg. 2011;81:650–2.
20. Behan F, Findlay M, Lo CH. The keystone perforator island flap concept. Sydney: Elsevier; 2012.
21. Behan FC, Rozen WM, Azer S, Gran P. Perineal keystone design perforator island flap for perineal and vulval reconstruction. ANZ J Surg. 2012;82:381–2.
22. Behan FC, Paddle A, Rozen WM, et al. Quadriceps keystone island flap for radical inguinal lymphadenectomy. ANZ J Surg. 2013;83:942–7.
23. Shayan R, Behan FC. Re: the keystone concept: time for some science. ANZ J Surg. 2013;83:499–500.
24. Behan F. Surgical tips and skills illustrating the keystone principle. Sydney: Elsevier Textbook Churchill Livingstone; 2014.
25. Klaassen MF, Brown E, Behan F. Simply local flaps. Cham: Springer; 2016.
26. Lo C, et al. Keystone island flap effects of islanding on vascularity. Plast Reconstr Surg. 2016;4(2):e617. https://doi.org/10.1097/GOX.0000000000000607.
27. Behan FC. Keystone perforator island flap: a clinical summary of 28 melanoma cases. Austral J Plast Surg. 2018;1:49–57. https://doi.org/10.34239/ajops.v1i1.66.
28. Behan FC. A keystone solution for major head and neck reconstructions. Austral J Plast Surg. 2019;2:154. https://doi.org/10.34239/ajops.v2n2.154.
29. Behan FC. Dupuytren's disease: modified keystone techniques to improve vascular dynamics in fasciectomy. Austral J Plast Surg. 2019;2:134. https://doi.org/10.34239/ajops.v2i1.134.
30. Rodriguez-Unda N, Abraham J, Saint-Cyr M. Keystone and perforator flaps in reconstruction. Clin Plast Surg. 2020;47(4):635–48.
31. Potet P, De Bonnecaze G, Chabrillac E, Dupret-Bories A, Vergez S, Chaput B. Closure of radial forearm free flap donor site: a comparative study between keystone flap and skin graft. Head Neck. 2020;42:217–23.
32. Behan FC, Sizeland A. Keystone perforator island flaps in major head and neck surgery – the P.A.C.E. perspectives. World J Surg Surg Res. 2021;4(1):1293.
33. Behan FC. Keystone perforator island flap in lower limb reconstruction. Austral J Plast Surg. 2021;4(2):105–7. https://doi.org/10.34239/ajops.v4n2.341.
34. Behan FC. A simple solution to mallet deformities – a patient's perspective. Austral J Plast Surg. 2022;126(5):1624–9.
35. Klaassen M, Burton I. Atlas of extreme facial cancer, challenges and solutions: keystone flap concepts. Cham: Springer; 2022.
36. Behan FC. Perforator flaps: anatomy, technique, & clinical applications. In: Part D: the keystone perforator island flap. 3rd ed. New York: Thieme Publishers; 2022.

GPSR Compliance

The European Union's (EU) General Product Safety Regulation (GPSR) is a set of rules that requires consumer products to be safe and our obligations to ensure this.

If you have any concerns about our products, you can contact us on ProductSafety@springernature.com

In case Publisher is established outside the EU, the EU authorized representative is:

Springer Nature Customer Service Center GmbH
Europaplatz 3
69115 Heidelberg, Germany

Batch number: 10732801

Printed by Printforce, the Netherlands